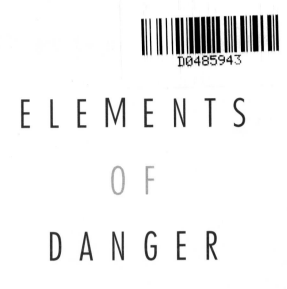

ELEMENTS

OF

DANGER

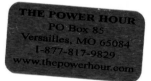

Also by Morton Walker, D.P.M.

ELEMENTS

OF

DANGER

Protect Yourself Against the
Hazards of Modern Dentistry

Morton Walker, D.P.M.
Foreword by Julian Whitaker, M.D.

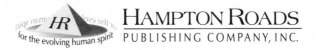

HAMPTON ROADS
PUBLISHING COMPANY, INC.

Cover design by Marjoram Productions
Cover photography by Jonathan Friedman

For information write:

Hampton Roads Publishing Company, Inc.
134 Burgess Lane
Charlottesville, VA 22902

Or call: 804-296-2772
FAX: 804-296-5096

e-mail: hrpc@hrpub.com
Web site: http://www.hrpub.com

If you are unable to order this book from your local
bookseller, you may order directly from the publisher.
Quantity discounts for organizations are available.
Call 1-800-766-8009, toll-free.

Library of Congress Catalog Card Number: 99-71623

ISBN 1-57174-146-1
10 9 8 7 6 5 4 3 2 1

Printed on acid-free paper in Canada

Dedication

To Stanley Machenberg, D.D.S., the entire Walker family's excellent dentist for thirty-six years, who upon his retirement from practice in 1989, has remained my personal friend and confidant these many years.

Table of Contents

Disclaimer and Disavowal of Responsibility

This book has been written and published strictly for informational purposes and in no way should be used as a substitute for advice from your own health care professional. Therefore, you must not consider educational material found here as replacing consultation with dental or medical practitioners. Most of the facts in this book come from laboratory or clinical studies, scientific publications, interviews with informed health care personnel, or patients who have experienced chronic fatigue, low levels of wellness, subclinical illness, or outright disease resulting from dental impairment and the so-called orthodox or standard treatment techniques as taught in dental school.

Unless indicated otherwise as by footnotes, the identities of patients, including their occupations, residences, or locations, and their direct quotes are fictional in this book. However, the research scientists quoted and the mercury-free, biocompatible, holistic, or biological dentists or medical doctors who offer patients' case histories are authentic. Direct quotes of health care professionals are taken from tape-recorded interviews conducted by the author or from published research papers and press clippings that they contributed for inclusion here. Eager to share their clinical experiences with treating patients' illnesses, certain dentists and medical doctors have provided scientific information, case reports, and published or unpublished laboratory or clinical investigations. Even so, none of the information imparted should be considered the practice of dentistry or medicine. This book's author, consultant, and publisher are providing educational material and nothing more.

If information gleaned here raises questions about your own or a loved one's dental care, you should consult Jerome S. Mittelman, D.D.S., any of the holistic dentists contributing information for this book, or a listed member of the holistic (biological) dental professional organizations cited in appendix C. The author, Morton Walker, D.P.M., is not an expert on dental or medical care but rather a full-time, freelance medical journalist, who depends on authorities or other experts outside of the areas of his medical/dental research and writing talents.

Please take the above message as a disavowal of all responsibility by the author, consultant, publisher, editorial content contributors, listed organizations, and product suppliers for any practice, procedure, diagnostic technique, or other information taken from this book and acted upon by a reader or other interested parties.

Foreword

Dr. Morton Walker is undoubtedly the most prolific and reliable writer of information about alternative healing methods, holistic medicine, and orthomolecular nutrition of the twentieth century. His seventy-three published books are invariably crammed with expertly researched medical facts, internal and external environmental truths, and other verifiable knowledge on medical topics. Equally important, however, is that what he investigates and reports on is a constant and almost relentless challenge to the often wayward orthodox thinking of modern medicine, podiatry, nutrition, and dentistry. Dr. Walker consistently points out the foibles and inconsistencies of conventional medical practices and procedures, as well as the economic interests that buttress the medical industry, the foot care industry, the nutrition industry, the cancer industry, and now the dental industry. Furthermore, Dr. Walker's lectures, media appearances, books, clinical journal articles, magazine articles, and other writings offer clear, workable alternative treatment techniques for a variety of degenerative diseases, dental disorders, and other unhealthy human conditions.

This newly created book of his, *Elements of Danger: Protect Yourself against the Hazards of Modern Dentistry,* is no exception. In these pages Dr. Morton Walker exposes the dangers that many of us face when we sit in the conventionally practicing dentist's treatment chair. We should be wary, but often we are not. Little do we know that feeling confidence in some dentist's skill and integrity may be the undoing of one's general health as well as dental health.

Still, all is not lost. As a dynamic medical journalist and author, Dr. Walker educates the reader on root canals and how they harbor pockets of infection that contribute to chronic illness with associated degenerative diseases. He alerts us to undetected cavitation, which insidiously eats away at the jawbone and causes severe bone deterioration. He discusses the fallacy of water fluoridation, the many fluoridated toothpastes, and dentist-applied fluoride, which expose the American population to a known toxin that attacks the brain, weakens the bones, and causes cancer. He also develops a sound case for the strong relationships between dental ailments and overall health and well-being.

However, it is "silver" mercury amalgams that Dr. Morton Walker goes after with both guns blazing. His exposé of the confused ethics of the American Dental Association (ADA) and why this organization and its members stubbornly insist on using mercury amalgams, which are banned in many countries around the world, is an eye opener. The ADA was originally formed to perpetuate the use of mercury amalgams. And as the primary patent holder of mercury amalgam, this same American Dental Association, although refusing to be open about collecting royalties each year from amalgam production, does indeed make money off of this dangerous substance! So you can see, the last place you should go to seek advice on the safety of mercury amalgams is the American Dental Association and its cadre of conventionally practicing member-dentists who follow the ADA party line.

Dr. Walker goes on to describe in voluminous scientifically documented detail the long-term health risks and dangers of dental amalgam fillings, other metallic substances installed into the oral cavity, root canals, cavitations, and fluoridation. There are nearly a thousand footnoted references in this book, many taken from the dentists' own scientific journals. And he doesn't just point out the problems—Dr. Walker offers solutions as well. He lays out the rationale for having mercury amalgam fillings replaced with safer materials and then guides the reader toward the appropriate resources for doing so. This struck a particular chord with me, as I personally have had all of my amalgam fillings removed a few years ago. It was my desire to prevent the dental amalgams' mercury from leaching out and making me chronically ill as they've already done to literally millions of North Americans, Europeans, Australians, New Zealanders, and others.

Finally, this superb medical journalist devotes several chapters to steps you can take on your own to ensure optimal physical and mental health by means of appropriate medical and nutritional procedures. Dr. Walker presents dietary guidelines that benefit the teeth and gums and details specific therapies for the treatment and prevention of periodontal disease. He introduces us to the growing field of holistic dentistry and invokes a new standard of dental care for all those unholistic and nonbiological health professionals who have something to do with the oral cavity—yours and mine.

Dr. Walker uses a lucid style of writing that is clear, concise, accurate, and easy to read. The information he provides herein is certainly usable. You should both benefit in your health and relish the education received from this book. My advice is to act on what you learn here in order to avoid the elements of dental danger lying in wait for all of us who aren't paying attention to our teeth. This book is a gem! You'll be taking it down from the shelf frequently to use as a good read, a shocking exposé, and for purposes of citation, substantiation, and quotation. It illustrates perfectly how a medical consumer's book of facts and story should be written.

My prediction is that this enlightening text, produced by one of the world's premier medical journalists and authors, is the handbook that will be referenced by numerous members of the legal profession to make the American Dental Association and its ADA member-dentists answer for the harm they have done to almost all of us.

Julian Whitaker, M.D.
Author/Editor, *Health & Healing* newsletter
Newport Beach, California
June 14, 1999

Introduction

Holism as It Relates to Dental Care

If you have ever had root canals installed or had dental cavities that were filled with dental mercury amalgams (known as "silver" fillings), consider that those mercury fillings could be

- leaching mercury vapors into your body and brain;
- causing your gums to ache and bleed after brushing;
- the reason you are beset by marginal gingivitis, hemorrhagic gingivitis, inflammatory gum enlargement, or periodontal infections;
- the source of ulcerations of the gums, lips, mouth, oral thrush, or other disorders of the mouth;
- the reason you suffer with mouth odor stemming from pyorrhea or another form of periodontitis;
- the cause of chronic, destructive periodontal pocketing containing broken-down bone;
- causing immune system suppression from bacterial toxins lodged in these same dead roots;
- causing your jaw to deteriorate from a hole in the bone (called a "cavitation"), producing chronic inflammation (osteitis);
- turning you or some family members into potential or true dental cripples;

Are you aware that your health difficulties from immune system suppression may have been foisted on you by your friendly family dentist?

Have you ever suspected that this dentist may be ignorant or noncaring about the overall harm that poor dental care is doing to your body and brain?

Are you familiar with the ever-popular slogan taught in dental school as the first piece of information students learn: "Know How to Drill, Fill, and Bill"?

Well, join the crowd, because you are not alone! More than 75 percent of North Americans, Australians, New Zealanders, and Europeans past age thirty-five may be the victims of oral cavity problems engendered by the same dentists who are supposed to save us from oral cavity diseases.

What You Receive for Your Dental Care Dollars

Our teeth and gums are active, blood-filled, living tissue—designed to heal and repair if given a chance. Our mouths are home to a highly complex ecosystem of many types of microorganisms. The types of microorganisms that populate that ecosystem directly affect the health of teeth, gums, and jawbones. By taking an ecologically systemic approach to our mouths, we're entitled to expect near-perfect dental health our entire lives. Yet such a circumstance is hardly the case for most of us who live in industrialized Western countries. And it's alleged that while residents of the United States receive the most technologically sophisticated dental care, it is, in fact, close to the worst in the world.

In 1979, for example, Americans spent a little more than $12 billion on their teeth.[1] By 1991 the costs to keep all of us chewing had risen to nearly $37 billion.[2] During those twelve years, what did dental patients receive for their increasing expenditures?

From society's conventionally trained dental care professionals, nearly all of whom are dues-paying members of the American Dental Association (ADA), people did receive mostly pain-free therapy. ADA dentists are good with applying local anesthetics. Dental services dispensed during those twelve years consisted of some skilled mechanics, progressively sophisticated technology, lots of surgical treatment for gum disease, and abundantly applied

---

1   B. H. Waldman, "Who Is Paying for Dental Care?" *Compendium Continuing Education in Dentistry* 8, no. 7 (July 1992).

2   H. J. V. Goldberg, F. J. Carberry, M. Somerman, L. J. Horowitz, and N. E. Jones, *Your Mouth Is Your Business: The Dentists' Guide to Better Health* (New York: Appleton-Century-Crofts, 1980). ix.

orthodontics, mostly in children, for the effects of underformed dental arches.

But added to such mechanical advances were numbers of other defective practices, which holistic (biological) medical and dental professionals believe have brought much harm to dental patients. For example, disadvantageous procedures still include such wrong-headed recommendations as:

- Fluoride applications to bring about decreases in tooth decay. These decreases have been falsely reported. (See chapter 14.)[1]

- Toxic metallic substances installed within, on, and around the teeth and various other parts of the oral cavity. (See chapters 4, 5, 6, 7, 8, 9, 10, and 11.)

- Allergy-creating orthodontics. (See chapter 3.)

- Cancer-causing bridgework. (See chapter 3.)

- Infection-producing root canals. (See chapter 12.)

- Bone-deteriorating cavitations. (See chapter 13.)

Largely unrecognized by dental consumers is that almost all such dental adjustments and other treatments are likely to have produced an immense amount of human immune system suppression, leading the way to a vast quantity of major illnesses. Most medical consumers in the United States are sicker than ever, and those dentists who conform to the ADA's prescribed ways of rendering dental care probably have contributed daily to the people's disabilities.

That was what we received for our dental expenditures from 1979 to 1991, but today the situation may be even worse! Dental treatment as dispensed by conventionally practicing American dentists seems to be more of the same but at higher prices to the body, psyche, and pocketbook.

---

1   "Is There Poison in Your Mouth?" *60 Minutes* (CBS television broadcast 16 December 1990), CBS News, 542 West 57th Street, New York, New York 10019.

Current allopathically minded ADA members possibly know better but tend to ignore the truth about the harm they are doing. They may be aware but they seem uncaring about the fact that they are installing materials that poison the body and brain of Americans at every age level. (See chapters 4, 5, 6, 7 and 11.) And care of the mouth is administered at higher financial costs. Consumers receive some relief through dental insurance, but the costs remain. You and your loved ones possibly are the recipients of unconscionable and poor—perhaps even criminal—professional dental malpractices. Dentists who use traditionally taught toxic methods of dentistry may deserve public condemnation and legal punishment.

For these reasons, I felt this book needed to be written by an investigative journalist, issued by a courageous publisher, read by the heads of households, and acted on by you for your loved ones.

The Movement toward Holistic Dentistry

Besides administering questionable dental care, something else is happening in dentistry too. There is a remarkable intraprofessional rebellion taking place against what some dentists conceive as the ADA's tyranny, dishonesty, blindness, and pigheadedness. A certain group of conscientious, holistically minded (biological, biocompatible, mercury-free) dentists exists. They are the honorable and high-principled members of four particular professional dental health care organizations:

1. The American Academy of Biological Dentistry

2. The Holistic Dental Association

3. The International Academy of Oral Medicine and Toxicology

4. The Environmental Dental Association

The book you are reading has been written largely predicated on information contributed by individual members—about twenty-eight dentists in all—of these four dental professional groups.

Infused with some revolutionary information about good dental practices, this book subsequently carries two main messages: first, major failings abide among those dentists who use poor health care procedures followed in ordinary conventionally administered modern dental practice, and, in contrast, concepts, techniques, procedures, and methods are finally being followed by the dentists involved in the profession's movement toward mercury-free, biocompatible, and holistic dentistry.

Biologically minded dentists in rebellion against certain toxic methods and policies of the ADA daily employ body and brain ecology—the administering of excellent dental care techniques. (See chapter 2.) They are offering sustained health and longer life to some people in the know—their informed patients who live mostly in North America, Australia, New Zealand, and Europe. The practice of biocompatible or holistic dentistry seems not yet to have reached South America, Central America, Asia, or Africa, but it is accepted especially well in a few countries of Europe such as Germany, Sweden, Hungary, and Great Britain. Also, mercury-free dentistry has traveled to the Pacific rim and settled into Australia and New Zealand. The dental professional a posteriori dinosaur (described below) obviously still remains strong in those less progressive areas of the world where holism has not found a home.

The A Posteriori Dental Professional Dinosaur

Paleontologists have described a dinosaur so huge that an attacker might have consumed half its tail before the big lizard's distant brain received any message and reacted to the emergency. Nature solved this problem, the paleontologists say, through evolution. It created a second brain, located near enough to the tail to provide a faster protective response. So what might be the ultimate result? In that way nature formed the first animal capable of reasoning a priori and a posteriori.

The dental profession, as practiced conventionally throughout the latter half of the twentieth century, is comparable to that same kind of a posteriori dinosaur. Invariably so large and unyielding is the organized dentistry "dinosaur" that it seems to function by guarding against attacks on its tail and lacks any ability to respond to real innovations or advances in dental science. The dental profession's politicians potentially remain locked in a rearguard action in philosophy and ethics (see chapter 8), and they appear to rule their members with an iron fist.

As an aftereffect to this reactionary thinking and perhaps out of fear of reprisals from their "labor union" (the American Dental Association), most orthodox dentists fail to respond to consumers' dental health requirements either with their brains or their backsides. These ADA members simply follow the party line and stay out of political trouble with their leaders. (Again, be directed to chapter 8's shocking exposé.)

Even larger, uglier, longer, and less caring than the a posteriori dinosaur described above, and with no posterior brain, the American Dental Association tends to respond sluggishly or not at all to any beneficial changes in the medical/dental environment.

Based on my research for this book, I must issue the following consumer warning: *accepting the services rendered by conventional dentists as they have been administered until now is potentially hazardous to your health and may be dangerous to your life.* It's not that I started out with such a belief; it has evolved from the journalistic investigations I have conducted. The information I uncovered in interviews with practicing dentists and by researching the dental and medical literature was teeming with questionable practices—one after the other—detrimental to the health of Americans of all ages, and sanctioned by the ADA. (See chapters 12, 13, and 14).

From these journalistic investigations, I came to the firm opinion that unquestionably organized dentistry promotes the onset of illnesses such as allergies, emotional instability, tremors, gingivitis, kidney failure, leukemia, hematopoietic dycrasias, epileptic seizures, Minamata disease, Parkinson's disease, multiple sclerosis, Alzheimer's disease, amyotrophic lateral sclerosis (Lou Gehrig's disease), peripheral neuropathies, and other neurological involvements.[1]

---

1   W. Shafer, M. Hine, and B. Levy, *A Textbook of Oral Pathology*, 4th ed. (1983), 578; D. Eggleston and A. Nylander, "Correlation of Dental Amalgam with Mercury in Brain Tissue," *Journal of Prosthetic Dentistry* 704 (1987), 58; I. A. Brown, "Chronic Mercurialism: A Cause of the Clinical Syndrome of Amyotrophic Lateral Sclerosis," *Archives of Neurology and Psychiatry* 72 (1954):

From its wrongheadedness on fluoridation (see chapter 14), organized dentistry has been accused of being responsible for some deaths too.[1] As I see it, the ADA's longtime prevailing attitude is "the public be damned!"

Supervised Dental Patient Neglect

How and why does such illness or possibly death occur for mistreated dental patients? This powerful American Dental Association, in its fossilized approach, perchance stifles originality in preventive dental care and is the guardian of an archaic dental status quo that perpetuates immune suppression of the population. Policies and dictates of the ADA appear to force the average dentist into application of crisis dental care or only cosmetic dentistry. The practices that could prevent illness as a result of dental impairment remain ignored, at overwhelming cost to the consumer but with big financial returns for organized dentistry. (See chapter 8.)

The editor of that consumer-friendly bimonthly newsletter, *The Holistic Dental Digest PLUS*, retired dentist Jerome S. Mittelman, D.D.S., IAPM, of New York City has stated: "In my opinion, the average dentist knows very little about the human bite. And when he or she makes a bridge for the patient, that's when the TMJ (temporomandibular joint) syndrome starts."[2] In TMJ syndrome the individual suffers mild to extreme pain in the facial muscles and joints of the jaws.

674–81, cited in J. D. Mitchell, "Heavy Metals and Trace Elements in Amyotrophic Lateral Sclerosis," *Neurologic Clinics* 5 (1987): 43–60; H. Huggins, "Proposed Role of Dental Amalgam Toxicity in Leukemia and Hematopoietic Dyscrasias," *International Journal of Biosocial and Medical Research* 84 (1989): 11.

1   J. A. Yiamouyiannis, "Water Fluoridation and Tooth Decay: Results from the 1986–1987 National Survey of U.S. Schoolchildren," *Fluoride* 23 (1990): 55–67.

2   J. W. Friedman, *Complete Guide to Dental Health: How to Avoid Being Overcharged and Overtreated* (Yonkers, N.Y.: Consumer Reports Books, 1991), 121.

Dr. Mittelman added, "At the preventive medicine academy, we label what orthodox dentists do as *supervised dental patient neglect.*" This studious, farsighted, and ultraholistic dentist is past president and fellow of the International Academy of Preventive Medicine (IAPM). The attitude expressed by Dr. Mittelman is a shining example of what honest, humane, and service-oriented dentistry should be. Consequently, I have asked him to be my dental professional consultant for this book.

Sitting in on our conversation, Dr. Mittelman's wife, Beverly Mittelman, B.S., C.N.C. (certified nutritional consultant), a well-experienced office administrator and former dental assistant, added, "With some dentists participating today in managed care programs, now you can label what's done to the policy holders' teeth as *institutionalized dental patient neglect.*" Holding a bachelor of science degree in medical technology, Mrs. Mittelman performed services adjunctive to her husband's when she dispensed nutritional counseling and myofunctional therapy during her sixteen years as a dental assistant.

Writing in the January 1998 *Townsend Letter for Doctors and Patients*, Robert B. Stephan, D.D.S., of Spokane, Washington, president of the Holistic Dental Association, warned: "Beware consumers, all is not right with dentistry. . . . The recent editorial attacks in leading dental journals on holistic and biological concepts are the dying quivers of those who live in an intellectual vacuum. Those who attack holistic dentistry lack insight and influence. The next few years will be trying times for us all as the paradigms of traditional dentistry shift to the tenets of biological concepts. It is hoped we will all take the high ground of truth into the future—our health depends on it."[1]

Consumers Have a Right to Good Dental Health

We who are the consumers of dental services are making our wishes known. Most of us very much want improvements in the

---

1   R. B. Stephan, "Biological Dentistry," letters to the editor, *Townsend Letter for Doctors and Patients* 174 (January 1998): 99.

delivery of dental care even though only a relatively few dentists—approximately 8 percent of dental professionals—have put themselves in a position to provide change for the better (see appendix C). The quest for holistic dentists who offer new therapies and aids to overall healing has never been more intense.

Do you realize that a modern-day dental revolution is in progress in our society? The ADA's member-politicians, who have tried to keep this profession steeped in doctrines from the dark ages, are on their way out. And we, the long-suffering medical/dental consumers, are destined to be the beneficiaries.

Medical/dental consumers are shouting loudly and clearly, albeit symbolically, "We don't want to be chronic patients anymore!" Not only do dental patients expect to be cured of their oral cavity diseases, but many believe they have a right to dental health. People in Western countries are assuming this right as they accept the concept that they are entitled to food, housing, clothing, freedom, and happiness.

Yet an ongoing stumbling block to furtherance of the right-to-dental-health concept remains. Organized dentistry itself—the twentieth century dinosaur—has presented a unified front of negativity when it comes to keeping people in a state of optimum dental health. Nonprogressive and narrow-minded actions of the dental politicians toward holistic or biological dentists, whose practices are mercury free, tend to make any observer such as myself feel disheartened and negative in turn.

The situation is a paradox, for the nature of dental care among industrialized nations has our dental health providers reacting to disease rather than keeping people's mouths functioning healthfully and well. This sort of crisis care does nothing to encourage good dental health and an overall healthy lifestyle among patients. It only has dentists applying skills and basic knowledge the way they are taught as novices in dental schools and in postgraduate dental training courses. No innovative whole-person procedures appear to be followed to encourage overall wellness. These dentists seemingly behave merely as "molar mechanics" and attempt no healing beyond the technical aspects of fixing a tooth or adjusting a bite.

If you want the best that dentistry has to offer, you must seek out the services of a dental professional who views the patient as a complete individual rather than as a walking oral cavity. You must find a holistic (biological) dentist who uses biocompatible, mercury-free material and who makes the concept of holism an integral part of his or her life. (See chapters 1 and 2).

The Hypothesis of Holism

Holism derives from the Greek *holos,* meaning *healthy, entire and whole,* and the first user of *holos* for treatment of the total person was Hippocrates, a Greek. The words *holy, health,* and *whole* all come from the same old English roots. To be holy, healthy, and whole means to be an individual filled with integrity: *integrated.* It also means to be in right relationships with self, others, and the universe. Its derivation is clear! The practice of this form of medicine and dentistry by doctors and the acceptance of this kind of personal health responsibility by individuals is known as *holistic.*

The hypothesis of holism is that the body is a holy temple sheltering the mind, which is sparked by the spirit or soul. The whole healthy person is made of all three: body, mind, and spirit, and their sum is greater than their parts. A now-out-of-print book of mine, *Total Health: The Holistic Alternative to Traditional Medicine that Stresses Preventative Care, Nutrition, and Treatment of the Whole Person,* which was published twenty years ago, was the first book to discuss holistic medicine and dentistry as a way to render excellent health care.[1]

In *Total Health* I wrote, "The person who views himself holistically takes into account every available judgment and skill for his or her growth toward harmony and balance."

As stated originally by Hippocrates, often cited as the father of modern medicine, holism means giving treatment to the person, not to the disease. It means using mild, natural methods whenever

---

1   M. Walker, *Total Health: The Holistic Alternative to Traditional Medicine That Stresses Preventative Care, Nutrition, and Treatment of the Whole Person* (New York: Everest House, 1979), xii–xv.

possible and engaging in the healthiest lifestyle available to enjoy the highest level of wellness and the fullest joy of living. Taking a holistic approach promotes the interrelationship and unity of body, mind, and spirit. They need to be integrated for the completeness of the whole person. The pursuit of holism encourages healthy, enjoyable activity on all levels of existence.

Holism means more than the total healthy individual and his acceptance of health responsibility: we who think in holistic terms find our personal path for social, political, economic, physical, psychological, and spiritual change. We look for ways to learn more about ourselves and our feelings, to find how to cope creatively with occurrences beyond our control. We let go of anger, confront pain, enjoy fun times to the fullest, relax tensions, sleep peacefully, have satisfying bowel movements, and do all the other "holy" things that help to keep us healthy and whole. Nature's plan is that we be integrated individuals.[1] Following this path, we can affect our functioning far more than we presently are aware. We influence our own health by using the tools and techniques of personal healing.

Holistic Dentistry Goes beyond Preventive Dentistry

There is a growing consciousness about this concept of holism as it relates to dental care. Many of today's dental consumers are looking for the holistic concept of dental care. Even so, many people don't know how to find it, where to get it, who furnishes it, what they have to do for it, or even why they feel the urge for dental holism. (See chapter 2.) The only thing most dental patients recognize is that they *sense* this gnawing need to change, to have something other than what they've been getting this past half-century in ADA-approved dental care.

A holistic dental practitioner in upstate New York, who is afraid the American Dental Association will attack him and remove his

---

1   J. Tate, "To Be Whole and Holy," *ME Newsletter of Oklahoma City* (March 1977).

license to practice if his colleagues learn his identity, describes how holistic dentistry goes beyond preventive dentistry. This truth-telling dentist has said: "In holistic dental practice, the emphasis is on the body's integrated self as if it's a whole piece of equipment and consciousness with all its parts functioning. Like a car, the body must be road worthy. The holistic healer's goal, be it in medicine, dentistry, or mental health therapy, is to treat the entire person and help him or her avoid degeneration and disease.

"The basic principle of holistic dentistry is that the mouth can be used as a diagnostic area for the body," continued the dentist. "Today we recognize that dental problems are the result of body imbalances. The condition of one's oral tissues is an excellent indicator of a body's total health. The mouth, while having its own form and function, being the first part of one's digestive system, is also a vital part of your early warning system. A patient's oral cavity, especially the gum tissue, is extremely sensitive to the changes the body is going through, including emotional stress.

"After years of practicing dentistry, I still feel surprise when I witness how sensitively responsive a patient's mouth is. I feel the weight of responsibility of how important my job has become as my patient's mouth guardian," assured this mercury-free dentist. "Still, I have found a dark side to the dental profession, in particular as it involves several items such as the dentist's reconstructive orientation, certain treatment modalities, periodontal surgery and its side effects, painkillers, and the rest of the dental paradigm. Being a guardian for my patient's mouth is not enough for me. I realize now that to be the best I can be at my chosen field, I must aim high and see myself as a healer—even as a dentist. In brief, my conclusion is that the fundamental principle of holistic dentistry is that the mouth can be used as a diagnostic area for the body overall.

"One of my favorite patients once commented that the amount of money he had spent fixing his teeth could just as easily have been spent buying a flashy new car. I noted aloud that, unlike the car, his body's response to good dental care could never be traded in for a replacement. The patient replied that, nevertheless, he was planning to treat his mouth with the same delicacy with which he behaved with a new car. In turn, I joked that, as his lead mechanic, I was going to ensure that his oral cavity gets the correct checkups, tune-ups, and overall care one would expect from a good mechanic. After all, what else is a 'Mr. Good Wrench' for?" the holistic dentist asked.

Speaking to his fellow dentists, Jerome S. Mittelman wrote as a contributor to the textbook of *Myofunctional Therapy*: "It is important to understand that in preventive dentistry, the overriding philosophy is simply that the effects of dental disease should not be treated until the causes have been removed. To rehabilitate by performing operative dentistry, orthodontics, or periodontal surgery before the causes for the need of the therapy have been removed is a disservice and invites recurrence of the very dysfunction that we treat. (The obvious exception to this is the dental treatment of emergencies.) If one is to perform conscientious, preventive dentistry, priority must be given to removing the causes of dental disease."[1]

Some ADA Party-Liners Could Be Incompetent, Dishonest, or Both

It's possible that some ADA party-line followers are fundamentally either incompetent or dishonest, or both. This was confirmed in February 1997, when *Reader's Digest* published its investigation that found a lack of diagnostic consistency, treatment competence, and pricing uniformity among fifty dentists studied. Dentists from twenty-eight states were randomly selected by an investigating journalist, William Ecenbarger, who told each dentist that he needed a new dental specialist. Then he opened his mouth and showed the individual doctor his teeth and a set of X-ray films that accurately depicted them.

Ecenbarger asked each practitioner for a written treatment plan and a cost estimate, saying that he needed them because his dental care was paid for by a direct-reimbursement insurance plan provided by his employer. Because every one of the dentists was supposedly hungry for this insurance-financed business, the potential "patient"

---

1   J. S. Mittleman, "Preventive Dentistry," in *Myofunctional Therapy,* ed. D. Garliner (Philadelphia: W. B. Saunders, 1993).

received these documents every time he asked for them during the semi-sting operation.

Before Ecenbarger started his investigation, the journalist had checkups of his teeth by his personal dentist and by three others who "had no financial interest" in his dental health. These four health professionals agreed that his oral cavity was in good shape with one exception, the number 30 tooth. Some also thought that number 18 needed attention, as well. The four dentists further agreed that if two crowns were recommended, the total cost should be under $1,500.

Ecenbarger's survey brought unexpectedly diverse and disturbing responses from the party-line dentists, leaving him to wonder, "What, then, can Americans do to protect themselves from so much overtreatment and overcharging?" According to his report, the following is the kind of incompetence or dishonesty to which this "typical dental patient" was exposed:

Only twelve of the fifty consulted dentists agreed with the findings of Ecenbarger's original disinterested panel of four dentists. Fifteen of the fifty missed his problem number 30 tooth completely; three of those fifteen dentists found no problems whatsoever. Most disturbing were recommendations for extensive and unnecessary treatments. For example, a Memphis, Tennessee, dentist told the journalist that he could "squeak by with a barebones approach, 'with absolutely no guarantees for the future,' at a cost of $5,000. But what he really ought to do . . . would be to crown all twenty-eight teeth. . . . Total cost: $13,440." In Salt Lake City another dentist told Mr. Ecenbarger that he needed a complete $19,402, full-mouth reconstruction.

As the number of dentists and competition for patient dollars increase, many ADA party-line dentists are seeking ways to increase profits. One sure way is to push expensive restoration work instead of simple fillings. Some dentists just set higher prices. Among the fifty dentists investigated by William Ecenbarger, examinations cost $20 to $141, and a porcelain crown would cost between $329 and $1,150. There was no uniformity of prices.[1]

---

1   W. Ecenbarger, "How Honest Are Dentists?" *Reader's Digest* (February 1997).

As the premier labor union for dentists, the American Dental Association holds a loose rein on its dues-paying members, except when they fail to follow the party line. Then, as you'll discover in reading the ensuing chapters (especially chapter 8), this health professional organization, supported financially by dental journal advertisements, toothpaste endorsements, product approvals, mouth appliance acceptances, sales of dental convention exhibit spaces, insurance company kickbacks, membership dues, patent royalties, special assessments, and other nefarious means of milking money from the public, assumes complete control of how the profession is practiced. The ADA does this by attempting to take away holistic dental livelihoods and individual dentists' integrity by lifting state licenses to practice the profession. No one seems able to stop what may be characterized as "the dental mafia" entrenched within the ADA.

The Final Analysis of Holistic, Biocompatible Dentistry

In the final analysis, all of us desire holistic health as the ultimate goal of preventive dentistry. However, it's more than just prevention that we're after. Holism goes beyond one's defensive reactions to the potential of disease and the chance of accidents. Rather, holism promotes the enrichment of health and the enhancement of life. What the individual patient must do is avoid toxic elements of dental danger and provide an optimal internal and external environment.

Holism in dentistry meets a near-similar criterion. It is founded on the belief that almost everyone has the inborn mechanism to remain in a state of optimal wellness and live the full number of humankind's allotted years (perhaps 120 or more). For the dentist who would practice holistically, the aim is to deprogram illness and eliminate it from the patient's experience by employing only biocompatible materials. This is readily achieved through the dispensing of holistic dental services and the adoption generally of a holistic (biological) approach to practice. It's an application of orthomolecular dentistry, a procedure we will explore in the first chapter.

One

Toximolecular Dentistry versus Orthomolecular Dentistry

A board-certified family practice physician, Bruce Shelton, M.D., Dr. Hom. (the doctor of homeopathy degree from England), is medical director of the Allergy Center in Phoenix, Arizona. At that clinic Dr. Shelton specializes in eliminating ear, nose, and throat allergies for patients through the application of homeopathy (among numerous other therapies). Of the many observations he has made during thirteen years of specialization in allergy and homeopathy, Dr. Shelton says that organized dentistry's use of mercury amalgams for filling cavities in the teeth "is as close as you can get to the center of the illness universe; dental amalgams have set us up for most of the health problems we see today. I'm convinced that 80 percent of my patients are here [in his Phoenix, Arizona Allergy Center] because of hidden dental problems."

This allergist is completely opposed to the toximolecular (poisonous element) dental techniques usually employed by conventionally practicing dental practitioners. Specifically, Dr. Shelton points to mercury amalgams, root canals, cavitations, fluoridation, and orthodontic braces, as the prime sources of health problems originating from the toxic techniques of dentistry.

Dr. Shelton points out that he condemns such toximolecular dental techniques because of true pathological processes that occur from them. For instance, he detests dentists placing amalgam fillings into patients' cavities because mercury vapors leach from those same mercury-filled cavities as a person chews on the filled teeth. Such vapors are distributed throughout the body and produce numerous symptoms of disease. Dr. Shelton says that metallic poisons from the dental amalgam material are forced into the mouth, where they create such illnesses as Parkinson's disease, amyotrophic lateral sclerosis (ALS), and other neurological pathologies.

Since fluoride is another poisonous substance, Dr. Shelton also opposes the mandatory fluoridation of our public water supplies, as well as tooth brushing with fluoride toothpaste.

"Root canals harbor hidden bacterial infections and block energy currents [and acupuncture meridians] that pass through the mouth and that are energetically connected with internal organs," states Dr. Shelton.

"Cavitations are areas of infected jawbone underneath defective root canals or remaining from [poorly managed] tooth extractions," he advises.

"Orthodontic braces in children affect the electrical balance in a patient's mouth," he says, "and thereby disturb electrical balances throughout the body."[1]

It may be assumed that almost all of the procedures a dental student learns in professional school are toximolecular in nature. This teaching is opposite to the orthomolecular (proper or correct element) types of services rendered by holistic (biological) dentists, who use biocompatible and mercury-free treatment methods. Out of the need to assuage their consciences as moral human beings and honest health professionals, many holistic dentists investigate, learn thoroughly, and apply the orthomolecular procedures of dentistry. They study holistic dentistry extracurricularly and on their own while in private practice. Then they teach each other on a one-to-one basis. Such conscious-ridden health professionals have gone on to form numbers of extracurricular study groups, as well. They work together outside of mainstream dentistry, often to the chagrin or vexation of politically minded leaders of the dental profession who run the various state dental societies affiliated with the American Dental Association (ADA).

---

1   R. Leviton, "The Ideal Clinic: Fibroids and Male Impotence," *Alternative Medicine Digest* 19: 46–53.

Occasionally the state ADA affiliate becomes so irritated with one of its holistic-minded members that charges are brought against the particular biological dentist. Such charges do frequently get filed with the state's board of dental examiners. Then the biological dentist's license to practice dentistry is in jeopardy, and a legal battle is likely to ensue.

It's rare that any holistic dentist escapes harassment and legal hassles involving the license to practrice. At the very least, threats of delicensure are made, and the dentist must decide if the requirement to practice honesty is more compelling than the need to earn a living. Those dentists possessed by strong ethical and moral principles attend investigative board hearings and occasionally end up in court, where they usually win against the state's dental board but at great cost in time, money, and mental duress for the dentist. It's a highly distressing situation. During the most recent decade, at least 220 mercury-free dentists have found it necessary to fight off legal attacks by state boards of dental examiners. Most have retained their licenses to practice, but some have not.

I must note that a number of biological/holistic-type dentists who wished to speak their minds by contributing information for this book were fearful of their identities being made known to the ADA. They did not want the harassment, threats, and potential loss of licensure that invariably comes with such honesty and exposure. Therefore, some dentists provided me with shocking information about the practice of ADA-type dentistry but made me promise not to reveal that they were the source.

Toximolecular and Orthomolecular
Dental Differences

What are the differences between the two types of dentistry: toximolecular and orthomolecular? First, we have the known quantity that most of us are acquainted with—a dentist who dispenses presently practiced conventional toximolecular dental services as propounded by the American Dental Association with its affiliated state organizations. Second, we have the other, contradistinctive type of oral cavity specialist who employs the orthomolecular philosophy and treatment methods of holistic, biological, biocompatible, and mercury-free dentistry.

Toximolecular means that the administering dentist is using toxic (poisonous) substances or molecular materials (elements or molecules) that cause conditions of severe and progressive illness. The illnesses may be devastating, even causing the death of the patient.2 Thus, toximolecular dentists are likely to kill people sooner or later.

If you want to experience a healthy and wellness-filled longevity, my recommendation is to avoid the services of any dentist employing the present toximolecular methods of oral cavity care that are defined in this book.

Paradoxically, condemnation of these toximolecular methods often inadvertently comes from the ADA itself. Its publicity people don't discuss how their members' services adversely affect the growth of children, aging of adults, midlife sexuality, psychological and emotional aspects of living, general activity level, genetics, toxic overload, drug usage, overall longevity, and quality of life. Instead, the ADA public relations department focuses strictly on teeth as if they are separate from the body. The public relations department condemns the quality of patients' teeth and talks about the public's neglect as if the organization's own members have nothing to do with such neglect.

The ADA unabashedly states that 75 percent of American adults older than age thirty-five are victims of gum disease. Aren't the periodontal specialists of dentistry supposed to be forestalling such disease? They are not!

It's known that more than a hundred million people in this country suffer from periodontal disease and other oral cavity illnesses. Dental and oral diseases are declared the most common but preventable health conditions afflicting people in the United States, but the toximolecular methods of conventional dentistry don't even solve those particular mouth problems to which dentists are supposed to administer and in which they are supposed to be expert.[1]

---

1   "Dental Armory," *Energy Times* (September 1997): 80.

In contrast, *Orthomolecular* means there is provision for mechanical, nutritional, and other components appropriate for overcoming problems with the oral cavity of the individual patient. Enlightened doctors practicing orthomolecular dentistry view the wholeness of the body in relation to dental disease.

The now deceased, two-time Nobel laureate Linus Pauling, Ph.D., a biological chemist and physicist, coined the term *orthomolecular* as it refers to orthomolecular psychiatry. In this mind/body connection, nutrients rather than drugs are used for healing mental illness. (Please see my coauthored book from Keats Publishing, Inc., *Putting It All Together: The New Orthomolecular Nutrition*, for which Dr. Linus Pauling wrote the foreword.)[1]

Quite simply, "ortho" means to be proper or correct or straight or upright. Dr. Pauling wanted to convey the basic idea that many illnesses could be corrected by straightening out, in effect, the concentrations of specific molecules so as to provide the optimum molecular environment for the body and mind. He wrote: "Only during the last few years has the field of orthomolecular medicine attracted much attention. . . . Good nutrition is important for the preservation of health and prevention of disease." Other than to admonish you about eating sweets, when was the last time your conventionally practicing toximolecular dentist asked you about your diet? Holistic dentists invariably do that as part of their diagnostic and treatment plans!

The mouth, although it has its own separate functions apart from the rest of one's physiology, shows symptoms of the body's imbalance. The holistic dentist looks in your mouth and sees a full story told by your oral cavity. The mouth reveals a great deal about your total health—indicated, for instance, by the condition of the teeth, the color and texture of the tongue, the color of the gums, and lots of other signs and symptoms. Using herbology, homeopathic remedies, aromatherapy, nutrient supplementation, diet, and a whole lot more that will be discussed in the next and later chapters, the biological

---

1   A. Hoffer and M. Walker, *Putting It All Together: The New Orthomolecular Nutrition* (New Canaan, Conn.: Keats Publishing, Inc., 1996), 14.

dentist who uses orthomolecular methods creates a new way of diagnosing, preventing, and treating infections of the teeth and gums. At the same time, this holistic health professional banishes the old stigma of conventionally practicing dentists who are known as being perpetual administrators of pain.[1]

Dental Exposures Wrought
by Hal A. Huggins, D.D.S., M.S.

Many anecdotes could be told that depicted situations in which the practice of orthomolecular dentistry saves lives. For example, there's the chest-pain situation for Janet Bartholemew, a seventeen-year-old patient attended by Hal A. Huggins, D.D.S., M.S. Young Jan had been hospitalized dozens of times during prior years by her family physician because of angina-like attacks that seemed to have no physical cause. Eventually, her heart symptoms were diagnosed by consulting psychiatrists as "nerves"—described to Jan's parents as no doubt being "all in her head." It was psychosomatic, they said.

But suddenly the patient's chest pains disappeared permanently. Why? Because Jan's mother refused to lock up her daughter in a mental institution as was suggested by one of the psychiatrists. Instead she brought the teenager to Dr. Hal Huggins for dental care. He investigated holistically and went to the source of the child's problem. He removed her mercury amalgams and replaced them with porcelain filling material. The procedure worked beautifully. "Jan was my first big exposure to the destruction of life through toxic metals, but far from my last," writes Dr. Huggins.[2]

At the Huggins Diagnostic Center, on a snowy Thursday morning, November 2, 1995, I interviewed Dr. Huggins; his wife, Rocky Huggins; and the center's consulting cardiologist, Thomas Levy,

---

1   "Dental Armory," 81.

2   H.A. Huggins, *It's All in Your Head: The Link between Mercury Amalgams and Illness* (Garden City Park, N.Y.: Avery Publishing Group, 1993), 12–15.

M.D., F.A.C.C., of Colorado Springs, Colorado. Dr. Levy readily fits the designation of "cardiodentologist," because he knows more about dental disease as it influences the body's physiology than any dentist who uses toximolecular oral treatment procedures.

Dr. Hal Huggins has been a pioneer in dental toxicity testing, as well as an advocate for safe, nontoxic (orthomolecular) dentistry. Also he has educated dentists and patients about proper nutrition and supplementation of nutrients specifically based on each patient's laboratory profile. His lectures and writings, which have been anathema to the American Dental Association for more than two decades, consistently warn against amalgam toxicity, other nonmercuric toxins, additional poisonous metals installed in the mouth, fluoride in all its forms, orthodontic procedures, careless tooth extractions that leave behind cavitations, root canal treatment that allows bacteria to remain in place, and much more. As a result, the Colorado Board of Dental Examiners and the state attorney general have been after him. In multiple ways they have been attacking him for more than twenty-two years. Recorded on audiotape, which I've stored in a safe place, Dr. Huggins told me that the Colorado Dental Association, an affiliate of the ADA, had "hit" men make an attempt on his life. He was forced to install bulletproof window glass in his office after bullets shattered his picture window and nearly killed him.

I arrived at the Huggins Diagnostic Center for interviews exactly one day after Dr. Huggins relinquished his license to practice dentistry in the State of Colorado. It's what he had to do to preserve his life and stave off the repeated legal attacks that have brought tremendous emotional upsets to him and Rocky Huggins, as well as to staff members at the Huggins Diagnostic Center. The ADA and Colorado State legal harassments were bankrupting the Huggins family.

"It irritates me when dentists *deny* that we in the profession are the biggest purveyors of toxins to humans in the world," says Dr. Huggins. "Obviously, the orthodox dental professional community is not happy with me because I am exposing to consumers what dentists are doing to them. As a result of the toxins we as a health profession promote throughout patients' bodies, individual dentists are the sources of breast cancer, multiple sclerosis, parkinsonism, and other major health problems. I possess autopsy reports which prove my statements."

Dr. and Mrs. Huggins are driven by the truth of their convictions, which are based on original clinical and laboratory research they've conducted. As a Feldenkrais therapist, Mrs. Rocky Huggins has worked with her husband's patients for years to overcome numbers of serious illnesses such as arthritis, backaches, bursitis, cerebral palsy, coordination problems, digestive difficulties, headaches, lack of endurance, multiple sclerosis, musculoskeletal disorders, polio, respiratory disease, stress-related disorders, and others.

Her Feldenkrais approach is distinct from any other form of therapy. It's a method of treatment that teaches participants to become aware of movement patterns and to improve body motion. This approach endeavors to correct bad habits, alleviate pain, reduce stress, and enhance self-image. Mrs. Huggins' clients learn to move with greater ease, spontaneity, and freedom, resulting in benefits to the mind, the emotions, and the entire body. A Feldenkrais therapist does not attempt to change the structure of a client's body through adjustment or manipulation. Rather, she instructs individuals to relearn proper body movements.[1]

"As described by my husband, how do those toxins escaping from tooth cavitations and poison substances placed in the mouth impact the patient's immune system?" asks Mrs. Huggins. "I've come to recognize a real flaw in the mechanical application of dental care. Unbeknownst to most consumers, by their doctors' following certain harmful dental procedures, the patients often experience problems with their immune systems. The dental society's publicity machine doesn't allow this information to be available to people and so the public lingers in ignorance.

"I'm a body practitioner, so that I look at the whole person and not just an individual body part, such as the teeth. My observation is that the usual dentist is taught in dental school to save teeth but at the cost of a patient's entire body and mind," affirms Mrs. Huggins.

---

1   L. P. Credit, S. G. Hartunian, and M. J. Nowak, *Your Guide to Complementary Medicine* (Garden City Park, N.Y.: Avery Publishing Group, 1998), 56, 57.

"Frequently the dental patient's immune system fails. The teeth are not separate entities; they are an integral part of the physiology. The result is that we at the Huggins Diagnostic Center are doing something different from routine dentistry. We are practicing the delivery of health care using integrated medical/dental multidisciplines. That is the pure practice of holistic orthomolecular dentistry."

Multiple Sclerosis Is Predominantly a Dental Disease

Multiple sclerosis (MS), also known as disseminated sclerosis, is a chronic disease of the nervous system affecting young and middle-aged adults. The myelin sheaths surrounding nerves in the brain and spinal cord are damaged, which affects the function of the nerves involved. The course of the illness is characterized by recurrent relapses followed by remissions. The disease affects various parts of the brain and spinal cord, resulting in typically scattered symptoms. These include unsteady gait and shaky movements of the limbs (ataxia), rapid involuntary movements of the eyes (nystagmus), defects in speech pronunciation (dysarthria), spastic weakness, and optic neuritis.[1]

Since its discovery around the mid-1830s, there has been endless speculation about the cause of MS. Now we've come to realize that the first reported appearance of the disease occurred only a few years after the original insertions of dental mercury as amalgam fillings in 1826. During our interview, Cardiologist Thomas Levy told me that Dr. Hal Huggins has researched this medical history and acted on it.

"Dr. Huggins has consistently witnessed improvement in MS patients undergoing amalgam removal. He observes clear symptomatic and laboratory test improvements in up to 85 percent of the patients. Until he relinquished his Colorado dental license, it was common to see wheelchair-bound patients discontinue use of their support chairs and take steps on their own once again," said Dr. Levy.

---

1   R. D. Adam and M. Viktor, *Principles of Neurology*, 5th ed. (1993), 778.

Multiple sclerosis recovery has happened repeatedly for patients so afflicted because they have undergone dental amalgam removal. Clinical observation confirms that multiple sclerosis is predominantly a dental disease.[1] It is brought on by dentists packing mercury and other amalgamated metals into the cavities of people with impaired teeth. Mercury amalgams have made people what holistic and mercury-free dentist Richard T. Hansen, D.M.D., of Fullerton, California, has described as "dental cripples." (Note: Dr. Hansen's holistic practice procedures are discussed at length in chapter 2. See the listing of his book on holistic dentistry in appendix B.)

The success rate of healing for MS patients increased with Dr. Huggins' discovery of fluoride in all its forms as a complicating factor in the disease. Fluoride must be scrupulously avoided by MS patients. They must not drink fluoridated water, brush with fluoridated toothpaste, or take fluoride dental treatments. Ingestion of this chemical retards the patient's clinical progress toward healing or even promotes frank clinical relapse of MS symptoms.

Dr. Huggins has MS. Since he has experienced its symptoms for many years, Dr. Huggins himself is all too keenly aware of the nuances and persistence of MS as a disease. But he keeps the symptoms largely in check by following a series of stringent lifestyle modifications, eating an excellent diet (the dental diet), and taking nutritional supplementation as part of his daily regimen.[2] It is well known that dentists push the use of fluoride products and fluoride drinking water on the public. By doing so, they are assuredly increasing the incidence of multiple sclerosis in the Western world. (See chapter 14.)

The brain and central nervous system (CNS) are strongly affected by the electrical current present in all people whose mouths contain metal. This phenomenon is readily recognized as "oral galvanism." Such electrical currents can be measured easily

---

1   T. Levy, "Teeth—The Root of Most Disease?" *Extraordinary Science* (April/May/June 1994).

2   Ibid.

with a probe and a microammeter. Amalgams, metallic crowns, and braces generally all register from 1 to 100 microamperes of current in a positive or negative polarity. The natural currents found in the brain are in the range of 7 to 9 nanoamperes, making the mouth currents anywhere from 100 times to 10,000 times more powerful. Keep in mind that the base of the brain is roughly an inch away from the upper teeth.[1]

The consequence is that MS patients and various other neurologically affected patients demonstrate improvement immediately with removal of this metallic electrical dental material. Their muscle strength and coordination improve and various symptoms decrease, including severe migraine headaches, chronic cough, jaw pain, muscle cramping, chest pain, and low energy levels. Even psychiatric and emotional depression disappear.

The Origins of Holistic (Biological) Dentistry

The connection of multiple sclerosis to the methods of modern ADA-practiced dental procedures is but a smattering of information uncovered by leaders in the movement to further holistic (biological) dentistry. This movement began in 1923 when Weston A. Price, D.D.S., M.S., former director of research for the American Dental Association for fourteen years, published his 1,100-page, two-volume treatise on dental pathology from microorganisms, *Dental Infections, Oral and Systemic (Volume 1)* and *Dental Infections and the Degenerative Diseases (Volume 2)*. The results of Dr. Price's research were profound, detailed, reproduceable, and truly scientific. For the first time ever, he proved that there was hardly any disease or pathological process that was not either primarily caused or worsened by dental infections.

Now we know that people's heart and circulatory systems are favorite target sites for the bacteria or their toxins coming from dental infections. Dr. Price observed that angina pectoris, phlebitis,

---

1   Huggins Diagnostic Center, *Position Papers: Amalgam Issue, Root Canals, Cavitations,* 15.

hypertension, heart block, anemia, and inflammation of the heart muscle are frequent side effects of root canal therapy. He also reported that he would sometimes see heart patients with outwardly normal-appearing root canal teeth resolve most or all of their symptoms upon removal of those dead teeth.[1]

To illustrate, the death of humorist Lewis Grizzard, who died of heart disease in March 1994 at age forty-seven, has been directly tied to heart valve problems stemming from infected teeth. (See chapter 15.) New research shows that dental infections are behind hardening of the arteries, heart attacks, strokes, and spontaneous preterm births. Dennis Mangan of the National Institute of Dental Research (NIDR) in Bethesda, Maryland, has pointed to dental difficulties as causing damage in body parts far distant from the mouth,[2] the source of dental infections.

The underlying premise behind the toxicity of root canals is the following: (1) the interior tubules of root canal teeth cannot be sterilized, (2) all root canal teeth demonstrate the presence of infectious bacteria, however normal they may appear clinically, and (3) the anaerobic (oxygen-lacking) environment root canals offer in the root tips allows otherwise benign, oxygen-using mouth bacteria to undergo a toxic transformation, causing the production of thio-esthers as a bacterial by-product. These thio-esthers are a million times more deadly than snake venom, and a billion times more potent than botulism. They can cause disease and death if released into the blood stream, and they are so released slowly over years in ever so tiny amounts.[3]

For this reason, my conclusion is that conventionally practicing endodontists (root canal specialists), along with their other dental colleagues, must take responsibility for causing a great deal of the immune suppression diseases (and autoimmune diseases)

1   H. A. Huggins, *The Price of Root Canals* (Colorado Springs, Colo.: Huggins Diagnostic Center, 1994).

2   S. Sternberg, "Chronic Tooth Infections Can Kill More Than Smile," *USA Today*, section D, 14 April 1998, 1D, 2D.

3   W. A. Price, *Dental Infections and Related Degenerated Diseases: Some Structural and Biochemical Factors* (Chicago: American Medical Association, 1925).

we are experiencing today among populations of industrialized Western nations. I believe that dentists bring on much of the difficulties related to cancer, rheumatoid arthritis, AIDS, chronic fatigue syndrome, the yeast syndrome, fibromyalgia, the seven forms of herpes infection, systemic lupus erythematosis, and so much more.

Cavitations as Another Result of Toximolecular Dentistry

A few dentists and physicians in the mid-1950s took note that certain long-established sites in the mouths of patients possessed sealed-over layers of tissue. The tissue covered the tops of openings that had been left behind when teeth were extracted. Under these seals were holes, or *cavitations*, where the roots of teeth used to be lodged. Articles appearing in dental and medical journals showed that cavitations, which penetrated the gum all the way down to, and sometimes through, a person's jawbone, were present because of a lack of healing where the lining of the tooth socket had *not* been removed.

When a tooth is extracted, proper procedure is to remove the layer of connective tissue between the tooth and the bone known by anatomists as the *periodontal ligament* or the *periodontal membrane*. Its presence indicates to the immune system that the tooth is in place in a normal manner and if this periodontal ligament is not removed appropriately at the time of tooth extraction, the bone will not regenerate to fill the space left behind after surgery. The empty tooth socket heals over the top with a thin layer of bone and some new gum tissue, but the socket never fills in with good solid bone. Therefore, a void remains in the bone and toxins escape from bacteria or pleomorphic microorganisms (see chapter 12) and gradually leach into the body fluids and bloodstream to bring on slow immune system suppression.

In contrast, the performance of orthomolecular dentistry involves a procedure to prevent cavitations from forming. The holistic (biological) technique of forestalling cavitations is simple, painless, and merely requires a single extra minute of attention from the extracting dentist to use the slow-speed drill to clean periodontal ligamentous material from the tooth socket and rinse it properly.

That's all! This is the way to save a dental patient from experiencing the leaching of toxins lodged in the socket of an unhealthy hole in the jawbone—an osteitis—and the resulting breeding ground for autoimmune disease.[1]

For dental patient welfare, the contrast in value between ortho-molecular dentistry and toximolecular dentistry is significant beyond measure. It's like the difference between health and disease or life and death.

Commentary from the Upstate New York Holistic Dentist

"Since its inception, dentistry has been a set of surgical practices designed for reconstructing the results of nutritional deficiencies on one's teeth and mouth. The field has moved from traveling itinerants yanking rotten molars to developing new smiles for tired faces—from the use of pliers and screwdrivers to dental lasers and implants," explained the holistic dentist from upstate New York who wants no name revealed because of worries about threatening behavior from dental society colleagues. "For many dental patients, the most impor-tant advancement in all this time has been the introduction of anes-thesia. For most of us in the dental field, the biggest change has been the quality of tools used to restore people's mouths back to full function.

"As a holistic dentist, I have found myself studying the blossom-ing worlds of nutrition, acupuncture, and other 'alternative' meth-ods of treatment now considered mainstream. I have seen how feelings affect people's immune systems and their physical well-being. I've also learned how to read my patients as full people, not just the open mouths we learned about in dental school. Com-bined with what I was learning about myself and others," says this biological dentist, "I realize that such knowledge is applicable to dentistry. Being a guardian for my patients is not enough; I know that to be the best I could at my chosen field of dentistry, I must

---

1   Huggins Diagnostic Center, *Position Papers*, 23, 24.

aim high. I have to see myself as a healer, with the tools of dental care as my medium.

"The more I study, the more I realize that this new form of holistic and orthomolecular dentistry is the only way to practice. There is a growing awareness among the public and my dental colleagues that each part of the body is part of an integrated self. The holistic healer's goal, no matter the specialty, is to treat the entire person and help him or her avoid degeneration and disease," concludes this colleague-wary dentist who treats his patients honestly.

Two

The Biological Procedures of Holistic Dentists

When she was sixteen years old, my granddaughter was awakened one morning with a terribly painful tooth. Her jaw was swollen, achy, and hot and any pressure on the tooth produced awful stabbing pain. The child's loving and consciencious mother immediately rushed this high schooler to the family's conventionally-practicing, nonholistic dentist for examination and treatment, who told her, "Your daughter needs a root canal performed or we must pull the tooth."

What is the parent to do? Being somewhat informed about the dangers of root canals (see chapter 12 for a detailed discussion), as opposed to viewing the consequences of her daughter's living with the hole left in her jaw from a missing tooth, what decision must my daughter-in-law come to? Should it be the tooth pulling or a root canal installation?

Writing in his well-documented consumer book, *Root Canal Cover-Up*, George E. Meinig, D.D.S., F.A.C.D., a founding member of the American Association of Endodontists and dentist for the Twentieth Century Fox film studio, discussed how and why root canals damage health by crippling the immune system. Dr. Meinig wrote: "Bacteria trapped inside the structure of the [root canaled] teeth migrate throughout the body. They may infect any organ, gland, or tissue and can damage the heart, kidneys, joints, eyes, brain, and endanger pregnant women." This endodontist went on to advise readers that tooth decay causes many patients to choose root canals, but an improved tooth extraction technique better supports health.[1]

---

1   G. E. Meinig, *Root Canal Cover-Up* (Ojai, Calif.: Bion Publishing, 1994).

Root Canal Information from
Richard T. Hansen, D.M.D.

For answers to the questions that had faced my daughter-in-law about her child's painfully infected tooth, I later talked to the respected holistic dentist, Richard T. Hansen, D.M.D., clinic director of the Center for Advanced Dentistry in Fullerton, California. Of course, Dr. Hansen's response came after my granddaughter, as permitted by her mother, had already gone through the endodontic procedure. Now this attractive young woman owns at least one gutta-percha root canal implanted in her jawbone.

Gutta-percha is the solid, rubbery sap of various tropical trees that's shaped into fine, tapered cylinders used for sealing prepared tooth cavities such as root canals. Because these cylinders are easily seen on X-ray films (from metallic salts added), dentists use gutta-percha points to probe tooth hollows to measure their depth. The gutta-percha cylinders are also fitted into root canals and left there.

Dr. Hansen stated, "No doubt the mother followed her dentist's advice and the girl's root canal was filled with gutta-percha. The dentist probably administered a course of antibiotics to rid your granddaughter of the massive infection lodged in her jaw. This is the standard procedure of conventional dentistry, and it's the underlying source of immense amounts of physical difficulties for the patient some years down the road. Modern, orthodox, allopathic-oriented dentistry demands this type of therapy, and it's wrong.

"In contrast, if the teenager's mother had consulted a practitioner who employs the old fashion type of traditional dental techniques, that dentist would have extracted the tooth, performed cavitational surgery, and left a hole where the tooth had been," Dr. Hansen says. "In this type of traditional procedure, the dentist replaces the extracted tooth with nothing—just allows a gap to remain between the teeth.

"However, today, nearly all dentists recognize that such a hole left by a lost tooth leads to the domino effect of catastrophic dental crippling disease. Dental crippling from a missing tooth is destined to strike later in life owing to the movement and shifting of the teeth," advises the Fullerton dentist. "A teenager undergoing the nonreplaced tooth experience will likely also go through a loss of bone early on. It's bound to be a disastrous occurrence for such a young person. Because of the potential of crippling dental disease, endodontic root canal therapy performed the correct way is superior to pulling the tooth. But the endodontic procedure must be done right, and much of the time it is not.

"Let me emphasize that most of the dental disease I see in adults is on dentally treated teeth which occurs in childhood. [Please see the next chapter, "Dentist-Treated Teeth as the Source of Systemic Disease."] If a person is in good nutritional health and faithfully takes care of the teeth, virtually no adult dental problem will arise. There won't be any pathology existing around a nondental-treated tooth! It's a fact that the only teeth in adults to manifest difficulties are those structures which have undergone manipulations by a dentist in the past," Dr. Hansen says. "These structures include root canaled teeth which collapse because they are too massive for the mouth's engineered load distribution. The materials of such root canals will break down and lead to more problems, including additional root canals, dental crowns, and partial or full bridges.

"But what other dental care choice did your daughter-in-law have for your granddaughter's long-term comfort?" asks Dr. Hansen, rhetorically. "An unscrupulous dentist might grind down two other adjacent and perfectly healthy teeth in the child's mouth and build a dental bridge made out of materials which eventually can go bad. Or, another bad alternative would be to install a titanium-based implant into the child's jawbone. That's an even worse mechanically therapeutic method than extracting the tooth and leaving a hole.

"Yet, there's a newer, better, more holistic and biological dental procedure for a massively abcessed tooth such as you've described, Dr. Walker. It involves dealing with the two existing conditions present in the jaw: (1) the patient's dental infection and (2) the necrosed [dead or dying] bone that is beginning to dissolve away as a result of the infection. Yes, the root canal will have to be done," confirms Dr. Hansen. "Additionally, the consciencious and skilled dentist must treat the cleaned and shaped central canal's tubules and membranes, and the bone surrounding and holding that tooth in place. All structures have to be treated: the root first, because that's the source of this patient's initial problem of a bacterial infection. According to the correct biological procedure, treatment is designed to stop any pumping of bacterial toxins into the tooth's tubules and bone."

Root Canal Procedures
Used by Holistic (Biological) Dentists

"Unlike the conventionally practicing dentist who just leaves the infecting bacteria permeating the tubules, a holistic dentist will go much further. He or she cleans out the affected dental site with a laser beam," Dr. Hansen says. (This sterilization procedure is in contrast to the commonly held belief in dentistry that bacteria become sealed into the root canal tip, and they couldn't be killed off anyway no matter what sterilization method is used. That belief has been proven untrue.) "Such a laser technique easily penetrates the dental tubules through the tooth root and its boney plate. That way the internal aspects of the root are sterilized, and the holistic dentist can then fill the central canal with a biocompatible filling paste such as Biocalex [See chapter 12.]

"Biocalex converts to a bacteriocidal agent having the basic pH of 9 (alkaline) which kills the invading acid-loving bacteria. The Biocalex also expands while its calcium-enriched mixture seals the tubule," explains Dr. Hansen. "If the patient's immune system is active and there are healing capabilities around the exterior of the tooth, as is usually the situation for a sixteen-year-old, her body will go ahead and repair itself locally and systemically.

"With an older person having an impaired immune system, the treatment circumstances may be different. Following the patient's undergoing a root canal procedure, probably a microsurgical technique will be carried out to eliminate the cavitational area. Required bone may be harvested from another area of the jaw that's then filled into the cavitation," Dr. Hansen advises. "Most times, if the cavitation is small enough, it doesn't need bone fill. The correcting dentist goes in with an instrument to clean out the junk products and creates a bleeding site. This causes a blood clot to come on and the body itself will fill in the cavitation with new bone. Just by the dentist's stimulation of bleeding, bone will replace the clotted blood. It becomes a matrix for creation of this new bone. Osteoblasts [bone-forming cells] migrate into the clot to form new bone. That happens in the small area around the end of the tooth's impaired root, especially if the patient's nutrition has been stable and wholesome."

Conclusions Arrived at by Dr. Richard Hansen

In conclusion, based on Dr. Hansen's explanation, my grand-daughter was treated correctly by the orthodox dentist, but only up to a point. Her dental abscess and root canal procedure took place before I conducted investigations to write this book, and our family was not aware of the advantages of biological dentistry. Bacteria were presumably allowed to remain lodged under my granddaughter's dental pulp replacement gutta-percha implant. Even as you read this, they may be leaching bacterial toxins into her body's fluids, produc-ing an ongoing low-grade but subclinical poisoning that is immune suppressive. This is the situation for nearly everyone who undergoes nonholistic root canal treatment.

(A personal note: I will attempt to educate my daughter-in-law and son, who is a medical doctor, about the use of homeopathic remedies [see chapter 17] and Enderlein pleomorphic therapy for overcoming the infection lingering under my grandchild's root canal tooth. The two parents know about and do take supplemental nutrients already. [See chapter 16.] To further my beautiful grand-daughter's state of wellness, I would want them to advance another step along the path of holistic dental health.)

As with my grandchild, subclinical toxicity lingers in the mouths of almost all Americans who own root canal implantations. From this circumstance, the incidence of immune suppression diseases is likely to have grown enormously in the United States. People are being struck more commonly with chronic fatigue syndrome, fibromyalgia, the seven known forms of herpes infections, AIDS, colds, flu, various degenerative diseases such as cancer and arthritis, and other chronic, debilitating health difficulties.

"Existing root canals are a major source of patient referrals to my Center for Advanced Dentistry," admits holistic dentist Richard Hansen. "The first thing we do to treat a long-established root canal is remove the bad stuff inside the tooth's central root. If a metal post is installed there, my clinic staff uses a high-energy ultrasonic device to vibrate and free-up the post so that it may be removed manually. This allows us to get to the inner portion of the tooth. Then, the gutta-percha is taken away by use of certain dental files designed for that purpose. Used judiciously, such files spiral and clean out the gutta-percha implant. We use visually enhanced X-ray films and other diagnostics to identify the lodged sites for this foreign material. My dental clinicians make sure that bleeding occurs at the end of the root by going through its ending tip with an instrument and penetrating into the cavitation that invariably is present.

"Sterilization of this area with the laser beam comes next. And then sealing with Biocalex must take place. It's essentially the same procedure followed for a longstanding root canal as that acute condition described for the sixteen-year-old girl," says Dr. Hansen. "Your granddaughter's root canal should be reopened and redone with laser sterilization."

Dr. Hansen suggests that children experiencing infected teeth should not undergo root canal treatment at all. His method is to first target any areas of tooth decay as the source of potential abscess; second, use the laser to vaporize whatever decay is present; third, weld together any separated portions of a tooth; fourth, remineralize the dentin naturally with intravenous infusions and nutritional supplementation; and possibly fifth, inject into tiny, pinpoint decayed areas the currently available glass-filled polymers. The dental structures that had been impaired will then remain solid and intact. When they reach adulthood, such treated children will never need more dentistry in the form of cavity fillings, root canals, crowns, or anything else.

"If at all possible," Dr. Hansen states, "keep dentists' fingers out of the mouths of children." My interpretation of his statement is that parents should avoid the services of pedodontists.

"Allow me to add an important piece of advice. Before engaging in any dental treatment, people must be sustaining themselves on good nutrition, including the taking of daily food supplements and eating an excellent diet. They have to maintain good calcium metabolism and use it as a basic factor for dental healing. And they must take high doses of vitamin C, including the undergoing of intravenous nutrient drips before and after dental therapy," Dr. Hansen emphasizes. "Moreover, the patients must accept adrenal support with adjunctive nutrients to enhance neurotransmitter mechanisms, which are required for healing dental trauma. They should be taking free radical quenchers such as OPCs [oligomeric proanthocyanidins] and coEnzyme Q10. A protocol for such nutritional support is an integral part of the biological procedures followed in holistic dentistry." (Please see chapter 16.)

What Is Holistic (Biological) Dentistry?

"Biological dentistry is first and foremost a comprehensive form of clinical and rational dental care for medical consumers," says Edward M. Arana, D.D.S., president of the American Academy of Biological Dentistry.

"The treatment and diagnosis of pathology in patients' teeth, jaws, and related structures are accomplished with an awareness of how such pathology may affect the entire human being. Since it is impossible to divide one's mouth from the body, it's usual for a holistic dentist to treat the whole person through his or her oral cavity.

"Biological dentistry can be categorized as *dentistry with a conscience* as well as with a consciousness of how treatment of the teeth and jaws will affect the total health of an individual. It also encompasses his or her immune system," Dr. Arana continues. "Holistic (biological) dentistry is aesthetic, relatively nontoxic, and individually biocompatible. It is accomplished by use of thermographic, physiologic, and electronic methods to locate chronic areas of disease that often are difficult to find by the currently used and standard dental methods of diagnosis.

"Incorporated in this field of bioecological dental medicine are those time-proven healing techniques we know as homeopathy, acupuncture, nutrition, physical therapy, and herbology. In holistic dentistry, they are combined with the more modern sciences of neural therapy, hematology, immunology, and electroacupuncture," adds Dr. Arana. "The scientific disciplines that encompass the field of clinical dentistry form the basis for holistic (biological) and biocompatible (mercury-free) dentistry.

"This is an emerging new field of probiotic dental medicine, which began to develop in Germany some thirty years ago. It's now being taught and practiced in various countries such as the United States, Austria, Germany, England, France, Switzerland, Australia, Taiwan, Sweden, Italy, and Colombia," Dr. Arana says.

"The Food and Drug Administration (FDA) regulates dental filling materials and implants as 'devices' (such as a crutch or a splint). Such a device has to undergo only very few safety checks, rather than something like an implant that is placed in the body, having a rather remarkable interaction with the body's immune, endocrine, and nervous system." This is how Chrystyne Jackson, formerly of Enderlein Enterprises Corporation, explained regulation of dental materials to two hundred health professionals attending a seminar sponsored by her company. Jackson was founding president of Pleomorphic Product Sales, Inc., known worldwide as the importer of the German-produced Sanum-Kielbeck line of homeopathic live organisms for eliminating dental infections and toxicity. (See appendix B.)

"Teeth, implants, and dental materials are erroneously considered to be something 'outside' the body!" Jackson continued. "In contrast, holistic (biological) dentistry has looked early on at the effects that dental interventions and dental illness bring on for the rest of the body. "There's a big difference between the two practice forms of dentistry."

"Holistic (biological) dentistry bridges the ever-widening gap between the biological principles of holistic medicine and the mechanical, technological approaches of modern dentistry. Dentists graduating from dental universities are excellent technicians, but they usually have little understanding of how the pathology of the teeth and jaw affects the rest of the body," Jackson concluded.

The Philosophical Concepts of Holistic (Biological) Dentists

Holistic (biological) dentists study the existing research, perform further studies, and then integrate all of the current diagnostic and therapeutic schools of thought for rendering professional dental services. Holistic dentists utilize state-of-the-art procedures in all aspects of patient dental care. They diagnose the conditions bringing on illnesses, and then find the most effective ways to treat them. They work closely with health professionals who render health care in almost all other disciplines to avoid massively destructive procedures, which lead to greater amounts of dentistry and create dental cripples out of patients.

The holistic dentist burrows into the root of the patient's oral problem (pun intended). He or she identifies how an impaired mouth is adversely influencing health. Such a harmonizing dentist works under the philosophy that dentistry cannot exist by itself—as in a vacuum—and the profession must integrate with skills and services provided by other health disciplines. A notion shared by these biocompatible dentists is that a biological basis for the mouth prevails, which throughout history has been considered "the golden pentagon." As the foundation for good health, this oral golden pentagon is a perfectly designed entity.

Every person's nutrition begins in the mouth. By means of salivation, chewing, and swallowing, nutrition incorporates the first stages of eating, digestion, and the breaking down of food for metabolism, overall nourishment, cellular repair, and physiological energy. None of this metabolic functioning could exist without oral health.

Treatment for Pathological Microbes in the Mouth

Microorganism entry to the body often happens from the oral cavity. Numerous bacterial pathogens lodge themselves in and around the teeth, and they can be transmitted to family members, friends, and neighbors. To rid someone's body of these pathogens, the holistic dentist sometimes must reluctantly put a patient on heavy doses of antibiotics: amoxicillin (Amoxil, Larotid, Polymox, Trimox, and Wymox), tetracycline (Achromycin V and Sumycin), metronidazole (Flagyl and Metryl) or ciprofloxacin hydrochloride (Cipro). Since antibiotic drugs often are allergenic or otherwise toxic for people, the treating dentist attempts to make use of other alternative and nontoxic means of antimicrobial therapy such as with the use of the nonprescription, over-the-counter nutritional supplement olive leaf extract, in the form of capsules, tablets, bulk powders, or solutions.[1]

With infections prevailing in the mouth, no matter what dental treatment is administered, the patient's jawbone will continue to dissolve. Lasers, devices producing very thin beams of

---

1   M. Walker, *Nature's Antibiotic: Olive Leaf Extract* (New York: Kensington Publishing Corp, 1997).

light in which high energies are concentrated, often are the therapies of choice for holistic dentists. The laser (an acronym meaning light amplification by stimulated emission of radiation) doesn't damage surrounding tissue but does sterilize an abscessed tooth.

A laser beam rids the mouth of its potential to be a small sewer that's filled with pathogens. The by-products of these bacteria, identified by Professor Boyd Haley, Ph.D., chief of the Department of Chemistry at the University of Kentucky, as thio-ethers, hydrogen sulfide, and other chemicals, become far deadlier than the mercury when mixed with the mercury in amalgam dental fillings. Mercury is the most poisonous single metallic substance known. The mercury-combined by-products turn into methylmercury, thiomercury, and other exceedingly deadly components. Thus, the mouth actually is a test tube in which hazardous chemicals are being mixed daily. Holistic dentists remove the existing mercury part of this chemical equation and never install dental amalgam fillings.

The Integration of Oral Health into Body Health

The human body functions properly as an alkaline environment. Thus the saliva should remain in an alkaline state to neutralize the acid-loving pathogenic bacteria. But the process of tooth decay and gum tissue breakdown are both known acidic processes. Bacteria produce an acid, electrolyte-enriched environment in which they combine with dentist-installed mixed metals and composite resins, many of which contain petrochemical bases such as metallic oxide, toluene, and other toxic materials. Together, they act as solvents to leach out metallic poisons bringing on electrogalvanism and a subsequent destructive electromagnetic force (EMF) reaction between metals.

Harmful elements leach into the mouth from all of these dental metals (for example, mercury, nickel, palladium, and gold) with EMF generation coming from each at a microvolt range. Being in the mouth, the emitting EMFs are located near the human brainstem, which carries the neurotransmitter mechanism. The potential result? Brain deterioration with the onset of dementia, senility, Alzheimer's disease, parkinsonism, and other central nervous system disorders! Thus metals in the mouth are believed by holistic medical/dental experts to be main sources of various mental and physical illnesses.[1]

Mouth metals interfere with the human electrical generations within the brain. Neurotransmitters are being altered not just by the chemical and material metallic absorption inside the oral cavity but also from the mouth's electrical conductivity. It is the same sort of brain interference and immune system suppression caused by the use of cellular phones, microwave generators, electric blankets, water beds, video display terminals, electric razors, hair dryers, and other such electrical appliances applied to the body and near to the brain. We who have metallic substances implanted in our mouths have another electrical generator working away inside the mouth. Thus the teeth tend to transmit electromagnetic frequencies just like television tubes, cellular phones, computers, or automobile batteries.

The Upstate New York Holistic Dentist Speaks from Experience

"Through my studies in holistic dentistry, I have found that the condition of a person's mouth explains a great deal about the health of that patient's body overall. For example, if someone consults me with the complaint of bleeding of the gums, I have come to recognize that he or she is the victim of a deficiency of several vitamins and/or minerals," reports the holistic dentist from upstate New York I had mentioned (who prefers not to be identified). "When the missing nutritional elements are restored, along with the application of proper oral hygiene, the patient's bleeding invariably stops.

"Holistic methods of dentistry utilize the body's own defenses and work to establish a patient's biochemical balance. Whenever

---

1   T. Warren, *Beating Alzheimer's: A Step towards Unlocking the Mysteries of Brain Diseases* (Garden City Park, N.Y.: Avery Publishing Group, 1991); T. Warren, "Beating the Diagnosis: The Case for Unlocking Brain Disease—Alzheimer's to Schizophrenia and Other Chronic Diseases," *Townsend Letter for Doctors and Patients* (April 1997), 50–60.

possible, I, as the treating dentist, use herbs, minerals, and other natural agents instead of man-made drugs. Let me draw you a parallel situation between standard operating dental procedure and holistic dentistry: today in organized dental practice there are two usual methods of treating periodontal disease. Both are established and remain well-accepted within the purview of orthodox dentistry," our anxious holistic dentist explains. "The dentists who perform periodontics love these two methods but most often their patients hate them. The main treatment technique involves periodontal surgery and entails cutting away the infected tissue. The second method requires that the treating dentist tie a string impregnated with tetracycline [an antibiotic] around the impaired tooth, and this string is allowed to remain in place for a few weeks.

"Among those patients who had engaged in periodontal surgery, it was firmly reported by a dental journal that they would never repeat the treatment, even if it was mandatory. Periodontal surgery just hurts too much and offers excessive numbers of complications such as ongoing bleeding. The patients wouldn't again allow the tetracyclined string to be retied on them either, since its antibiotic action is unlimited and doesn't merely affect the one dental area. The whole body feels a tetracycline overload. Thus, both of today's standard periodontal procedures get negative marks from patients," this biological dentist says.

"In contrast, the treating periodontists enjoy using the two techniques a great deal because both of them eliminate the patients' symptoms, although not their causes. The people's complaints stop—no more lamentations and moaning—at least for a time, until their periodontal diseases recur in five years or so," this patient-oriented dentist states. "But my method of biological dentistry for periodontal problems is more holistic. It's pleasant, highly successful, and happily acceptable to the patients. That method entails the use of a mouth rinse that contains the right combination of herbs and vitamins. It helps the body prevent the original periodontal disease from occurring. [See chapter 15 on periodontal disease therapy.]

"Beginning in 1979, I started applying herbal combinations for the prevention and healing of gum disease. At first I settled on a mixture consisting of the herbs goldenseal, myrrh, garlic, and cayenne pepper," the inventive dentist tells us. "Although the mixture brought together the right elements of blood cleansers, antibiotics, and tissue-tightening astringents for healing purposes, the result tasted terrible and turned one's teeth yellow. So, I went back to the drawing board and created other herbal combinations.

"My rinses and toothpastes have been used by people the whole world over, helping with bleeding gums and a variety of mouth problems. Many of my patients, and the patients of other holistic-thinking dentists using this treatment, are finding that they do not need any additional form of therapy other than teeth cleanings and good oral care," says my source. "My belief is that this growing emphasis on preventive dentistry of the holistic type will allow all of us in the field to enhance our reconstructive work tenfold.

"The difference in the entire natural dentistry approach is that more than the symptoms are being taken care of," he says. He adds that the herbs and vitamins he recommends not only stimulate the body's natural healing processes (see chapters 16 and 17), but also bring about a change in the chemistry of the mouth and body, creating the favorable alkaline environment.

Advanced Therapies of Holistic Dentist Ara Elmajian, D.D.S.

I interviewed Ara Elmajian, D.D.S., of Vancouver, British Columbia, about the biocompatible/biological procedures that he follows as a mercury-free and holistic dentist. After our discussions, I investigated further among his colleagues and learned that Dr. Elmajian is a most extraordinary and highly respected dental practitioner. In practice for two-and-a-half decades, he considers himself a "dental physician" and has working for him medical doctors, osteopaths, chiropractors, naturopaths, dentists, and other health care professionals. His is the ideal holistic dental practice, which patients have come to recognize—so much so that Dr. Elmajian is booked with appointments for the next four years. He takes no new patients except by health professional referral, but still functions actively ten hours daily during a six-day work week as a dental diagnostician, technician, therapist, and clinic supervisor.

"In this dental clinic," says Dr. Elmajian, "we evaluate the total patient—the whole self of an individual from top to bottom. That includes his or her psyche, function, structure, biochemistry, and more—not only the teeth. Dental discomfort may bring the patient to consult me, but I am aware that 80 percent of all body difficulties for people are connected to dental pathologies.

"We practice dental medicine here and conduct diagnostics, which include regulation thermography, biological terrain assessment, VEGA machine testing [electroacupuncture, according to Rheinhardt Voll, M.D., Ph.D.], structural examination, immune system evaluation, musculature observation, neurological trigger point checking as taught by Janet Travell, M.D. [at one time President John F. Kennedy's personal physician], and other physical, mental, emotional, and spritual determinants. Those are the diagnostics we conduct before giving the patient any therapy," says Dr. Elmajian.

"As for treatment, our dental clinic provides much more than drilling, filling, and billing, as taught in professional school. We stabilize loose joints for the patient by the use of prolotherapy [also known as reconstructive therapy], of course focusing our efforts on the TMJ [temporomandibular joint], but the overly flaccid joints of the neck, cranium and others are worked on too.[1] The patient's immune system is boosted, and then we fix the proprioceptor system. The individual's physiology is strengthened first, and then we move on to assist the structure," Dr. Elmajian explains. "Next, the patient's waste disposal system is improved; and finally we work on correcting the oral cavity.

"Starting with dental cleaning in a sequence of steps, we eliminate the patient's foci of infection, sterilize root canal teeth, correct cavitations, and remove heavy metals. The psyche—a patient's considered relationship to the world—gets profiled and dealt with properly. It's not just teeth that we fix in this dental practice; it's the entire person," says Dr. Elmajian. "People arrive at the door of my

---

1   W. J. Faber and M. Walker, *Pain, Pain Go Away* (Menlo Park, Calif.: Ishi Press International, 1990).

holistic dental practice when they've come to the end of the line with their many other therapies and doctors."

Dr. Ara Elmajian is among the most advanced of all the holistic (biological) dentists interviewed for this book. He often is called upon to lecture and teach his methods to colleagues who enroll for his presentations around North America.

The National Council Against Health Fraud

In New York City two dentists who practice as partners, Marvin J. Schissel, D.D.S., and John E. Dodes, D.D.S., brand holistic (biological) dentists as exemplified by Richard T. Hansen, our upstate New Yorker, and Ara Elmajian, with the expletive words: incompetents, quacks, and frauds.[1] Drs. Schissel and Dodes have been vice president and president, respectively, of the New York chapter of the National Council for Reliable Health Infomation, Inc. (NCRHI), formerly known as the National Council Against Health Fraud (NCAHF). Such NCRHI members compose what they think of as a health care watchdog group. By their aggressive tactics, including attacks on health professional licenses, name-calling, negative media campaigns, and other outrageous behavior, the national and local NCAHF groups are likely to sway observers' minds. Such erroneous persuasion is wrong, but it happens!

The NCAHF appears to be the ultimate mad-dog supporter of allopathic, pharmaceutically oriented, industralized Western medicine, and the absolute enemy of holistic/alternative/complementary methods of healing.

They earmark as "quackery" any modality, regimen, or practice that their group decides is out of the medical mainstream.

The NCAHF techniques of aggression are used not only against holistic (biological) dentistry but also just as often against other commonly employed procedures. These include nutritional

---

1   M. J. Schissel and J. E. Dodes, *The Whole Tooth* (New York: St. Martin's Press, 1997).

supplementation with vitamins and minerals; diagnostic procedures like electroacupuncture; certain health care services such as reflexology; manually administered methods of diagnosis like applied or behavioral kinesiology; healing devices such as thermotherapy for prostate enlargement; truly beneficial techniques exemplified by chelation therapy; salutary thinking such as prayer; medicinal herbs like gingko biloba; non-Western treatment as with self-administered traditional Chinese Qigong; and anything else *unrelated* to chemotherapy, radiation therapy, surgery, or allopathic, drug-based medicine.

Three

Dentist-Treated Teeth
as the Source of Systemic Diseases

"In dentistry, we health professionals use a lot of substances that are 'bad' for the human body. Nickel is just such a commonly employed metallic substance, which some dentists put in the mouth in the form of crowns and braces. For instance, pedodontists [dentists specializing in the care of children's teeth] often install stainless steel crowns; orthodontists attach stainless steel braces into the mouths of preteens, teenagers, and some adults to reposition their teeth. Both crowns and braces are made stainless by incorporating nickel into the metallic combinations making up alloys for these dental appliances. My own son underwent an adverse experience with nickel as a result of his orthodontic treatment," Mark Breiner, D.D.S., told me.

Dr. Breiner, a member of the International Academy of Oral Medicine and Toxicology (IAOMT), practices mercury-free and biocompatible, holistic (biological) dentistry in Orange, Connecticut. The IAOMT is one of four dental professional organizations (listed in appendix C) comprised of members who endorse ortho-molecular methods of dental practice. Because Dr. Breiner provides his patients with this form of nontoxic dentistry, his license to continue practicing is being attacked by the Connecticut Dental Association.

"As an infant, my son had suffered from chronic ear infections, which my wife and I finally managed to clear up by having him treated with homeopathy. His ear symptoms disappeared completely, but more than a decade later they resumed again because of his need to wear dental braces. When the child was twelve years old, his mother and I decided that he needed some orthodontic treatment. Thus, we authorized my favorite orthodontist to attach two stainless steel bands to our son's teeth. Subsequently, for the first time in eleven years, the boy came down with a new bout of ear infections," says Dr. Breiner. "We had them treated again by an otolaryngologist [ear, nose, and throat doctor], but his ear problems did not go away. Suspecting that there could be some connection to his new dental braces, I had the orthodontist remove those two stainless steel bands.

"Upon reflection over time, however, I came to the conclusion that I was overly conscious of the concepts of holistic-biocompatible dentistry. Perhaps this awareness as it related to my son was allowing my imagination to run rampant, I thought. It struck me that the problem might be 'all in my head' and not in his. So I asked the orthodontist to reattach the two metal bands to straighten the boy's teeth. A short time later, he came down not only with infectious involvements of both ears but also my son was struck by bacterial pneumonia. I realized then that the stainless steel had so reduced his immune system's ability to ward off bacteria that he became vulnerable to serious infections," advises Dr. Breiner. "As much as I knew about biological factors in dentistry, this personal occurrence to a member of my family shocked me.

"To check this clinical finding, therefore, I sent a sample of my boy's blood to Douglas Swartzendriper, Ph.D., M.D., who is immunology department chief and head pathologist at the medical laboratory of the University of Colorado. From assaying the boy's blood against various dental metal components, this immunologist reported that my son was definitely reacting to nickel molecules present in the stainless steel of his orthodontic braces," says Dr. Breiner. "The nickel had shut down my son's immune system, and stainless steel orthodonture no longer was an option acceptable for him."

The lesson from this case history offered by Dr. Breiner is easily learned. Because of the traumatic dental techniques administered or the toxicity of dental substances applied, even holistic (biological) dentists or their families may experience difficulties with dentist-treated teeth.

Dentist-Treated Teeth Cause
Thirty Different Disease Symptoms

Over the course of four years, ending in February 1996, the Toxic Element Research Foundation (TERF) in Colorado Springs, Colorado, conducted an investigation among 1,320 dental patients engaged in treatment or medical consultation for heavy metal toxicity. These people had undergone orthodonture, root canals, dental restorations, periodonture, dental implants, dental cavity fillings, or otherwise had their teeth manipulated by conventionally practicing general dentists or dental specialists who commonly employed the profession's recognized orthodox procedures.

It turns out that dentistry's standard use of toxic substances, especially those involving heavy metals placed in the mouth, such as cobalt, cadmium, chromium, gallium, beryllium, titanium, palladium, mercury, nickel, gold, silver, tin, copper, zinc, and others were the source of discomforting symptoms or outright illnesses for these 1,320 medical/dental consumers. Data from that research documents that symptoms from a total of thirty different diseases developed among the patients. This information is available by telephone from the Toxic Element Research Foundation. (See appendix A for the listing.)

In table 3-1 (shown next), the symptoms listed comprise physical, mental, or emotional difficulties arising from metallic substances implanted into patients mouths by dentists. Such illnesses may include fibromyalgia, arthritis, the yeast syndrome (systemic candidiasis), parasitic infestations, sensitivities, allergies, chronic fatigue and immune dysfunction syndrome (CFIDS), or worse (AIDS and various cancers). (Note: in the United Kingdom, CFIDS has for a long time been designated as *myalgic encephalitis* [ME]).

These symptoms are most often reported to attending holistic medical doctors, osteopaths, chiropractors, naturopaths, homeopaths, acupuncturists, and other enlightened health professionals by patients diagnosed with autoimmune or immune system suppression illnesses. In contrast, a health professional locked into the lessons of medical orthodoxy will probably diagnose a patient adversely responding to metallic toxins as having psychosomatic problems. Frequently, doctors administering strictly orthodox medicine don't even acknowledge the existence of some of the above-listed conditions.

Table 3-1

Order of Occurrence, Frequency, and Percentages of Symptoms from Oral Implantation of Heavy Metal Toxicity

Presented in the order of frequency and percentage of occurrence for 1,320 patients poisoned by heavy toxic metals, these were their disease manifestations:

Symptom Shown	Patient Percentage
1. Unexplained irritability	73.3
2. Constant or very frequent periods of depression	72.0
3. Numbness and tingling in the extremities	67.3
4. Frequent urination during the night	64.5
5. Unexplained severe chronic fatigue	63.1
6. Cold hands and feet, even in moderate/warm weather	62.6
7. Bloated feeling most of the time	60.6
8. Difficulty with remembering or use of memory	58.0
9. Sudden, unexplained or unsolicited anger	55.5
10. Constipation on a regular basis	54.2
11. Difficulty in making even simple decisions	54.2
12. Tremors or shakes of hands, feet, head, etc.	52.3
13. Twitching of face and other muscles	52.3
14. The experiencing of frequent leg cramps	49.1
15. Constant or frequent ringing or noise in ears	47.8
16. Getting out of breath easily	43.1
17. Having frequent or recurring heartburn	42.5
18. Feeling excessive itching	40.8

Symptom Shown	Patient Percentage
19. Experiencing unexplained rashes, skin irritation	40.4
20. Having constant or frequent metallic taste in mouth	38.7
21. Feeling jumpy, jittery, nervous	38.1
22. Fighting off a constant death wish or suicidal intent	37.3
23. Having sleepless nights and frequent insomnia	36.4
24. Undergoing unexplained chest pains	35.6
25. Feeling constant or frequent pain in joints	35.5
26. Experiencing tachycardia (100 heart beats per minute)	32.4
27. Showing unexplained fluid retention	28.2
28. Having burning sensation on tongue	20.8
29. Getting headaches just after eating	20.1
30. Experiencing frequent diarrhea	14.9

No Meeting of the Minds between Orthodoxy and Holism

To recap, almost all of the symptoms listed in table 3-1 are recognized by the holistic medical/dental community as potentially coming from teeth overly stressed by dental manipulations. In contrast, almost none of these symptoms are accepted by conventionally trained and practicing allopathic physicians and dentists as symptomatic of teeth stress.

As indicated from the additional quotes offered below by Dr. Mark Breiner, the difference in thinking at this time between members of the four holistic (biologic) dental groups and the orthodox allopathic dental community seems just too great to overcome. It may take another thirty years for conventional dentistry to become enlightened. During that time, the personal body pollution of patients from their mouths will continue unabated, and those unfortunate medical consumers who receive diagnoses and treatment from the orthodox/establishment dentist types will pay the price in ill health and potential death for such differences of opinion.

Dr. Breiner says: "Holistic dentists such as myself are working from a different paradigm than the ordinary, conventional dental practitioners [who follow the ADA party line]. Simply because we holistic docs cannot talk with a common language to the party-line docs, there is no way for the two paradigms to meet. Nearly all biological/mercury-free dentists experience licensure problems with their state boards of dental examiners. The state board members—who represent conservative orthodox/establishment dentistry—are totally unconscious about dental material biocompatibility or keeping patients free of amalgam mercury toxins or avoiding troubles with root canals or correcting cavitations or that fluoride is a poisonous substance."

"Silver" Dental Amalgam Toxicity

Recognizing that having so-called "silver" amalgam dental fillings in your mouth is definitely dangerous to your health and life, Sweden has declared mercury-containing dental amalgam to be an environmental hazard and, in 1992, permanently banned its use in pregnant women by dentists anywhere in that country.[1] On January 1, 1999, the Reformed Dental Compensation Act took place in Sweden. There now is better general dental compensation there for patients, who have seen their costs rise considerably in recent years. For medical/dental consumer safety, the Swedish compensation act states, "No financial compensation will be given for the placement of amalgam fillings. The compensation for amalgam fillings is abolished. The aim is a total ban of the use of dental amalgam in approximately two years."[2]

---

1   G. Drasch and others, "Mercury Burden of Human Fetal and Infant Tissues," *European J. Pediatrics* 153 (1994): 607–10.

2   APMA, "APMA Director's Report," *Townsend Letter for Doctors and Patients* 180 (July 1998): 138, 139.

Being a resident of North America and an American citizen, I must wonder about the two exemplary health-minded countries of the United States and Canada. They usually behave protectively of their citizenry. Concerning the toxicity arising from dental amalgam fillings, however, these two nations are hardly as protective as is Sweden. Why? Canada is beginning to wake up, but not enough! The United States has a long way to go as yet, and that's a reason my research and writing of this book has been necessary. Mercury amalgams must be banned from use.

Accordingly, for chapter 5, I have included the case history of Jaro Pleva, Ph.D., of Hagfors, Sweden, a metal materials chemist and expert in corrosion science. He is in large measure responsible for the banning of any orally placed amalgams in Sweden. Dr. Pleva's series of illnesses are typical of literally over a billion dental patients in Western industrialized countries (at least two hundred million in the United States alone) who, according to the evidence, are presently being poisoned by their dental amalgam fillings. These uninformed people don't recognize that physical and mental symptoms do come from this circumstance.

Edward M. Arana D.D.S., president of the American Academy of Biological Dentistry, holds some definite opinions about the adverse effects of dentist-applied oral substances. In a report he prepared for this third chapter, Dr. Arana writes,

> The most tragic example of misstated biocompatibility of dental materials is organized dentistry's position of advocating a known poison, mercury in amalgam fillings, just because amalgam has been used for 150 years. In doing so, dentists have been misled and the truth obfuscated concerning the fact that mercury does indeed cause ill effects when placed as an implant in the body. Organized dentistry clouds over the issue even to the point of denying that a filling in a prepared tooth cavity is an implant.
>
> Mercury and other heavy metals from dental fillings contribute to all chronic disease states as do multiple chemical sensitizing exposures. From environmentally ill patients there is clinical evidence that the heavy metals from dental fillings and multiple chemical exposures act synergistically to intoxicate and stress the patient, thus causing disease.
>
> The first area of concern in biological dentistry is the toxicity of metals and their release from the fillings and prostheses used

in dentistry. These metal ions disassociate from their masses to diffuse, migrate and become absorbed in the tissues altering the electrochemical character of the immune system concomitantly changing the ratios and populations of the blood cells and the cells of the immune system.

The direct electrical currents generated by the dissociation of dissimilar metals in the human body's electrolyte medium—described as "oral galvanism"—carry disruptive metallic ions to opposite poles in the mouth's galvanic batteries. How much oral galvanic power is necessary to change organic function, to change membrane permeability, to interfere with the power of thought and recall, or to initiate degenerative change?

As dentists, we just don't know! But we do know that oral galvanism does change from electronegative to electropositive and acts as a blockade in the meridians or bioenergetic circuits associated with the teeth. The blockade causes dysfunction in the organs, endocrine systems, vertebrae, muscles, nerves, and nerve reflexes.

With just about any restorative material used in dentistry there will be a reaction by the body if the immune system is still functional because the tooth is an open and dynamic living organ. Biological dentistry is concerned with treatments that cause the least disturbance to the human immune system.

As described by Dr. Edward M. Arana, therefore, the metals that compose amalgams produce circumstances of electromagnetic galvanism in the teeth. This information brings me to the case history of naturopathic physician Victoria Zuppa, N.D., of Darien, Connecticut, who experienced her own set of circumstances with oral galvanism.

The Oral Electromagnetic Galvanism of a Naturopath

"I was exceedingly nervous and what I must describe as 'wired' since the teen period of my life. I was the victim of a disquieting type-A personality. I'm forty years old today, and it was only recently that the solution to my keyed-up characteristics fell into place," Dr. Zuppa said during our interview.

"Seven years ago I heard an authority speaking on the radio about silver dental amalgam fillings and the electromagnetic charge they produce in the mouth. He called it 'oral galvanism,' and I realized at once that I met the criteria of symptoms the speaker was describing," explained Dr. Zuppa. "Criticism of me by family members and friends was always being leveled with the statements that I was distressed too much and constantly creating stress for those around me. I remember a dentist telling me that stress was causing me to grind my teeth.

"But from listening to that radio program—a health show—I began to wonder if my overly high-strung difficulties were not stress at all but rather the electrical charges coming from my dental amalgams. Was my personality being altered by oral galvanism? I was loaded with a minimum of twelve or more mercury-filled cavities, and some other metals were in my mouth as well. So I went looking for and found a test that measures the electromagnetic waves in one's mouth. A holistic dentist had a galvanometer as one of his pieces of dental equipment. Three teeth that I sensed possessed excessive vibratory charges, indeed, were filled with mercury while at the same time showing the highest electromagnetic vibrations," Dr. Zuppa said. "I therefore proceeded to have Howard Hinden, D.D.S., of Suffern, New York, remove my amalgam fillings. As an alternative to amalgams, I went through blood testing to learn what composite substances should be substituted as filling material.

"Following the procedures taught by Dr. Hal A. Huggins, Dr. Hinden first removed amalgams from the two worst areas in the right upper quadrant of my jaw. Immediately I noticed a subtle improvement in my temperament. Upon his taking out the amalgams from the left lower quadrant, I suddenly felt like somebody had pulled me out of a light socket," Dr. Zuppa described. "My state of being wired-up turned down remarkably! I got rid of my overcharging tenseness. Friends, neighbors, family, and other people commented upon meeting me again that I was much calmer. Getting rid of those dozen or so dental amalgam fillings did it for me.

"I feel really well now, although I still do work on myself, such as following up with chemical detoxification. [See chapter 9.] I'm trying to neutralize not only oral galvanism but also chemical sensitivies. I have done a lot more work on myself by following the teachings of Dietrich Klinghardt, M.D., the holistic/biological physician and teacher located in Seattle, Washington," specified Dr. Victoria Zuppa.

Dentist-Stressed Teeth Encourage Cancerous Growth

Medical consumers possessing dentist-stressed teeth are probably more predisposed to coming down with cancer, according to board-certified clinical oncologist Vincent J. Speckhart, M.D., of Norfolk, Virginia. Dr. Speckhart, participating in a panel discussion on cancer causation, diagnosis, and therapy during the May 1998 scientific conference of the American College for Advancement in Medicine, spoke before an audience of medical colleagues who routinely use holistic, alternative, and complementary methods of healing.

I sat in this audience listening to "Clinical Prospectives on Cancer Therapies" and heard Dr. Speckhart state the following:

> Several years ago it became obvious to me that administering treatment to a patient's lump and bump wasn't going to do it for cancer management. I had been only a short time into prescribing chemotherapy when it also was apparent that this sort of treatment was not impacting on survival either. Therefore, at the request of my patients, I gradually got into dispensing alternative therapies and other ways of looking at cancer.
>
> I didn't realize that I was acting the role of an alternative [holistic or complementary] physician until my patients pointed to this changed manner of thinking. I had thought I was just helping out my friends with life-threatening illnesses. I had realized then that treatment should focus on the host [the patient with cancer], not only in terms of nutrition but also as to the individual's internal environment.
>
> Thereafter I became acquainted with a biofeedback device [the computron] which determines galvanic skin resistance—surface characteristics of acupuncture points. The device produces a signal identity of various internal events the patient is undergoing. I set up a computer spreadsheet to establish my database and captured the biofeedback of various disease states. Although this machine is not a diagnostic instrument itself, it does provide an electromagnetic biofeedback identity.

I recently completed the review of 660 cancer patients derived from 1310 files [some patients had multiple diseases] over an eighteen-month period. Among the most common of [cancer] signals are dental metals. They are a big issue in cancer, including gold. Dentists consider gold to be a noble metal, but it has a profound effect systemically. Among the biofeedback data I collected, methylmercury, an outgas form of mercury amalgam, presents itself in that data. Methylmercury makes up 100 percent of the local area cancer signals, and it affects acupuncture points [along the body's meridians] of the [immune system's] B-cells, T-cells, lymphocytes, monocytes, and splenic macrophages.

Mercurus vivus is one of the compounds escaping from mercury amalgams. It shows a 38 percent nonlocal expression [of cancer production]. And, another toxic form [of mercury vapor leaching from dental amalgams] has a 44 percent expression outside of the teeth. This means that there is a biophysical effect in the mouth from these dental metals. Other things can also be found [from the acupuncture points' biofeedback mechanism]. Meridian effects from each one of these oral metals have allowed me to identify fifty-five different acupuncture points [offering pathology]. These points will be related to a tooth and the problem within the tooth; so it isn't happening just once in awhile when you must have a tooth worked on. Rather, the entire role of dentistry is key to the internal environment of an individual. My progressive belief is that patients never really get better [healed from cancer] until all of the metal is out of their mouths. There is no place for metal in the mouth.[1]

Being a clinical oncologist, Dr. Vincent Speckhart was most interested in the cancer-stimulating effect of dentist-stressed teeth and the substances installed as part of oral therapy. My understanding from his presentation is that dentist-installed metallic substances definitely encourage the production of cancerous growths. In my opinion, metal in the mouth should be avoided at all costs. (See chapter 11)

---

[1]   M. Schacheter, R. Atkins, D. Brodie, F. Speckhart, and J. Stoff, "The Hot Seat Panel," *Clinical Prospectives on Cancer Therapies,*" American College for Advancement in Medicine, 1998 spring conference, Ft. Lauderdale, Florida, May 1998.

Two Major Federal Regulators Label
Fluoride a Poison

Most people are aware of the wars waging between organized dentistry's politicians, who advocate the fluoridation of teeth, and others—predominantly medical/dental consumers—who oppose involuntary addition of fluoride to our public water supplies. Among the opponents are members of the Safe Water Coalition of Washington State. (See appendix A for its address.) Well, the U.S. Food and Drug Administration (FDA) has joined the fray on the side of those fluoridation opponents, who have declared fluoride to be a deadly poison. The FDA agrees! (Ordinarily the chemical is extensively spread as a rat poison inside the slum sections of inner cities and around farmyards.) Now, as of March 1998, the FDA requires that all fluoride toothpaste containers, even the ADA-endorsed Crest toothpaste, carry a poison warning label.

Some of organized dentistry's representatives think this labeling is an unnecessary move. "The label is overkill," says Christopher Hughes, D.M.D., chairman of pediatric dentistry at Boston University's School of Dental Medicine. An FDA spokesperson disagrees with Dr. Hughes. She says, "Since there was significant risk that a child might accidentally ingest an entire tube of toothpaste, the label was warranted."[1]

The Environmental Protection Agency has joined the FDA in taking a stand against fluoride compounds. At the 1997 Kyoto (Japan) Climate Conference, the U.S. EPA was able to win some international limitations to the use of three particular aerosol pollutants: hydrofluorocarbons, perfluorocarbons, and sulfur hexafluoride. With the three aerosols containing one poisonous chemical pollutant in common, *fluoride*, scientists are worried that this fluoride element (along with carbon dioxide, methane, and nitrous oxide) could provoke a global warming that would shift patterns of rainfall, raise sea levels, and increase weather variability.

---

1   "A Brush with Poison," *Natural Health* (March/April 1998): 19.

While U.S. governmental agencies recognize the hazards of fluoride compounds domestically and globally, the state and national dental associations steadfastly bring political pressure on federal and state health departments to continue to promote adding fluoride to public drinking water at taxpayers' expense. Dentists continue to sell fluoride treatments for the prevention of tooth decay. Industrial fluoride polluters, represented by fluoride legislative lobbyists, support the dentists with financial contributions in their advocating of the poisoning of Americans. Such fluoridation proponents ignore recent scientific studies that link the long-term drinking of fluoridated water and the brushing with fluoridated toothpastes to diminishing intelligence quotients in children, bone cancer in young males, hip fractures among the elderly, mottled teeth, caries, gingivitis, and a general reduction in one's feeling of well-being.[1] (For proof of these statements about water fluoridation, please see chapter 14.)

Extracting Dentists Leave behind Painful NICO Lesions

Do you or a loved one suffer with any facial pain such as neuralgia or trigeminal neuralgia? More than likely pain like this is connected to the teeth, and dentists have classified the difficulties as coming from one or more cavitations, which, as I have discussed, is the destruction of the section of bone where a tooth has been removed—a type of osteonecrosis that's localized, pathologic, and results when there has been an impairment of blood circulation to the specific region of bone surrounding the extraction site. As also mentioned, one thing that is definitely important if any tooth is being removed, no matter whether it is a live tooth, a dead tooth, or a root canal tooth, is that the periodontal ligament be removed during or directly after the

---

1   Safe Water Coalition of Washington State, "Kyoto Climate Conference Limits Fluoride," *Townsend Letter for Doctors and Patients* 180 (July 1998): 30.

extraction. If not, awful consequences can result in the form of neuralgia-inducing cavitational osteonecrosis (NICO); this situation happens to dental patients more often than you might imagine. More than 70 percent of atypical facial neuralgias come from cavitations; 23 percent of phantom pain and headaches are related to NICO lesions, and 10 percent of trigeminal neuralgias arise from NICO.[1]

Painful neuralgia-inducing cavitational osteonecrosis lesions are a form of jawbone osteomyelitis, which results from poorly cleaned-out cavities created during tooth extractions and root canals. If you are left with a NICO lesion, it's unlikely that you'll be able to tolerate the associated bone destruction without some health consequences. It is very unlikely to have osteomyelitis and not feel your body complain about it. NICO lesions are produced by poorly trained or unskillful or uncaring extractionists who leave behind a septic site filled with bacteria to breed in the environment from which they've extracted teeth. Breeding bacteria may bring on jawbone dissolution, disabling pain, and potentially death. Most holistic dentists agree that leaving behind a cavitation is the worst kind of dentistry to which a patient may be exposed.[2]

Not only does bone disintegration occur in the surrounding area of an extracted tooth, but the myelin sheath for the nerve that runs through the jawbone also becomes involved. And when the periodontal ligament is not removed along with the tooth, NICO results so that complete bone healing almost never takes place. (See chapter 12.)

Generally, such a NICO involvement causes an ongoing, low-level infection that affects one's overall well-being and health. It pulls you down with subclinical illness. Certainly the underlying dental infection leaches toxins into the blood stream, which brings

---

1   P. Bennett and P. Brawn, "Toxic Teeth," transcribed from the Northwest Naturopathic Physician's Conference, 18–20 April 1997, *Townsend Letter for Doctors and Patients* 169/170 (August/September 1997): 144–48.

2   L. G. Casura, "Sick of Being Patient: Continuing the Hard Work of Healing: Part 3," *Townsend Letter for Doctors and Patients* 157/158 (August/September 1996): 74–81.

on immune system suppression and potential autoimmune disease, often manifested by the variable symptoms of chronic fatigue syndrome, the yeast syndrome, and many other even more serious illnesses.[1]

1   P. Yutsis and M. Walker, *The Downhill Syndrome* (Garden City Park, N.Y.: Avery Publishing Group, 1997); J. P. Trowbridge and M. Walker, *The Yeast Syndrome* (New York: Bantam Books, 1986).

Four

Mercury Poisoning
from Your Amalgam-Filled Teeth

As illustrated by what occurs to the amalgam-filled teeth of dead persons, "silver" dental amalgam fillings are dangerous to the health of any living being.[1] Cremation had traditionally been considered one of the safest and most sanitary methods of disposing of human corpses. But researchers now have discovered that the mercury amalgam dental fillings lodged in the mouths of dead persons that become exposed to the high heat of a crematorium release highly toxic mercury vapors. Gases escaping from melting mercury dental fillings pollute the environment and poison those livingin the crematorium's vicinity.

According to the calculations of Allan Mills, Ph.D., senior lecturer in the Department of Geology at the University of Leicester in England and the author of a paper on the research, each year a busy crematorium releases vapors carrying as much as twenty-four pounds of mercury into the ambient air and surrounding atmosphere.

"The use of mercury is controlled in industry because of the known danger to health of the living, while the crematorium across town is producing a large quantity of mercury vapor," Dr. Mills said. "None of the investigators involved with the environment seem to have considered the final destination of filled teeth when they are melted down with the rest of the cremated corpse."[2]

1   S. Ziff, "Dental Offices Polluting the Water Supply with Mercury?" *Dental & Dental Facts* 2, no. 6 (1989): 2.

2   "Cremation Pollution," *New York Times*, 21 August 1990.

Conventional Dentistry Is Hazardous to Your Health

Mercury, a verified toxic heavy metal, is packed by nonholistic but rather conventionally practicing dentists into over four-fifths of all dental cavities that 98 percent of the North American population develops. It has been confirmed that in the United States alone, approximately a hundred million amalgam fillings get implanted into the teeth of dental patients each year. A minimum of two hundred million Americans are wearing them, and it's probable that unrecognized subclinical illnesses from mercury poisoning frequently are the result.

What are some of the more minor symptoms of mercury toxicity arising from what's packed into people's teeth? The ubiquitous dental amalgam syndrome—those signs and symptoms of mercury poisoning—includes another syndrome: persistent overall fatigue and a feeling of being "run-down" or just plain tired all the time. Associated with this chronic fatigue syndrome (CFS) are weakness, drowsiness, adverse alterations of vision, heart palpitations, breathing troubles, headache, chills, dizziness, anxiety, depression, nervousness, bad breath, metallic taste, immune system compromise, allergies, various urinary tract problems such as pain on urination (dysuria), anemia, gastrointestinal disturbances, arthritis-like joint achiness and inflammation, skin eruptions, premature aging changes, and numerous conditions the causes of which have been erroneously labeled by some ignorant or misunderstanding health care professionals as being "all in your head" or "psychosomatic."

Scientific studies, which go back nearly seventy years and are being carried out even more convincingly today, show that there *definitely is* a correlation between most of these CFS symptoms and the so-called "silver" dental amalgam fillings. To emphasize again, silver accounts for only 33 percent of the amalgam filling; mercury makes up over 50 percent of the total. So, toxic mercury is the main component in the alloy. The other metals in a dental amalgam are copper, zinc, tin, and sometimes nickel.

Not infrequently, gold, a sixth metallic dental component not mixed into the amalgam alloy, offers its own pathologic consequences of exposure to these many oral materials implanted by conventionally practicing dentists. (See chapter 10.)

Harmful Electrical Qualities of Amalgam

A homeopathic authority advises that dentists are inflicting a true health hazard on their patients by refusing to acknowledge the adverse electrical qualities of the metals placed permanently in teeth as amalgams or alloys. The homeopath, F. Fuller Royal, M.D., H.M.D., of Las Vegas, Nevada, who treats patients poisoned by those majority of dentists continuing to implant mercury amalgams, points out that the body's internal energetic control systems are subtle. They operate with minute amounts of electromagnetic energy.

Dr. Royal writes:

> Our body cells respond to energy in the form of electron transfer, also called electricity. Galvanic electricity, coming from the metals in dental fillings or crowns, results in the emission of metallic ions from the positive electrodes which are quite toxic to cells. Also, cells are damaged by the heat generated by electrical currents in excess of the body's currents. The water within the tissues will be subjected to electrolysis, a process in which the water molecules are broken apart, producing gases such as hydrogen, that are extremely toxic to cells. Small amounts of pulsed electrical current have major effects upon the highest functions of the brain.[1]

Certain cells in the body, such as bone marrow, hair follicles, the gastrointestinal mucosa, and fibroblasts, have the ability to dedifferentiate and grow into new tissue under controlled conditions. Cells that turn into cancer, classified as oncogenes, also have this capability and grow from 300 to 1500 percent faster in the presence of 10-microampere (mcA) of localized current.[2] Metals in teeth frequently generate galvanic currents of from 20 to 107 mcA. When the visible metal in the tooth displays a negative (-) electrical current, the opposite side

---

1   F. F. Royal, "Are Dentists Contributing to Our Declining Health?" *Townsend Letter for Doctors and Patients* (May 1990): 311– 14.

2   H. Fukata, "DC Electrical Current Increases DNA Synthesis in Cancer Cells," *Report of the Japan Committee of Electrical Enhancement of Bone Healing*, Abstract no. 8 (1981).

deep within the tissues of the tooth is positive (+). This means that ions of copper, mercury, tin, zinc, silver, and nickel when present are continually being released from the amalgam filling and are driven into the body tissues, including the nerves, bone, blood, and lymph, producing a toxic effect on cells. Cancer and autoimmune disease with associated symptoms of CFS, also known as chronic fatigue and immune dysfunction syndrome (CFIDS) must result.[1]

Mercury gas vapor escaping from dental fillings finds its way into the bloodstream and gradually poisons the body tissues. This circumstance occurs especially when fillings on the grinding surfaces of teeth are subjected to pressure and abrasion from chewing. Clinical dental/medical researchers concluding twelve separate investigations, one of the more significant ones performed within the last eight years at the University of Calgary, and another conducted at Oral Roberts University report in the *Journal of Dental Research* that the level of mercury after chewing is fifteen times greater in the breath of people with silver amalgam fillings than in subjects who do not possess such fillings.

The University of Calgary's Faculty of Medicine reported that mercury from amalgam fillings placed in the teeth of adult sheep made its appearance in various organs and tissues of these animals within twenty-nine days of the implantation.[2] Radioactive mercury ($Hg2O3$) used in the amalgam was found in the sheep jaw, lung, and gastrointestinal tissues. High concentration of mercury rapidly localized in the kidneys and liver, those sites where autoimmune disorders are known to occur.

Recognizing that the ADA and other groups representing organized dentistry in North America were lying to the public to protect themselves from being defendants in a multibillion dollar class action

---

1   J. Phillips, W. D. Winters, and J. Rutledge, "Exposure to 60-Hz Electromagnetic and Magnetic Fields Increases Rate of Growth of Human Cancer Cells," *International Journal of Radiation Biology* 49 (1986): 463.

2   L. J. Hahn, R. Kloiber, M. J. Vimy, Y. Takashashi, and F. L. Lorscheider, "Dental 'Silver' Tooth Fillings: A Source of Mercury Exposure Revealed by Whole-Body Image Scan and Tissue Analysis," *The FASEB Journal* 3 (1989): 2646.

law suit filed by dental patients from all over the continent, the Calgary University authors concluded with an obvious statement. The renowned research scientists wrote: "Our laboratory findings in this investigation are at variance with anecdotal opinion of the dental profession that amalgam tooth fillings are safe. . . . From our results we conclude that dental amalgams can be a major source of chronic mercury exposure."[1]

Dentists Are Shown to Pollute the Earth

Today, dentists are extending mercury pollution beyond their offices and their patients' mouths to the overall Earth environment. For example, the Arizona Department of Environmental Quality and the EPA discovered in 1990 that water treatment plants near the two Arizona cities of Tucson and Phoenix were discharging high levels of mercury into river systems.[2] Testing done in Pima County (Tucson) resulted in the closure of seven dental offices and the fining of the responsible polluting dentists. Such penalties were levied as a result of discovering that toxic mercury was being dropped by the dentists down their sink drains or allowed to be leached into the earth around their offices. Rain water running off the dentists' properties polluted the drinking water supplies of the two cities.

Such irresponsible actions by conventionally practicing dentists are not confined to members of the ADA alone. For example, it was discovered that one hundred dental offices in Hamburg, Germany, routinely contribute 0.4 tons of mercury to the water system of that city each year.[3] The result is that Hamburg residents are experiencing hair loss and other more serious autoimmune diseases from mercury toxicity. The conclusion that any person with common sense must come to is that whether you still retain dental amalgams in your

---

1   Ibid.

2   Op. cit. Ziff, "Dental Offices Polluting with Mercury." 1989.

3   Ibid.

mouth or not, the unthinking practices coming from some members of conventional dentistry truly are dangerous to your health.

History Shows Dentistry Personifies Original Quackery

In 1848 all members of the American Society of Dental Surgeons (ASDS) were required to sign pledges promising not to use mercury in the fillings of the teeth because the majority of these conscientious dental surgeons acknowledged then that patients were being poisoned by implantation of dental amalgams. Some ASDS members violated their pledges, however, and subsequently were suspended from the dental society in New York City. The written charge against the errant dentists was that they were persisting in their pursuit of "malpractice by using silver mercury fillings."[1]

The suspended fellows refused to give up their toxic ways because working with mercury offered them an easily malleable filling material that required much less time and effort to fill into a patient's teeth. Silver mercury fillings, therefore, continued to be used not to benefit patients but rather for the work production advantage of the dentists. This strife, internal to the dental profession, led to the formation of a new and competitive dental organization, the one we know currently as the American Dental Association. Today, the leaders of this modern professional trade union organization not only do not oppose the use of mercury, but many ADA state societies now actually *demand* its application. Moreover, most ADA state societies threaten their members and nonmembers alike with violation of the ADA code of professional ethics if such dentists tell patients they are implanting the mercurial poison in their teeth. Some holistic-type biological dentists have lost their licenses to practice, because out of their need for professional integrity, they've communicated such information to a few patients.[2]

---

1   M. Ring, *Dentistry: An Illustrated History* (New York: Harry N. Abrams Publishing, 1985).

2   J. H. Berry, "Questionable Care: What Can Be Done about Dental Quackery?" *Journal of the American Dental Association* 115, no. 5 (1987): 679.

In the United States, mercury is alternatively called *quicksilver*. But in many European countries such as in Germany and Austria it is referred to as *quecksilber* or *quacksalver*. Derived from the *quack* part of this quacksalver word is *quackery*, and a quack is one who pretends to cure disease but does not. In fact, the quack may create more of a disease process for the patient. Coming from the *salve* part of quacksalver, a salve is a supposedly healing substance for application to wounds or sores. The derogatory term *quack* was first used in reference to anyone using mercury preparations on the skin to "cure" diseases such as syphilis. When the skin lesions of syphilis were treated with mercury salves, the skin eruptions would disappear, resulting in the deeper penetration of the dread disease to the organs and nervous system, and a painful death (the ultimate quackery).

I hope this book will convince you that using mercury amalgams is as much a fake cure today as it was one hundred and fifty years ago.

Dental Amalgams Help to Create Chronic Fatigue Syndrome

Going back over seventy years, investigations during the decade following 1926 offered a very clear picture of mercury intoxication, both from amalgam fillings and industrial sources.[1] The early symptoms of chronic mercurialism are exactly duplicated in those suffering victims of CFIDS, the chronic fatigue and immune dysfunction syndrome. (As stated, CFIDS is also identified in North America as *chronic fatigue syndrome* and in Europe as *myalgic encephalitis*). Poisoning from one's amalgams and other forms of mercury toxicity result in largely subjective devastating effects. You may wish to compare the symptoms of mercury poisoning to this cited chronic fatigue and immune dysfunction syndrome and be amazed by their similarity.

---

1   A. Stock, "Die Defaehrlichket des Quecksilberdampfes," *Agnew. Chem* 39 (1926): 461; A. Stock, "Die Chronishce Quecksilber und Amalgamvergiftung," *Arch. Gewerbepath* 7 (1936): 388; A. Stock, "Die Milkroanalytische Bestimmung des Quecksilbers und Irre Anwendugng auf Hygienische und Medizinishe Fragen," *Svensk Kem. Tidskr* 50 (1938): 242.

Mercurialism causes the beginning mental difficulties of severe tiredness that seems always to be part of the symptoms. There is ever present "difficulty in getting up in the mornings," reduced energy, lack of disposition for intellectual work, inner unrest (what we today would call type-A behavior as expressed in chapter 3 by Victoria Zuppa, N.D.), mental or emotional depression, irritability, shyness, and loss of memory (mainly short-term memory).

Subsequently, mercury toxicity progresses to more objective somatic (physical) symptoms. The symptoms appear in chronic mercurialism as increased salivation, chronic catarrhs in the nose and upper airways, inflammations in the oral mucosa, easily bleeding gingiva, temporary loosening of teeth, "nervous heart" (palpitations), disturbed digestion, loss of appetite, sudden diarrheas, slight intestinal bleeding and pains, skin manifestations (including eczema, dermatitis, or urticaria), hearing difficulties, changes in vision with dimming of eyesight or double vision and speech and writing difficulties.

In addition to the symptoms and signs already mentioned, there may be more serious pathologies, such as an abnormal increase in the number of lymphocytes in the blood (lymphocytosis), weakness and numbness in all the peripheral nerves (polyneuropathy), joint pains (arthritis), sexual disturbances, fetal damage, thyroid changes, elevated LDL cholesterol, increased frequency of caries, chronic ear sounds (tinnitus), Meniere's disease, a higher general susceptibility to disease, and the predisposition to death (mortality).

For a summary of the many conditions related to mercury poisoning showing complications of the dental amalgam syndrome, please refer to table 4-1 below. The signs and symptoms of dental amalgam syndrome are listed in this table not necessarily in the order of their frequency. Also, not all of the discomforts may occur in each poisoning victim. These symptoms and signs are grouped according to body systems.

Each person implanted with silver dental amalgams will likely be hit at his or her weakest point of physiology by the toxic effects of the amalgamated mercury. Be aware that the poison in your mouth or the mouths of your loved ones is escaping slowly as a vapor or gas over an extended period. Most especially, this vapor seeps into the brain, blood, lymphatics, and other body tissues so gradually that the disease indicators make themselves known only subclinically. That is, you or your loved ones will not immediately show signs and symptoms of illness. Rather, somebody's subclinical or low level of wellness from sickness may be suspected, but it's probably not sufficiently developed to produce definite debilitation in the patient.

Table 4-1

Signs and Symptoms of the Dental Amalgam Syndrome

A series of difficulties characteristic of mercury toxicity affecting the eyes:

- Bleeding from the retina of one or both eyes
- Dim vision, especially after exercise
- Slow and poor accommodation to changes in vision distances
- Inability to fix one's gaze
- Uncontrollable eye movements
- Eyes drawn to one side
- Imaginary geometric figures appearing in the visual field, which migrate in a few minutes from the periphery toward the center and slowly disappear
- "Film" seeming to appear over the eyes
- Dry eyes
- A gray ring forming permanently around the cornea (known as *Arcus senilis*)

One or more heart difficulties:

- Irregular heartbeat (palpitations), often together with anxiety
- Strong pains in the left part of the chest come on

Problems in the upper respiratory tract:

- Asthmatic breathing troubles, such as a feeling of not being able to inhale
- A "cracking" sound in the lower part of the pleural sac, forcing one to cough
- Red irritated throat
- Inflammation in the upper airways and pleurisy appearing about a year after the dental treatment with amalgams
- Difficulties in swallowing

Psychological troubles come on such as:

- Severe amnesia
- Constant feelings of tension and strain
- Anxiety
- Irritability
- Difficulty and even impossibility to control behavior
- Indecision
- Loss of interest in life
- Mental or emotional depression

Conditions of the brain, including:

- Tiredness nearly all the time
- A feeling of being "old"
- Resistance to intellectual work
- Reduced capacity for work, both for intellectual and physical tasks
- Reduced powers of comprehension because information does not come through
- Increased need for sleep
- Headache about once a week. The headache often is migrainelike, especially induced by weather changes and by prolonged sleep in the mornings

Neurological complications can come on like:

- Vertigo (dizziness)
- Facial paralysis, usually on the right side, that is partly permanent
- Damage to balance and hearing
- A painful pull at the lower jaw toward the collar bone

Oral discomforts make their appearance such as:

- Increased salivation
- Often-present sour metallic taste
- Bleeding gums at toothbrushing

Numbers of other symptoms gradually showing up, including:

- Joint pains, especially increasing about a year after receiving the implantation of amalgam fillings
- Pains in the lower back
- Weakness of the muscles with a slowing down of muscular action
- Feelings of pressure, pains, and paresthesia ("pins and needles") in the region of the liver
- Gastrointestinal irritation
- Paresthesia in the region of the lymph nodes under the arms and in the groin
- Eczema or other skin eruptions

Sources: Stock, "Die Defaehrlichket des Quecksilberdampfes"; F. Gasser, "Quecksilberbelastung im Menschlichen Korper durch Amalgam," *Med.-Biol. Arbeits und Forschungsgemeinsch* (Baden-Baden, Germany: Dtsch. Zahnarzt., 1976); K. D. Jorgensen, "The Mechanism of Marginal Fracture of Amalgam Fillings," *Acta Odont. Scand.* 23 (1965): 347.

Amalgam Corrosion Leaches Mercury

Using a scanning electron microscope with diagnostic X-ray capability, Jaro Pleva, Ph.D., manager of the Corrosion Section of the Steel Research Division of Uddenholm AB, a metals manufacturing company in Hagfors, Sweden, performed an energy dispersive analysis of corrosion attacks and composition of his own and other persons' pieces of amalgam fillings. These fillings had been removed in 1982 and saved by Dr. Pleva for purposes of analysis. He carried out the analysis himself because his own dental amalgams were producing truly debilitating symptoms of mercury poisoning. Dr. Pleva's much detailed case history starts off the next chapter. It offers an exciting example of self-help sleuthing for the source of one's health problems. Dr. Pleva's self-discovery was partly responsible for Sweden's outlawing dental amalgam filling material.

Dr. Pleva performed a number of tests on the corroded amalgams he held in storage. What is visible to the naked eye when any used amalgam fillings removed from the patient's mouth are observed is that surfaces toward the tooth cavities are largely black with corrosion at the margin of the filling. These surfaces are corroded most severely near the margins toward the outer electrolyte (the saliva), a feature that is characteristic for crevice cell corrosion (Dr. Pleva's specialty). In the metallographically complexed amalgam there is dissolution of the least corrosion resistant phase, and this characteristic has been seen and reported many times before.[1] Amalgam corrosion like this releases metallic mercury that can either ionize, evaporate, or partly react with the other phases of amalgam to form new corrodible phases. Then the attack on a patient's immune system will commence or continue, a condition that has been documented.[2] The deteriorating filling becomes porous, which enhances further corrosion and causes the margins to crack.[3] Severe corrosion is likely to be seen, not only between the filling and the tooth, but also on the free surface towards the cheek.

Corrosion is an electrochemical or galvanic process that can be separated into a two-part reaction, (1) an anode process (at the positive pole), which brings about dissolution of the metal, and (2) a cathode process (at the negative pole). Both reactions proceed simultaneously and cause corrosion in such metals as aluminum, stainless steel, and dental amalgam.[4] It has been verified that amalgam of every known composition corrodes[5] so that crevices between tooth and filling cause the filling to become brittle and force the margins into cracking.[6] The entire surface of the filling then corrodes rapidly. If there is contact between amalgam and gold or other noble

1 C. E. Guthrow, L. B. Johnson, and K. R. Lawless, "Corrosion of Dental Amalgam and Its Component Phases," *J. Dent. Res.* 46 (1967): 1372; N. K. Sarkar, G. W. Marshall, J. B. Moser, and E. H. Greener, *"In Vivo* and *In Vitro* Corrosion Products of Dental Amalgam," *J. Dent. Res.* 54 (1975): 1031; S. Espevik, "Dental Amalgam," *Ann. Rev. Mater. Sci.,* 7 (1977): 55.

2 K. D. Jorgensen and T. Saito, "Structure and Corrosion of Dental Amalgams," *Acta O dont. Scand.* 28 (1970): 129.

3 G. Wrangle, Metallers Korrosion Och Ytskydd (Stockholm: Almqvist and Wiksell Publishers, 1967).

4 Espevik, "Dental Amalgam"; I. C. Schoonover and W. Souder, "Corrosion of Dental Alloys," *J. Am. Dent. Ass.* 28 (1941): 1278.

5 R. S. Mateer and C. D. Reitz, "Corrosion of Amalgam Restorations," *J. Dent. Res.* 49 (1970): 399; Jorgensen, "The Mechanism of Marginal Fracture."

6 Schoonover and Souder, "Corrosion of Dental Amalgam."

metals, the anode/amalgam will be polarized toward more positive potentials and the rate of corrosion increases considerably. The gold then takes over the function as a cathode.[1]

If someone with dental amalgams chews on a salad prepared with dressing containing vinegar and salt, an electrolyte solution is created in the mouth. Considerably increased conductivity and a lowering of the pH will result. Both of these factors produce higher corrosion currents and a concomitant increased release of mercury. Exactly such a case was described in the medical/dental literature of chronic inflammation of the mouth, nose, and throat. The symptoms were rapidly increasing after acid food was consumed. This patient had both gold and amalgam in his mouth. After elimination of the amalgam, however, the symptoms disappeared.[2]

How Amalgam Gets Transported throughout the Body

Since no amount of mercury in the body and brain is a safe substance or belongs there, the smallest concentration causes pathology. And its half-life for excretion from the brain is about thirty years. Therefore, Alzheimer's disease is a possible result of dental amalgams.[3] For additional explanations about mercury as a source of Alzheimer's disease, please see *Toxic Metal Syndrome: How Metal Poisonings Can Affect Your Brain*, by coauthors H. Richard Casdorph,

---

1   J. A. Fraunhofer and P. J. Staheli, "Gold-Amalgam Galvanic Cells," *Brit. Dent. J.* 132 (1972): 357; T. Till and G. Wagner, "Untersuchungen zur Loslichkeit der Bestandteile von Amalgam-Fullungen Wahrend des Kau- und Trinkaktes. I Teil," *Zahnarztl. Welt* 82 (1973): 945; G. Wagner and T. Till, "Untersuchungen zur Loslichkeit der Bestandteile von Amalgam-Fullungen Wahrend des Kau- und Trinkaktes. II Teil," *Zahnarztl. Welt* 82 (1973): 1004; G. Wagner and T. Till, "Untersuchungen uber den Temperatureinfluss auf Elektrochemische Vorgange an Metallishen Zahreparaturmaterialien," *Zahnarztl. Welt* 83 (1974): 980.

2   A. Rost, "Amalgamschaden," *Zahnarztl. Prax.* 27 (1976): 475.

3   H. R. Casdorph and M. Walker, *Toxic Metal Syndrome* (Garden City Park, N.Y.: Avery Publishing Group, 1995).

M.D., Ph.D., and Morton Walker, D. P. M. (See the title's listing in appendix B.)

In chapter 6 of this book, I discuss at length the findings of Professor Boyd Hailey, Ph.D., chief of the Chemistry Department at the University of Kentucky. Giving uncontestable proof, Dr. Hailey ties "silver" amalgam dental fillings to Alzheimer's disease. Dr. Hailey and my *Toxic Metal Syndrome* coauthor, Dr. H. Richard Casdorph, never met, but they've reached the same scientific conclusion: that amalgamated mercury in your mouth causes Alzheimer's disease.

Current research also shows that inorganic mercury is taken up by nerve endings and is transported toward the central nervous system by retrograde axonal transport. Mercury vapor is also transferred from the nasal mucosa to the brain in nerves or in blood vessels. Consequently, a variety of neurological diseases like multiple sclerosis, lung diseases such as asthma, and cardiovascular diseases, including heart arrhythmia, may occur from their connection with these pathways of pathology.

Mercury from amalgam can be taken up by the body and brain quite handily in three different but specific ways. They are:

1. **Inhalation of mercury vapor and absorption in the lungs.** Mercury becomes an integral part of the involved individual's inspiration and expiration. Both old and recent studies have shown considerable amounts of mercury in respired air during the dental cavity-filling process[1] and from people with amalgam fillings already in place.[2] Fifteen times higher mercury levels in respired air was recorded for amalgam carriers after chewing, compared to a group without amalgam. The mercury level in exhaled air was proportional to the number of fillings and reached levels of 87 micrograms (mcg) per cubic meter (m3)

---

1   K. O. Frykholm, "Mercury from Dental Amalgam: Its Toxic and Allergic Effects and Some Comments on Occupational Hygiene," *Acta Odont. Scand.* 15 (1957): supplement 22.

2   Stock, "Die Chronische Quecksilber"; C. W. Svare, L. C. Peterson, J. W. Reinhard, D. B. Boyers, C. W. Frank, D. D. Gay, and R. D. Cox, "The Effect of Dental Amalgams on Mercury Levels in Expired Air," *J. Dent. Res.* 60 (1981): 1668.

of air after chewing.[1] The industrial maximum level of mercury permitted according to EPA regulations for eight-hours, five-day-a-week exposure is 50 mcg/m3. Thus people with amalgam in their mouths are functioning in a subclinical state of perpetual illness because they are exposed twenty-four hours a day to about 75 percent more toxic mercury than the U.S. government allows.

2. **Oxidation of mercury and gastrointestinal tract absorption.** All soluble mercury compounds dissociate easily into mercuric ions in the intestine. The reaction leads to absorption through mucous tissues so that the mercuric poison becomes a part of every cell in the body and brain since it is transported as part of nourishing fluids.

3. **Absorption of mercuric ions diffusing through the teeth.** Released and ionized mercury is taken up by tissues and nerves beneath fillings and possibly in root canals.[2] Mercury is absorbed by nerve endings and gets transported towards the central nervous system in the same way as lead, only mercury is even more poisonous than lead.[3]

In my opinion, anyone who allows dental amalgam fillings to remain as part of his or her oral cavity has elected to commit slow but steady suicide by mercury poisoning. All evidence indicates that dental amalgams should be removed from your mouth in accordance with the techniques set forth by any of the four holistic dental groups. Since this is not a book dedicated to teaching dental technique,

---

1   Svare and others, "The Effect of Dental Amalgams."

2   K. O. Frykholm and E. Odeblad, "Studies on the Penetration of Mercury through the Dental Hard Tissues Using Hg203 in Silver Amalgam Fillings," *Acta Odont. Scand.* 13 (1955): 157; T. Till and K. Maly, "Zum Nachweis der Lyse von Hg aus Silber-Amalgam von Zahnfulungen," *Der Praktische Arzt* 32 (1978): 1042.

3   J. K. Baruah, C. G. Rasool, W. G. Bradley, and T. L. Munsat, "Retrograde Transport of Lead in Rat Sciatic Nerve," *Neurol.* 31 (1981): 612.

the methods of removing dental amalgams are touched on only peripherally in chapter 9. To learn such amalgam removal techniques or to acquire a listing of dentists who practice holistic dentistry, contact one or more of those professional mercury-free dentist membership organizations listed in appendix A.

All dentists are not created equal in knowledge, skill, and integrity just as all auto mechanics are not the same. Discerning dentist Don H. Lowrance, D.D.S., M.S., of Corpus Christi, Texas, admonishes us to beware of bargains "in parachutes and dentistry." Dr. Lowrance says, "Dental materials used to replace amalgams are very technique-sensitive; and a dentist who does not specialize in their use is a poor choice in placing them. The absolutely worst thing a patient can do is choose a dentist who does not believe amalgam is a health hazard. The basis of a patient-doctor relationship should be common objectives achieved with integrity. A *non*-mercury-free dentist can never provide this."[1]

Removing Amalgam Fillings Is Significant

Do you wonder why the American Dental Association refuses to admit that mercury amalgam fillings can affect health even though scientists have known for decades that mercury harms the human immune system, kidneys, reproductive system, brain cells, central nervous system, and beneficial mouth and colon bacteria? I believe you'll be shocked by the specific reasons for this ADA denial when I present them to you in chapter 8. Meanwhile, know that dentists who advocate removing mercury amalgams risk harassment, censure, loss of referrals, and finally, loss of state licensure to practice dentistry for promoting amalgam replacement. It's a costly procedure for the patient and a politically risky one for the holistic dentist. The ADA mainstream dental politicians say that dental amalgam removal has no scientific basis. From reading this book,

---

1   D. H. Lowrance, "Mercury Poisoning and Detoxification," *Townsend Letter for Doctors and Patients* 168 (July 1997): 95.

however, you will discover that amalgam removal preserves one's health and life.

In a recent study published in the *Journal of Orthomolecular Medicine*, proper amalgam removal reduced or eliminated 80 percent of the symptoms associated with chronic mercury poisoning in 118 patients. This study is separate and divorced from the investigation conducted by the Toxic Element Research Foundation reported on and listed under table 3-1 in chapter 3. The second survey listed thirty-eight symptoms reported by the involved patients before their fillings were removed. A total of 83 percent of those surveyed experienced disabling fatigue, 76 percent had poor concentration, 65 percent reported poor memory, 64 percent showed irritability, 62 percent suffered muscle fatigue, and 61 percent had a metallic taste in their mouth all the time.

In addition, half of the patients complained of bloating, headache, joint pain, throat pain, allergies, and poor appetite. After their mercury amalgams were taken out, these discomforts disappeared for massive numbers of the survey participants.

Before amalgam removal, researchers tested each patient's serum globulin reaction to thirty-four different metals and dental materials so that replacement fillings would be biocompatible with each individual.

Amalgam filling replacement followed the protocol recommended by the dental pioneer, Hal A. Huggins, of Colorado Springs, Colorado. The Huggins protocol includes the use of antioxidants, vitamins, minerals, and dietary guidelines (see chapter 16) to support the immune system and the use of proper ventilation and oral suction to lessen contamination from mercury and mercury vapor during its removal. Add homeopathic remedies (see chapter 17) to the Huggins protocol, and you can be certain of receiving the best possible procedure for ridding yourself of poison in the mouth.

One to four years after mercury (and, in some cases, other metal) fillings were removed, the subjects in the above-reported survey were given the same list of thirty-eight symptoms and asked to indicate whether their complaints had improved, disappeared, or remained unchanged. The thought-provoking response? Among these patients, 48 percent of symptoms were reduced, 31 percent were eliminated, and 21 percent were unchanged. Those patients whose blood serum tests showed a strong globulin reaction to amalgam metals "did not recover as favorably as those with mild reactions," wrote the dental investigator, Harold Lichtenberg, D.D.S. Thus, if protein changes have already occurred in the blood from longstanding mercury toxicity, people cannot easily throw off the effects of what those amalgam-using, conventionally practicing dentists have done to them.[1]

---

1   H. Lichtenberg, "Symptoms before and after Proper Amalgam Removal in Relation to Serum-Globulin Reaction to Metals," *Journal of Orthomolecular Medicine* (Fourth Quarter 1996).

Five

Do "Silver" Dental Mercury Amalgams Create Illnesses?

From the time he was twenty years old, in the 1960s, Jaro Pleva[1] had his cavities repaired, with the exception of the front teeth, with so-called "silver" dental amalgam fillings. Except, in 1963 a gold bridge was placed in the left side of his lower jaw to replace two missing teeth. By 1976 one of the supporting teeth for this bridge needed treatment for caries. The hole in the tooth was temporarily filled with amalgam through an opening drilled in the gold. The final treatment was delayed for a year and then the tooth was root-filled through the same opening in the gold. The cavity was again filled up with mercury amalgam. Thus within the gold bridge, Dr. Pleva had dissimilar metals combined together. This is the sort of dental work destined to create illnesses, but he did not know it at the time.

This information about young Jaro Pleva's teeth is significant because this man became an important scientific investigator of damage to the human body and brain caused by dental amalgam fillings. His story, among others, is the reason the government of Sweden, on February 18, 1994, publicly announced the final timetable for the banning of mercury/silver amalgam as a dental filling material. The use of amalgam was totally banned for children and adolescents up to the age of nineteen on July 1, 1995,

---

1   Jaro Pleva's is a true identity in the public domain. Dr. Pleva's health history has been previously published in Sweden, other European countries, and the United States.

and for adults in the spring of 1997. By January 1, 1999, no more amalgam was being allowed into Swedish dental offices.

Jaro Pleva went through undergraduate college and university graduate training. He earned his doctorate in chemistry and took employment as a physical chemist specializing in the corrosion science of metals. Twenty years after the initial placement of his gold bridge and its eventual permanent amalgam filling, Jaro Pleva, B.S., Ph. D., uncovered significant information about the poisonous character of mercury and its responsibility for massive amounts of illness in the industrialized Western nations.

Dr. Pleva reported before assemblies of his colleagues that this toxic metal escapes from the corroded surfaces of dental amalgams as a vapor. Then the dental substance leaches its toxic fumes and other forms of mercury into the bodies and brains of over two-and-a-half billion persons around the globe who have been treated by means of the tooth-filling methods of conventionally practicing organized dentistry.

As mentioned in the prior chapter, Dr. Pleva is chief chemist and manager of the corrosion science section of the multibillion Krona Steel Research Company, Uddenholm AB, in Hagfors, Sweden. Techniques of investigation available to the chemists at such a large steel research facility allowed Dr. Pleva to perform analyses of saved silver amalgam fillings taken from himself and numerous other dental patients. He showed that these amalgams were badly corroded. Documented corrosion attacks on every aged amalgam filling prove that the dental profession's assurances about amalgam being a stable alloy can be dismissed as so many lies.

To clarify: statements from dentists and politicians representing organized professional dentistry that amalgam is not harmful may be considered to be unfounded and based erroneously on short-term considerations. Galvanic coupling of gold and amalgam guarantees that the dental patient will experience mercury poisoning within a relatively short time.

Dr. Pleva proved the dangers of dental amalgam fillings by first examining his own health problems and then looking at others.

The History of Illness Experienced by Dr. Pleva

Starting in the late 1960s, after undergoing his first treatment with dental amalgam, Jaro Pleva experienced bodily discomforts in the form of stress and occasional migraine headaches. The migraine was most often precipitated by weather changes, especially from low pressures in the atmosphere. He related the feelings of stress to his driving ambition and a lack of balance between office work and physical activity. Dr. Pleva concluded that he worked too hard.

A few months after his final dental implantation in 1977, when his tooth was root-filled permanently with amalgam through an opening in the gold bridge, Dr. Pleva was surprised by being struck with strong, unexplainable symptoms. He began to awaken habitually during the night feeling intense anxiety and an irregular heartbeat. Each time, for a few minutes, he believed that those were the last minutes of his life. At the same time, other acute symptoms increased in frequency and severity.

He was constantly in a state of indescribable tiredness, stress, emotional depression, and anxiety. Performing simple tasks, joining discussions, talking and being sociable, even thinking clearly, required considerable effort. During his consultations with doctors about these symptoms, he mainly complained of his irregular heartbeat because this was something tangible and physical that he could pinpoint. He was examined for heart arrhythmia, which was not found. Results of medical tests, administered by several physicians, were in general normal except for a slightly elevated blood cholesterol level. The result was an entry in each doctor's records that the patient "imagines his troubles." In short, Dr. Pleva was labeled by the health professionals as having "psychosomatic" illness. They were convinced that it was "all in his head."

To be helpful, the patient did volunteer to several of the doctors that there was an amalgam filling bonded into his gold bridge. As a corrosion expert, he was aware of this filling's deterioration. A few months after its implantation, he had noticed the filling became black and rough, which indicated corrosion and dissolution of the amalgam had taken place. Still, hearing Dr. Pleva's evaluation of the corroding metal in his mouth, no doctor examined his oral cavity or even showed any interest in this factor.

The patient's many discomfitures continued. Because of eye troubles that developed next, he visited an ophthalmologist who found hypertension and bleeding in the retina, but prescribed no treatment. Instead, the eye specialist sent him back to a general practitioner for treatment of his high blood pressure. High blood pressure medication was prescribed, but Dr. Pleva experienced the same results as before—nothing changed in his various symptoms.

Then, a few months later, pains in his chest forced him to seek medical attention once again. The patient underwent more medical tests, including an electrocardiogram (ECG) conducted during rest and exercise. But the ECG showed a normal heart condition. Dr. Pleva's gastrointestinal system was X-rayed and examined for an entire day, but no diagnosis resulted. Mercury analyses of the man's urine and blood, performed on his urgent request, showed that mercury values in the fluids, while elevated somewhat, were below the danger mark of industrial limits. Nothing seemed to indicate that he was being sickened by the poison in his mouth. He began to wonder if, indeed, it was "all in his head."

Dr. Pleva Disregards His Personal Scientific Knowledge

Repeatedly Dr. Pleva was offered the diagnostic projection from his medical consultants that all of the symptoms came from stress on the job or from strained relations in his family. This guesswork he could not take seriously, inasmuch as he knew that it wasn't such a stressful period for him, and his family life was a real pleasure. Therefore, the patient reevaluated his health problems strictly from a scientific bent and again came around to examining his dental fillings.

He noticed that the surface of the amalgam filling (about 4 millimeters by 4 millimeters [mm] in size) within the gold bridge (whose surface measured 670 mm2) rather quickly had become black and rugged. As a corrosion expert he was fully cognizant of this metallic area being a galvanic cell wherein the more noble gold acted as the cathode and the potentially toxic amalgam was the anode. This meant that the anode/amalgam was dissolving and that the metals ionized as cations. Yet for too long a time Dr. Pleva did not fully believe in his own scientific studies. He ascribed little significance to the ionization effect, deciding that the process of corrosion certainly could not result in dangerous amounts of dissolved mercury since those university-trained dentists had twice shown not the slightest hesitation in putting amalgam in direct contact with gold.

Ignoring the truth of his personal knowledge proved to be Dr. Pleva's undoing, for he suffered in physical and mental torment from his disabilities: chronic and devastating fatigue, sleepiness almost to the point of narcolepsy, ever present depression and anxiety, repeated heart palpitations, chest pain, dim vision and other retinal troubles, headaches, dizziness, joint pains, "pins and needles" sensations in both armpits and both groins, an odd pulling of the lower jaw toward his collarbone, muscle weakness, eczematous skin eruptions, bleeding gums, metallic taste, a ring around his cornea called *arcus senilis*, and more.

Suffering severely for another eighteen months with help nowhere in sight, he finally chose the path that now seems self-evident. In earnest, Dr. Pleva studied mercury poisoning. He visited medical libraries and read toxicology and pathology books in which he found his symptoms clearly connected to chronic mercury intoxication coming from his teeth.

The next vital step he took was to consult a holistic dentist and have the amalgam in contact with his gold bridge exchanged for plastic composite. After about three weeks it became evident that this action had him moving in the right direction and that he really was mercury poisoned. The stinging sensations in both his armpits and groins and the eczema on his skin disappeared first. Then many of the subjectively strongest symptoms began to diminish, but not all of them and not completely.

About three months after the exchange of the filling material in the gold bridge Dr. Pleva suffered a stroke-like paralysis in the right half of his face; his balance and hearing was also affected. He consulted several doctors, and a tentative diagnosis by the first one indicated that he had a rare, tropical disease, imported from abroad. Of course, this diagnosis was wrong.

A second physician diagnosed the facial paralysis with damage to balance and hearing as manifestations of herpes zoster otis (shingles of the ear), which was based on the discovery of a small area of skin eruptions on the right ear. There was no pain or itching in the affected area, although the hearing, balance, and paralysis troubles were considered unusually severe, and the ear damages have stayed with him permanently. Again, the diagnosis was wrong. He did not have shingles.

The chemist's imbalance straightened itself out eventually when Dr. Pleva acted with more thought about the many other dental amalgam fillings that were crowding his oral cavity. The solution to his many health problems, this highly educated chemist finally discovered was to return his oral cavity to as natural a state of repair as is possible.

Finally the Patient Has All Dental Amalgams Removed

By autumn 1981, three years after elimination of the gold-amalgam galvanic cell, many sets of symptoms still remained, such as chronic fatigue syndrome, muscle pains, joint pains, breathing difficulties, and mental or emotional anxiety. Consequently, Dr. Pleva returned to the text books and studied the literature on dental amalgams even more fully. His knowledge of metal instability and corrosion mechanisms led to his decision, finally, to have all amalgam material removed from his mouth, and this was done during the summer of 1982.

Immediately after the first replacements of amalgam by dental filling substitutes, the patient's symptoms improved to the point of disappearance. For example, when the fillings opposite the gold bridge were removed, every tendency to headache or migraine went away permanently. Then his chronic fatigue eliminated itself and a resurgence of energy came back so abruptly that Dr. Pleva found himself needing only six hours in bed nightly instead of his usual twelve. Almost simultaneous with removal of two amalgam fillings in the lower jaw, the painful pulling and strain from the lower jaw toward the collarbone left him completely.

When all amalgam fillings had been removed and substituted with composite plastic, every physical symptom such as joint pains, chest pains, bleeding gums, paresthesias, paralysis, asthmatic breathing troubles, eye trouble from arcus senilis, and others, disappeared for Dr. Pleva.

His mental or emotional difficulties, including both depression and anxiety, seemed to abate more slowly however, for mental functions became more difficult to quantify. Some symptoms that he thought resulted from other causes than amalgam toxicity also disappeared, especially backache, which he had once related to office work and his height (six foot, five inches). Also pains below his ribs, which were thought by doctors to be remnants of a hepatitis infection twenty years earlier, eliminated themselves. In December 1982 the patient found that small vesicles and exfoliation of the skin on the sole of one foot and on the insides of his hands went away completely.

The well-being that he felt then was tremendous, the man reports. Improvements in his health could not be related to any factor in his surroundings such as work, home, personal relations, or diet, since these had remained unchanged. The disappearance of Dr. Pleva's symptoms clearly falls into that period of his dental amalgam removal. Mercury was gone from his oral cavity and so were his symptoms of illness.

Only three months after the final dental treatment had taken place, the associated chronic fatigue syndrome he had been experiencing was totally gone. Dr. Pleva regained a feeling of peace and calmness as well as an appreciation of smells, details, and gradations in his environment, something he hadn't been able to do for the twenty-five years or more in which he had retained amalgam in his mouth.

Today, at age fifty-five, Jaro Pleva no longer accepts that age-related symptoms of chronic tiredness, headache, or pains in many body parts must be part of everyday discomforts. A prerequisite for health is that corroding amalgam alloys with their potential for oral galvanism, releasing highly toxic heavy metals, must be removed from the oral cavity.

More Illnesses from Dental Amalgam Toxicity Reported

One of the amalgam's manufacturers inserts a precautionary notice into every new container of dental amalgam for use by the dentist to mix into alloy cavity filling material. This notice from the L. D. Caulk Division of Dentsply International, Inc., of Milford, Delaware to the dentist reads:

WARNING, THIS PRODUCT CONTAINS MERCURY

- Prior to use, read the material safety data sheet.
- Use in a well ventilated area.
- Avoid contact with the skin.
- Wear safety glasses and gloves.
- Exposure to mercury may cause irritation to skin, eyes, respiratory tract, and mucous membranes.
- Mercury may also be a skin sensitizer, nephrotoxin, neurotoxin, and pulmonary sensitizer.
- Mercury has also been reported to be associated with a wide variety of adverse health effects, including reproductive toxicity.

As to *reproductive toxicity*, mercury concentrations that came from dental amalgam fillings were measured in various tissues of fetuses obtained from medically necessary abortions and children who had died, mainly from sudden infant death syndrome. The concentration of mercury in the kidneys and liver of fetuses and in the kidney and cerebral cortex of infants correlated significantly with the number of dental amalgam fillings in the mother.[1]

Holistic physician and clinical journal columnist Alan R. Gaby, M.D., of Seattle, Washington, in commenting on the finding you've just read, wrote in his monthly column: "Mercury is one of the most toxic elements on earth. Small amounts of mercury vapor leach continually from dental amalgams and the potential dangers of this constant exposure have been debated vigorously. The present study suggests that fetal tissues accumulate mercury that leaches from the mother's dental amalgam."[2]

---

1   G. Drasch and others, "Mercury Burden of Human Fetal and Infant Tissues," *European Journal of Pediatrics* 153 (1994): 607–10.

2   A. R. Gaby, "Mothers Amalgam-Mercury Accumulates in Fetus," *Townsend Letter for Doctors and Patients* 147 (October 1995): 19.

Holistic dentist Gary A. Strong, D.D.S., further connects mercury amalgams to reproductive difficulties for women. The Billings, Montana dentist wondered in print: "Does mercury from dental amalgams contribute to reproductive disorders? Medical research data show that mercury plays a role in menstrual dysfunction, infertility, miscarriages, and birth defects. Then Dr. Strong cited a dozen references that link numbers of reproduction troubles with dental mercury amalgams.[1]

Amalgams Responsible for Infertility, Miscarriage, and Birth Defects

Since amalgam dental fillings consist of 50 percent or more of mercury, numerous studies now document chronic toxic metal release through elemental mercury vapors, inorganic mercury from electrogalvanic corrosion, and abraded mercury particles. All of this metallic poison in the mouth often exceeds the limits set for occupational exposure by the Environmental Protection Agency and the World Health Organization (WHO).[2] The WHO states that "the general population is primarily exposed to mercury through diet and dental amalgam, with dental amalgam providing the greatest degree of exposure."[3]

In two studies using the orally administered mercury chelator and removal agent, 2,3 dimercapto-1-propane sulfonic acid (DMPS), challenge doses demonstrated significant increases in urine mercury excr0etion, which correlated to the amount of intraoral amalgams (amalgams implanted into the teeth). One group of investigators concluded, "release of mercury from fillings represents

1   G. A. Strong, "Does Mercury from Dental Amalgams Contribute to Reproductive Disorders?" *Townsend Letter for Doctors and Patients* 118 (May 1993) 467–68.

2   EPA Office of Health and Environmental Assessment, "Mercury Health Effects Update Health Issue Assessment," final report, EPA-600/8-84-019F.

3   World Health Organization, "Environmental Health Criteria," *118: Inorganic Mercury* (Geneva 1991).

the main source of mercury exposure in subjects with amalgam fillings.[1]

The EPA states: "Women chronically exposed to mercury vapor experienced increased frequencies of menstrual disturbances and spontaneous abortions; also, a high mortality rate was observed among infants born to women who displayed symptoms of mercury poisoning."[2]

Two collaborating groups of researchers at separate Swedish universities exposed pregnant squirrel monkeys to mercury vapor. Early abortion, premature birth, and low birth weight with a perinatal death were observed. Behavioral studies of the offspring have revealed persistent deviation from the controls and also after neonatal exposure.[3]

A U.S. National Institutes of Health study of 418 registered dental assistants proved significant. All of these young women had become pregnant during the four years before starting work in their occupation, proving they were, indeed, fertile. When they then exposed themselves to pollution from mercury amalgam used in their dental offices, reduced fertility resulted. The young women had great difficulty in getting pregnant again. Measurements taken by the investigators showed that fecundity of the mercury-exposed women was only 50 percent of that for another unexposed group of female assistants.[4]

When stillbirths and birth defects were evaluated by gynecological researchers, it was found that mercury levels from amalgam

---

1   H. V. Aposhian and others, "Urinary Mercury after Administration 2,3-Dimercapto Propane-1-Sulfonic Acid: Correlation with Dental Amalgam Score," *FASEBJ* 6, no. 6 (1992): 2472 76; D. K. Zander and others, "Studies on Human Exposure to Mercury 3DMPS Induced Mobilization of Mercury in Subjects with and without Amalgam Fillings," *Zentralbaltt fur Hygiene und Umwelmedizin* 192, no. 5 (1992): 447–54.

2   EPA, "Mercury Health Effects Update."

3   M. Berlin and others, "Prenatal Exposure to Mercury Vapor: Effects on Brain Development," Abstract 245, *The Toxicologist* 12, no. 1 (1992).

4   A. Rowland and others, "Reduced Fertility among Dental Assistants and Occupational Exposure to Mercury," Abstract 246, *The Toxicologist* 12, no. 1 (1992).

fillings present in maternal blood and placental blood "exhibited significant positive correlation with background mercury levels."[1]

Researchers discovered that mercury vapor from amalgam fillings in pregnant women passes into the placenta and poisons fetuses. They wrote: "The blood-brain barrier is known to discriminate against ionic mercury but to allow transit of the dissolved vapor. Our results indicate that the placenta has similar properties. Thus mercury vapor now shares with the short-chain alkylmercurials the ability to pass across two important diffusion barriers in the body."[2]

Five women who had had dental amalgam fillings removed were studied by dental researchers. The dentists reported, "This study showed there was a reduction in blood-mercury levels when existing dental amalgam restorations were removed and replaced with a nonmercury-containing restorative material."[3]

Amalgam Poisons Are Following the Same Path as Lead Poisoning

Don Galloway, Ph.D., a scientist with the FDA's Center for Devices and Radiological Health in Rockville, Maryland, speaking at a Seattle meeting of the Society of Toxicology, drew parallels between the evidence against lead poisoning twenty-five years before and the evidence against mercury amalgam poisoning today. More than three thousand toxicologists listened to Dr. Galloway, who pointed out that lead has since been proven harmful to humans and has been removed from paint,

---

1   W. D. Kuntz and others, "Maternal and Cord Blood Background Mercury Levels: A Longitudinal Surveillance," *American Journal of Obstetrics and Gynecology* 143, no. 4 (1982): 440–43.

2   T. W. Clarkson and others, "The Transport of Elemental Mercury into Fetal Tissues," *Biological Neonate* 21 (1972): 239–44.

3   K. R. Snapp and others, "Contribution of Dental Amalgams to Blood Mercury Levels," Abstract 1276, *Journal of Dental Restorations* 65 (Special Issue, March 1986): 331.

pipes, and many other materials, including gasoline. In the United States and Europe, amalgam poisoning is following along the same path of proven toxicity as had lead poisoning twenty-five years ago. Only today, dentists implanting mercury amalgams, rather than lead-based paint, are the source of patients' illnesses.

While lead is an acknowledged poison in children—causing them to show lowered intelligence—mercury does even more damage by making them mentally ill. Have you ever heard the phrase, "mad as a hatter"? It comes from the use of mercury in hat manufacturing; hatters who handled mercury went crazy early in life. Many of the hatters were children.

Other speakers at that same toxicology panel in Seattle presented significant information on amalgam-produced diseases. Definitely, the presenters supported the contention that dental amalgams pose a health risk. For example, toxic metal researcher Fritz Lorscheider, M.D., from the University of Calgary in Alberta, said, "Dental amalgam is a major source of mercury in the general population. There is an impairment in kidney function in animal studies. And," he added, "certain regions of the human brain appear to concentrate mercury."[1]

Discover If You Have Mercury/Toxic Metal Sensitivity

The same sequence of health difficulties experienced by Jaro Pleva could happen to anyone who has mercury amalgams implanted in their mouth. Without knowing the source of your diverse symptoms, mercury/toxic metal sensitivity may be affecting you.

As an investigating medical journalist, I believe and flat out declare that under any circumstance, if you are one of those 98

---

1   T. Paulson, "Scientist Parallels Dental Amalgams and Lead Poisoning," *P-I Reporter (Seattle)*, in *Townsend Letter for Doctors and Patients* 107 (June 1992): 446.

percent of the American people with amalgams packed into your dental cavities, you should have them removed and replaced with harmless materials. If you are receiving dental services from one of the 92 percent of dentists, using amalgam materials, who are afraid of losing their license to practice or who remain nonbelieving, uncaring, or unenlightened about the effects of mercury amalgams, my advice is to change your dental health professional. Mercury amalgams disguised with the false name of "silver" dental fillings must never be allowed to remain as part of a person's oral repair work. Moreover, if certain nonobvious (subclinical) symptoms are present that you've not recognized as related to mercury toxicity, my recommendation is that with all speed seek out a mercury-free, holistic (biological) dentist and have your mercury amalgams replaced with nontoxic biocompatible dental substances.

Test yourself with the "Mercury/Toxic Metal Sensitivity Questionnaire" in table 5-1 below. The questionnaire was created by health and legal professionals. Leading the list is Keith W. Sehnert, M.D., a private practice holistic/complementary/alternative medicine physician located in Minneapolis, Minnesota. The second questionnaire creator is Gary Jacobson, D.D.S., a former practicing holistic dentist and founder of the Airport Dental Clinic located near the Minneapolis-St. Paul International Airport. Dr. Jacobson was denied the right to continue practicing dentistry in Minnesota since his state dental society declared him unethical and malpracticing because he told patients about the dangers of dental amalgams. The third leading exponent of discovering one's need for amalgam removal is Kip Sullivan, J.D., research director for a citizen economic issues organization located in St. Paul. Their questionnaire was published in the October 1995 issue of the *Townsend Letter for Doctors and Patients* for duplication and use by those clinicians or patients who suspect that mercury amalgams are creating subclinical symptoms of various illnesses.[1]

---

1   K. W. Sehnert, G. Jacobson, and K. Sullivan, "Is Mercury Toxicity an Antoimmune Disorder?" *Townsend Letter for Doctors and Patients* (October 1995): 134–37.

Attorney Sullivan reported that because of his experiencing colitis and numbers of additional nondescript but discomforting symptoms, he had his fifteen amalgam fillings removed by Dr. Jacobson during the spring of 1991. The patient's colitis disappeared completely within two months. Over the next three years, Dr. Kip Sullivan wrote: "numerous other health problems that first appeared in my teens and twenties have either gone away or improved greatly."

As regarding the licensure removal of Dr. Gary Jacobson, the Minnesota Board of Dentistry admonished him for warning patients about the toxic effects of mercury found in amalgam fillings. When Dr. Jacobson continued to educate his patients even in the face of the dental board's notification, his peers removed his license to practice dentistry. Shocked at the unfairness of this action and the dental board's "consumer health-be-damned" attitude, one of the defendant's lawyers is quoted as saying: "Tom Vasaly, assistant attorney general of Minnesota, admitted that the Board of Dentistry ordered him to take Dr. Jacobson's license. Why? Because of this dentist's antimercury stance."[1]

The Mercury/Toxic Metal Sensitivity Questionnaire shown in Table 5-1 is for your personal application. The three researchers who devised the questionnaire have already tested its diagnostic efficacy on more than three hundred persons carrying mercury amalgams in their mouths. The questionnaire served those patients and their medical doctors quite well as an alert when any single patient answered "yes" for five or more of the thirty questions. Such patients were then referred by their physicians to holistic dentists with special knowledge of mercury amalgam removal so that their fillings could be replaced with nontoxic composites or other less harmful dental materials.

You and your loved ones should consider answering the survey questions to make a determination as to whether any of you are being adversely affected by the mercury vapors or particles escaping from amalgam fillings.

---

1   "Board Investigates Mercury-Free Dentistry," *FDA Hotline* (October 1995).

Table 5-1

Mercury/Toxic Metal Sensitivity Questionnaire

If you have mercury amalgam "silver" fillings in your teeth and must reply to five or more of the following questions with "yes" answers, you should be alerted to the likelihood that you are being poisoned by these dental amalgam fillings.

1. Have you had sore gums (gingivitis) often over the years?   Yes   No

2. Have you had mental symptoms such as confusion or forgetfulness?   Yes   No

3. Has severe depression been a frequent problem?   Yes   No

4. Has ringing in the ears (tinnitus) been present?   Yes   No

5. Have TMJ (temporal mandibular joint) problems been a concern of yours?   Yes   No

6. Have you had unusual shakiness (tremors) of your hands or arms or twitching of other muscles?   Yes   No

7. Do you have "brown spots" or "age spots" under your eyes or elsewhere in the skin of your body?   Yes   No

8. Have you tended to have more colds, flu, and other examples of infectious diseases than "normal"?   Yes   No

9. Have you had food allergies or intolerances?   Yes   No

10. Have you been to many doctors for your health problems? And have they usually said, "There is nothing wrong"?   Yes   No

11. Do you feel numbness or burning sensations in your mouth or gums?   Yes   No

12. Do you feel numbness or unexplained tingling in your arms or legs?   Yes   No

13. Have you developed difficulty in walking (ataxia) over the years?   Yes   No

14. Do you have ten or more "silver" dental fillings?   Yes   No

15. Do you often have a "metallic" taste in your mouth?   Yes   No

16. Have you ever worked as a painter or in manufacturing/chemical or pesticide/fungicide factories (fungicides with methyl mercury ingredients) or in pulp/paper mills that used mercury?   Yes   No

17. Have you worked as a dentist, hygienist, or dental assistant?   Yes   No

18. Have you ever had Candida-Related Complex (CRC) or yeast infections (vagina, mouth, or GI tract)?   Yes   No

19. Do you have a lot of bad breath (halitosis) or white tongue (thrush)?   Yes   No

20. Have you frequently had low basal body axillary temperature (below 97.4 degrees F) over the years?   Yes   No

21. Do you experience problems with constipation?   Yes   No

22. Do you have heart irregularities or rapid pulse (tachycardia)?   Yes   No

23. Do you have unexplained arthritis in various joints?   Yes   No

24. Is it common for you to see a lot of mucus in your stools?   Yes   No

25. Do you have unidentified chest pains even after ECG's, X-ray, and heart studies are normal?   Yes   No

26. Is your sleep poor or do you have frequent insomnia?	Yes	No
27. Have you had frequent kidney infections or do you experience significant kidney problems?	Yes	No
28. Are you extremely fatigued much of the time and never seem to have enough energy?	Yes	No
29. Do you have irritability or dramatic changes in behavior?	Yes	No
30. Are you on antidepressants now or have you been in the past?	Yes	No

Source: K. W. Sehnert, G. Jacobson, and K. Sullivan, "Is Mercury Toxicity an Autoimmune Disorder?" *Townsend Letter for Doctors and Patients* (October 1995): 134–37.

Drs. Sehnert, Jacobson, and Sullivan have come to the conclusion that mercury toxicity brings on autoimmune disorders, as discussed in an article written by Dr. Sehnert and published in *Advance* magazine.[1] The wide range of symptoms created by mercury toxicity from "silver" dental amalgam fillings can only be accounted for by multiple adverse effects on a person's immune system, nerve tissue, and connective tissue in general. Chronic fatigue and immune dysfunction syndrome (CFIDS) is the main generalized manifestation of such autoimmune dysfunctioning.

Often accompanying CFIDS is fibromyalgia, a myofascial pain syndrome, or fibromyositis. It consists of a group of common nonarticular rheumatic disorders characterized by achy pain, tenderness, and stiffness of the muscles, fibrous tissues, tendons, ligaments, and other "white" connective tissues. It hits especially in the areas of tendon insertions, and in adjacent soft-tissue structures. These painful fibromyalgic sensations may be the individual's primary generalized

---

1   K. W. Sehnert, "Autoimmune Disorders," *Advance* (January 1995): 47, 48.

problem or be concomitant with another associated or underlying condition such as CFIDS.[1]

Canada and Germany Act against Amalgam Fillings

Both syndromes, CFIDS and myofascial pain, are associated with amalgam-filled teeth. Canada has become aware of the amalgam controversy and its tie-in to chronic fatigue syndrome and fibromyalgia. In late January of 1994, therefore, the Ontario government demanded a probe of mercury dental fillings. Ontario Health Minister Ruth Grier asked Health and Welfare Canada to investigate the safety of mercury tooth fillings and restrict their use, if warranted. Minister Grier warned that if allegations are correct and that Canada's dental profession is ignoring the fillings' potential health hazards, the health of many citizens could be at risk.

These allegations had been made by informed medical researchers, dentists, and citizen groups opposed to the amalgam fillings. Today, the controversy remains unresolved in Canada. Although much research has been conducted at Canadian universities, government bureaucrats are still debating the issues. Meanwhile, mercury intoxication from dental amalgam continues to make the citizenry sick.

The government of Germany has acted more responsibly. In 1987 Germany's Federal Department of Health (BGA) issued an advisory warning against the use of "silver" dental amalgam in pregnant women. On February 2, 1992, following an extraordinary congress or conference on dental amalgam sponsored by the International Academy of Oral Medicine and Toxicology (IAOMT), the BGA banned the manufacture and sale of low-copper conventional amalgam. Shortly thereafter, the BGA issued a document further restricting the use of amalgam, including the high-copper, non-gamma-2-amalgam. Thus, dental amalgam materials are no longer allowed to be implanted into the mouths of Germans in their country.

---

1   M. Walker, *Nature's Antibiotic: Olive Leaf Extract* (New York: Kensington Publishing Corporation, 1997), 85, 86.

Amalgam Scrap Is a Hazardous Waste

Considering that the United States regards amalgam materials removed from patients' mouths as a hazardous waste, why does our government allow it to be implanted into people in the first place?

The Council on Dental Materials, Instruments, and Equipment of the American Dental Association warns its members through the *Journal of the American Dental Association* (JADA): "All amalgam scraps should be salvaged and stored in a tightly closed container.... The scrap should be covered by a sulfide solution such as X-ray or photographic fixer solution."[1]

"Dental amalgam is classified as a hazardous material by the Office of Safety and Health Administration," reports the *ADA News*.[2]

The Garfield Refining Company of Philadelphia, Pennsylvania, an EPA-approved treatment storage processing facility, warns dentists not to handle this amalgam scrap. In one year, an average dentist produces a pound of scrap metals left over from filling cavities and forming replacement teeth and bridges, advises Donald Farley, D.D.S., a dentist practicing in Springfield, Massachusetts, and former president of the Valley District Dental Society. The incorrect disposal of these wastes could bring heavy penalties levied on dentists by the EPA in the form of fines.[3]

As it happens, Dr. Farley's newspaper remarks relate to a Connecticut salvage operation in which dentists sold scrap amalgam taken out of their patients' mouths to the Northeast Chemical Corporation during the years between 1969 and 1984. The EPA cleanup that resulted from the chemical company's mishandling of this scrap cost American taxpayers $450,000. The "Superfund" law, meaning the Comprehensive Environmental Response Compensation and Liability

---

1   "Recommendations in Dental Mercury Hygiene," *Journal of the American Dental Association* 109 (1984): 617–19.

2   "OSHA to Begin Enforcing 'Hazard' Rule," *ADA News*, 1 August 1988, 1.

3   "Sales of Dental Waste Could Bring Penalties," *Bridgeport Sunday Post*, 27 September 1987, A17.

Act (CERCLA) came into play, and the dentists were prosecuted under the CERCLA.

This Superfund law governing the disposal of hazardous substances defines four classes of parties liable for disposal, advises attorney Jeremy Firestone of EPA's Boston office. These parties include (1) those who own the dumping site at the time the hazardous material is deposited on it, (2) the current owners, (3) those who transport the material, and (4) those who arrange for its disposal or treatment. Some sixty dentists in Massachusetts and Connecticut were classified under the fourth category, and they were penalized.

The contaminated dental amalgam material was discovered by children exploring a dump site with their metal detector. The Connecticut Department of Environmental Protection informed EPA, which has removed contaminated topsoil from 19,000 square feet of ground since 1984. People were poisoned during the fifteen years the amalgam lay on the ground at the dump site. Some Connecticut residents probably died but nobody had traced their deaths to the old filling materials taken from people's teeth.[1]

---

[1] "EPA, Dentists Settle in Mercury Cleanup Case," *ADA News*, 1988, 1.

Six

Devastating Diseases Derived from Dentist-Implanted Mercury Amalgams

In 1959 nineteen-year-old Murlene Brake began suffering from diarrhea each month at the onset of her menses.[1] The episodes of diarrhea gradually worsened so that by 1984 Mrs. Brake was experiencing loose and explosive bowel movements up to twenty times daily for twenty-five days out of every month. Today it is known that her devastating gastrointestinal pathology derived from dentist-implanted "silver" mercury amalgam dental fillings, but the woman went through a terribly hellish experience until she learned the correct reason for her condition.

In 1980 Mrs. Brake was misdiagnosed for the first time as being affected by *Crohn's disease*, a long-term swelling bowel disorder of unknown cause, which most often affects the lower part of the small intestine (the ileum), the main part of the large intestine (the colon), or both structures. Crohn's disease is marked by frequent attacks of diarrhea, severe stomach pain, nausea, fever, chills, weakness, depression, appetite loss, and weight loss. Murlene Brake had all of these symptoms and more. Usually the diagnosis is based on the patient's clinical history, X-ray studies, and a special test (an endoscopy). Crohn's disease may easily be confused with ulcerative colitis and is alternatively called *regional enteritis*.

---

1   Murelene Brake's is a true, public domain identity. Her health history has previously been published in her organization's newsletter.

Later, the same physician decided Mrs. Brake was showing inconsistencies with symptoms and signs , and put her through a number of uncomfortable clinical examinations and laboratory tests. At their conclusion, he changed his diagnosis to *irritable bowel disease* (IBD). But IBD is not a true clinical entity, unless it's the misnomer for *mucous colitis*, also known as *spastic colon*.[1]

She lived with this incorrect label for a while. Then, having moved to New Mexico, the unlucky woman found other physicians who took more tests. Then she was rediagnosed as experiencing *irritable bowel syndrome* (IBS). That doctor also suspected she had an unidentified respiratory illness, *multiple sclerosis* (MS), and *spasmodic torticollis*.

Irritable bowel syndrome involves abnormally increased motility of the small and large intestines, often found with emotional stress. Victims complain of diarrhea and, sometimes, pain in the lower abdomen, often stopped by moving the bowels. But there is no organic disease in irritable bowel syndrome, and no specific treatment except for the use of bulk-producing agents in the diet.

"I had such severe adverse reactions to medications usually prescribed for Crohn's disease, IBD, and IBS that eventually I was forced to accept my condition without the aid of any medication," explained Mrs. Brake.

As for her other misdiagnoses, MS is characterized by loss of the protective myelin covering of the nerve fibers of the brain and spinal cord. The first signs are numbness, or abnormal sensations in the arms and legs, muscle weakness, dizziness, and sight disturbances. Mrs. Brake was experiencing all of these symptoms as well. The loss of muscle control in multiple sclerosis may cause difficulty with urinating and bowel movements.

Unrelated to diarrhea, spasmodic torticollis is marked by attacks of spasms of the neck muscles, which last briefly and have no known physical cause.

Obviously, Murlene Brake was an exceedingly unfortunate woman. Physicians guessed at her condition but all her symptoms

---

1   J. F. Balch and M. Walker, *Heartburn and What to Do about It* (Garden City Park, N.Y.: Avery Publishing Group, 1998), 40, 41.

tied in to the potential of mercury poisoning. Mercury toxicity turned out to be her health problem all right, but it went unrecognized to that point. So, for nearly a decade, the question remained unanswered: What was the cause of this woman's health difficulties? Nobody knew; her doctors made more guesses.

"I was told that stress was a causal factor, but after taking an in-depth look at my life, I came to the conclusion that the only stress I had was the very real fear of 'soiling' myself in public," Mrs. Brake told me during our interview.

Murlene Brake Goes through a Living Hell

"My condition became so bad that I had to abandon my career. The adverse impact on my life was terrible! I could not travel. I was afraid to accept dinner invitations. I left many a filled grocery basket in the supermarket aisle and ran home to clean up. In general, my life was 'in the toilet' [pun intended]. And, I was plagued with bouts of extreme fatigue, heart palpitations, esophageal spasms, kidney infections, respiratory infections, flu, colds, sinusitis, and hay fever," she said. "I had allergies, subnormal body temperature, laryngitis, weak leg muscles, muscle spasms, aches and pains that came and went, short-term memory loss, mental confusion, and a body that would not cooperate with my brain.

"Then depression reared its ugly head. I felt guilty all the time. My limitations kept my husband and me from enjoying life and doing almost everything. I was afraid that my condition would eventually drive my husband away. I couldn't stand to live with me—how could he?" Murlene Brake wondered aloud. "But in 1984, my daughter listened to TV news about a small Maryland community totally sick from mercury contaminating its water supply. The townspeople's symptoms were just like mine, but this community regained its health when the contaminated water cleared.

"So I acquired information about mercury poisoning from several U.S. governmental agencies, and learned that every sign and symptom I had been suffering from was on the list of mercury toxicity. That's when I asked myself, how was I being exposed to mercury?"

The Patient's Mercury-Free Dentist
Returns Her to Health

In Albuquerque the patient consulted a dentist for the first time to have her teeth cleaned. As it happens, Bill Wolfe, D.D.S., whose office Mrs. Brake visited, is a biocompatible (mercury-free) dentist who educates his patients. Dr. Wolfe advised her that she had twelve silver amalgam fillings implanted, and the letter he routinely gives to patients explains that amalgams contain 50 percent mercury by weight. Mrs. Brake underwent a "eureka experience!"

"I made an appointment with my gastroenterologist to discuss the possibility of mercury toxicity from my amalgam fillings. When I introduced the subject, he became annoyed, got up and walked out on me, saying, 'That dentist is just trying to get your money.' So there I was left—no one to discuss mercury with, virtually hopeless," the woman said. "Later, after discussions with my husband, I decided that all I had to lose was money if the procedure didn't work, but maybe amalgam removal would be the answer to my many illnesses.

"The last amalgam came out on December 6, 1985. All of my symptoms stopped immediately. During the next two years, my strength gradually returned so that I became healthy once again. Most of my adult life I had been ill, so it took me a while emotionally to recognize that I was not sick anymore. Now, in 1999, I am healthier and more active than I was in my twenties," said the patient. "My quality of life is excellent and the only physical limitations I am experiencing comes from a cavitation [see chapter 13], soon to be corrected. Truthfully I can say that over 90 percent of my life-long health problems have been caused by bad dental work."

Mrs. Murlene Brake is a founder of Dental Amalgam Mercury Survivors (DAMS), Inc., the international organization that represents victims of the dental amalgam mercury syndrome. She became its first two-term president, and is the current newsletter editor. For referrals to mercury-free dentists, newsletters, and a great deal of other information on issues in dentistry, please see appendix A for the location listing of DAMS, Inc.

To help those seeking information concerning the whole issue of "silver" dental amalgam/mercury, DAMS, Inc. was formed in the mid-1990s by a group of people affected by mercury amalgam toxicity. Almost all DAMS members have been made physically ill from poisoning by dental amalgams. Their organization is interconnected with several other groups that are counteracting fraudulent practices by organized dentistry. For instance, a notice in the *International DAMS Newsletter* advises:

> Dentist-injured patients who cannot find legal redress or proper dental corrections should contact the American Association of Dental Victims (AADV), 3320 East 7th Street, Long Beach, California 90804, or an Arizona chapter, The American Association of Dental Victims at Post Office Box 42051, Tucson, Arizona 85733. These two AADV chapters offer legal assistance in bringing malpractice claims against dentists who use amalgam restorations.

"People everywhere are suffering every day from the insidious, ever progressing health problems that, like mine, are caused by the unscientific dental practices of yesterday and today. How much longer will the public stay unaware of the devastation that can be laid directly at the feet of dentistry? And how much longer will the public tolerate 'the art of dentistry' rather than insist instead on 'science in dentistry'?" asks Murlene Brake.

Most of Mrs. Brake's story was taken from her own published report in the quarterly newsletter that she produces. The *International DAMS Newsletter* affirms to its readers: "The hidden progress of mercury toxicity is not often revealed until significant pathology has occurred."[1] Such pathology not uncommonly can end for amalgam-implanted patients in devastating diseases and possibly in death, such as for those who develop cancer, peripheral neuropathies, amyotrophic lateral sclerosis (Lou Gehrig's disease), multiple sclerosis, Parkinson's disease, and Alzheimer's disease.

---

1 M. Brake, "Insidious Progression," *International DAMS Newsletter* 4, no. 2 (Spring 1994): 8, 9.

Alzheimer's Disease Arising from Dental Amalgam Fillings

Boyd E. Haley, Ph.D., a professor of medicinal chemistry and biochemistry, provided me with irrefutable written proof that Alzheimer's disease (AD) arises from the mercury escaping out of dental amalgam fillings. Data Dr. Haley submitted in his as yet unpublished paper show that orally placed amalgams are a main source of mercury toxicity. Dr. Haley is chief of the Division of Medicinal Chemistry and Pharmaceutics at the University of Kentucky Medical Center in Lexington, Kentucky.

"Mercury must be considered as a contributor to the condition classified as AD. This is especially true when mercury is present in combination with other heavy metals such as zinc, cadmium, and lead," wrote Dr. Haley. "Mercury is much more toxic to individuals with other heavy metal exposures. As I have been sent numerous laboratory reports [for evaluation] on levels of elements in the hair and other tissues of suspected mercury toxic patients, I have noticed that many show exceedingly high levels of lead, cadmium, copper, zinc, etc. It is my opinion that the major questions left to be answered concerning the toxic effects of mercury is 'does the combination of mercury with various heavy metals lead to different clinical observations of toxicity?'

[Note: Chapter 11 discusses the cases of industrial workers who are exposed to lead or cadmium and who also carry amalgam fillings in their teeth, and are most predictably going to get Alzheimer's disease.]

"There can be little doubt that the elevated levels of other heavy metals increases the toxicity of mercury. Further, the reaction of oral mercury from amalgams and the reaction of this mercury with toxic thiols produced by periodontal disease bacteria very likely enhances the toxicity of the mercury being released. This makes any claim regarding the determination of safe levels of mercury as obtained under controlled [laboratory] conditions (for example, in a system where other heavy metals are excluded) very suspect when discussing toxic mercury effects in the uncontrolled environment that humans are exposed to," Dr. Haley concluded.[1]

---

1   B. Haley, "Results from the Boyd Haley Laboratory Relating the Toxic Effects of Mercury to Exacerbation of the Medical Condition Classified as Alzheimer's

This professor of medicinal chemistry studied mercury as an inhibitor of tubulin, a protein found in every brain and body cell. In nerve cells, tubulin is an element of the microtubules, described by one group of scientists as "neuronal railroad tracks, transporting molecules between the cell body and nerve terminals."[1] AD brains cannot use tubulin to make microtubules, because mercury creates this defect in neurons. Thus, the characteristic symptoms of Alzheimer's disease develops.[2] Such AD symptoms invariably become duplicated in those people poisoned by mercury.[3]

Amalgam, invented in England and perfected in France around 1820, became widely used throughout Europe and North America by approximately 1850.[4] That's when Parkinson's disease, multiple sclerosis, and amyotrophic lateral sclerosis were first described in the medical journals. In 1906 the German psychiatrist Alois Alzheimer, M.D., announced his finding of a "strange disease of the cerebral

Disease," personal communication, 9 June 1998.

1 K. Iqbal and others, "Defective Brain Microtubule Assembly in Alzheimer's Disease," *Lancet* (1968): 421–26, cited in J. C. Pendergrass and B. E. Haley, "Mercury-EDTA Complex Specifically Blocks Brain Tubulin-GTP Interactions: Similarity to Pathology Observed in Alzheimer's Disease," International Amalgam Symposium, Otzenhousen, Germany, 29 April to 1 May 1994.

2 S. Khatoon and others, "Aberrant Guanosine Triphosphate-Beta-Tubulin Interaction in Alzheimer's Disease," *Annuals of Neurology* 26 (1989): 210–15; E. F. Duhr and others, "HgEDTA Complex Inhibits GTP Interactions with the E-Site of Brain Beta-Tubulin," *Toxicology and Applied Pharmacology* 122 (1993): 273–80; J. C. Pendergrass and others, "Mercury Vapor Inhalation Inhibits Binding of GTP to Tubulin in Rat Brain: Similarity to Molecular Lesion in Alzheimer's Diseased Brain," *Neuro Toxicology* (January/February 1997).

3 P. A. Neal and R. R. Jones, "Chronic Mercurialism in the Hatters' Fur-Cutting Industry," *Journal of the American Medical Association* 110 (1938): 337–43; I. I. Maghazahi, "Psychiatric Aspects of Methylmercury Poisoning," *Journal of Neurology, Neurosurgery, Psychiatry* 37 (1974): 954–58; R. L. Siblerud, J. Motl, and E. Kienholts, "Psychometric Evidence That Mercury from Silver Dental Fillings May Be an Etiological Factor in Depression, Excessive Anger, and Anxiety," *Psychological Reports* 74 (1994): 67–80; G. E. Fagala and C. L. Wigg, "Psychiatric Manifestations of Mercury Poisoning," *Journal of American Academy of Child and Adolescent Psychiatry* 31 (1992): 306-11.

4 K. O. Frykholm, "Mercury from Dental Amalgam: Its Toxic and Allergic Effects," *Acta Odontal Scand.* 15 (Supplement 22): 9, 10; J. R. Mackert, "Dental Amalgam and Mercury," *Journal of the American Dental Association* 122 (1991): 54–61.

cortex" in which an autopsy of his demented patient's brain revealed numbers of plaques and tangles that eventually were to be considered the defining symptoms of AD.[1]

Now, as depicted in my book, *Toxic Metal Syndrome: How Metal Poisonings Can Affect Your Brain*, the signs and symptoms of Alzheimer's disease are making their appearance more frequently than ever before in the form of a mercury amalgam syndrome.[2] The typical American adult of today carries ten amalgams in his or her mouth. These weigh a total of about ten grams,[3] of which often more than five grams is mercury. (Note: the Silmet U.S.A. Corporation of Miami, Florida, which manufactures dentistry's most popular amalgam, *Nogama 2*, advertises that its branded amalgam product offers an average mercury to alloy ratio of 1:1.1, or 52 percent of mercury.)[4] Canadians carry a near-equivalent mercury content in their teeth. For instance, the average Canadian over eighteen years of age had a mouth filled with 9.05 dental amalgams during the years 1985 and 1986.[5]

The Pathology of Alzheimer's Disease Involving Mercury

Alzheimer's disease (AD) being an inflammatory disease brought about by the body's reaction to an infection or environmental insult, "fits the paradigm of the idiopathic rheumatic disorders," my coauthor and I wrote. "An unknown set of circumstances results in an initial insult triggering an inflammatory reaction in the brain.

---

1   B. Bogerts, "Image in Psychiatry," *American Journal of Psychiatry* 150 (1993): 12.

2   H. R. Casdorph and M. Walker, *Toxic Metal Syndrome: How Metal Poisonings Can Affect Your Brain* (Garden City Park, N.Y.: Avery Publishing Group, 1995).

3   G. M. Richardson, *Assessment of Mercury Exposure and Risks from Dental Amalgam* (Ottowa, Ontario, Canada: Medical Devices Bureau, Environmental Health Directorate, Health Canada, 18 August 1995).

4   "Nogama 2," product brochure, Silmet, Ltd., 18968 Northeast 4th Court, Miami, Florida 33179; (800) 228-4390.

5   Richardson, *Assessment of Mercury Exposure.*

The inflammation becomes self-propagating, or it continues because the obscure inciting factors persist." The scientists argue that the acute phase response augments production of beta-amyloid, the protein found among the plaques in AD brains. They conclude that "cytokines, acute phase proteins, activated microglia, and complement," all mechanisms that are triggered by the acute phase response of the immune system, are involved with AD, either as causes or consequences.[1] Mercury derived from amalgams is one of those "obscure inciting factors" that triggers the inflammatory response.

During an interview, Dr. Haley disputed my assertion that beta-amyloid is responsible for the Alzheimer's disease pathology. Rather, Dr. Haley pointed to a blood protein called *apolipoprotein E type-four* (apoE4) as the source of AD pathology. Ordinarily the apolipoproteins transport cholesterol out of the brain as one of their main functions. Backing up Dr. Haley, Duke University researchers have confirmed that people possessing two apoE4 genes have eight times the risk of developing late-onset Alzheimer's disease as those with two apoE3 genes. Moreover, those fortunate folk carrying two apoE2 genes have an even lower to nonexistent risk of coming down with AD.[2]

Dr. Haley advises that apoE4 is unable to transport mercury out of the brain at the same time it is carrying cholesterol; consequently, mercury lingers there, creating its neuronal damage. ApoE3 is moderately effective at moving mercury out of the brain. ApoE2 is highly effective at carrying mercury from the brain and dropping it into the physiology's waste disposal system. That's because apoE2 contains two cysteine amino acids; in apoE3 one of its cysteines has replaced arginine; and with apoE4 both cysteines have arginine substitutes. Because arginine contains no sulphur, it cannot bind mercury, which

1   P. S. Aisen and K. L. Davis, "Inflammatory Mechanisms in Alzheimer's Disease: Implications for Therapy," *American Journal of Psychiatry* 151 (1994): 1105–13.

2   E. H. Corder and others, "Protective Effect of Apolipoprotein E Type 2 Allele for Late-Onset Alzheimer's Disease," *Natural Genetics* 7 (1994): 180–84; A. T. Talbot and others, "Protection against Alzheimer's Disease with ApoE2," *Lancet* 343 (1994): 1432–33; P. Cotton, "Constellation of Risks and Processes Seen in Search for Alzheimer's Clues," *Journal of the American Medical Association* 271 (1994): 89–91.

has a high affinity for sulphur. Since cysteine does contain sulphur, apoE2 protein pulls out mercury from the brain but apoE4 protein and apoE3 protein are ineffective or less effective, respectively, in removal of brain-Hg.[1]

Dr. Haley's hypothesis is that mercury builds up more rapidly in the brains of people with the apoE4 gene; rising levels of brain mercury eventually cause the destruction of microtubules, which leads to neuron death; ever-rising mercury levels trigger an inflammatory response that accompanies brain cell death. Yet AD afflicts some who don't carry the apoE4 gene, signifying that an intolerable level of mercury can build up in people possessing amalgams regardless of their apoE status. This intolerable level may be reached with a reduced ability for the person to cope with mercury for the following five reasons:

1. An elevated exposure to high levels of mercury—more than the average number of mercury amalgam fillings

2. Pollution from other metallic toxins such as aluminum, cadmium, lead, arsenic, iron, manganese, nickel, and so forth

3. The contamination from chemical stressors like pesticides, herbicides, petroleum products, and so forth

4. Genes other than those controlling apoE status

5. Some combination of all these conditions

Kip Sullivan, of Minneapolis, Minnesota, the attorney I had cited in the last chapter as providing information for the Mercury/Toxic Metal Sensitivity Questionnaire shown in table 5-1, went on to furnish a literature review on "The Evidence Linking Silver-Mercury Fillings to Alzheimer's Disease." Attorney (Dr.) Sullivan's article gives an excellent overview of the dental component in dementia production among those poisoned by mercury leaching from their "silver" dental amalgams.[2]

---

1   Haley, "Results from the Boyd Haley Laboratory."

2   K. Sullivan, "The Evidence Linking Silver-Mercury Fillings to Alzheimer's Disease: A Literature Review," *Townsend Letter for Doctors and Patients*

The Amalgam Link to Amyotrophic Lateral Sclerosis

Evidence implicating amalgam mercury as a cause of amyotropic lateral sclerosis (ALS), known by the public as Lou Gehrig's disease, is documented in more magazine and clinical journal articles offering anecdotes than articles citing clinical or laboratory studies. Still, the published reports are compelling reading and stimulate an informed person to avoid dental amalgams, if for no other reason than their linkage to ALS.

In 1869 the original description of ALS appeared in the medical literature, and it showed a linkage to elevated mercury accumulating in the blood.[1]

Thereafter at least five articles were published describing the appearance of ALS symptoms in people after they were exposed to organic mercury and mercury vapor. For some of these victims described in the articles, the symptoms ceased when amalgam fillings were removed.[2]

1954 was the year that attention was most closely drawn to ALS, by an article describing a thirty-nine-year-old farmer who absorbed organic mercury from a fungicide he used on oat plants.[3]

Another report discussed ALS symptoms that started in eleven Iranians who ingested bread made from wheat treated with a fungicide containing ethyl mercury.[4]

169/170 (August/September 1997): 74–83.

1   M. T. Felmus, B. M. Patten, and L. Swanke, "Antecedent Events in Amyotrophic Lateral Sclerosis," Neurology 26 (1976): 167–72.

2   L. P. Rowland, "Amyotrophic Lateral Sclerosis and Autoimmunity," New England Journal of Medicine 327 (1992): 1752–53.

3   I. A. Brown, "Chronic Mercurialism: A Cause of the Clinical Syndrome of Amyotrophic Lateral Sclerosis," Archives of Neurology and Psychiatry 72 (1954): 674–81, cited in J. D. Mitchell, "Heavy Metals and Trace Elements in Amyotrophic Lateral Sclerosis," Neurologic Clinics 5 (1987): 43–60.

4   A. D. Kantargian, "A Syndrome Clinically Resembling Amyotrophic Lateral Sclerosis Following Chronic Mercurialism," Neurology 11 (1961): 639–44.

Then there were two men coming down with ALS following their exposure to mercuric oxide and mercury vapor in a factory that manufactured mercuric oxide.[1]

Another published piece told of a male patient (a hobo) who developed ALS three-and-a-half months after he had spent two days gathering liquid mercury from old thermometers.[2]

A 1994 article coauthored by Jaro Pleva described the recovery from ALS by a twenty-nine-year-old Swedish woman. The neurology department at the University Hospital in Umea, Sweden, made the diagnosis originally. Then, this same department pronounced her free of ALS in August 1984, five months after her amalgam fillings were removed. Nine years later the woman was still free of ALS symptoms.[3]

Mercury was implicated in studies examining health histories of groups of people diagnosed with ALS. In one such group of ALS patients, it was found that they were exposed to mercury and lead; but for another group not so exposed no such ALS pathology developed.[4]

At the University of Kentucky medical investigators found that seven deceased ALS victims showed more mercury in their brains, upon autopsy, than did nine deceased controls who did not have ALS. Also, the blood cells of forty living ALS patients contained more mercury than the blood cells taken from thirty-one living control patients.[5]

---

1   T. E. Barber, "Inorganic Mercury Intoxication Reminiscent of Amyotrophic Lateral Sclerosis," *Journal of Occupational Medicine* 20 (1978): 667–69.

2   C. R. Adams, D. K. Ziegler, and J. T. Lin, "Mercury Intoxification Simulating Amyotrophic Lateral Sclerosis," *Journal of American Medical Association* 250 (1983): 642–43.

3   R. Redhe and J. Pleva, "Recovery from Amyotrophic Lateral Sclerosis and from Allergy after Removal of Dental Amalgam Fillings," *International Journal of Risk Safety Medicine* 4 (1994): 229–36.

4   Felmus and others, "Antecedent Events."

5   S. S. Khare and others, "Trace Element Imbalances in Amyotrophic Lateral Sclerosis," *Neuro Toxicology* 11 (1990): 521–32.

Peripheral Neuropathies Affect Dentists Using Mercury Amalgams

"It is common knowledge within the health insurance industry that dentists have one of the highest utilization rates of medical insurance," reported medical claims reviewer, David Eddleston, M.D., in the *Newsletter of the Pacific Coast Society of Prosthodontists.* "The role of mercury has to be suspect, in light of the increased prevalence of polyneuropathies, which include tremors of muscles that perform fine-motor functions," amongst dentists.[1]

By definition, *polyneuropathies* is the general term denoting functional disturbances or pathological changes in the peripheral nervous system. In virtually all governmental publications, medical school textbooks, material safety data sheets, and research articles describing the effects of mercury poisoning, *tremors* is listed as one of numerous characteristic symptoms caused by chronic mercury exposure.

"Some 298 dentists had their mercury levels measured by an X-ray fluorescence technique to determine the relationship between cumulative exposure to mercury and chronic health impairment," wrote two clinical investigators. They discovered that "Electrodiagnostic and neuropsychological findings in the dentists with more than 20 mcg/g of tissue mercury levels were compared with those of a control group consisting of dentists with no detectable mercury levels. Among the high mercury dentists, 30 percent were affected by polyneuropathies; while no polyneuropathies were detected in the control group. Additionally, the high mercury group had mild visuographic dysfunction; they also had more symptom-distress than did the control group. These findings suggest that the use of mercury as a dental restorative material is a health risk for dentists."[2]

---

1   D. Eggleston, "Dental Amalgam—To Be or Not to Be," *Newsletter of the Pacific Coast Society of Prosthodontists* 9, no. 2 (1988): 4–10.

2   I. Shapiro and others, "Neurophysiological and Neuropsychological Function in Mercury-Exposed Dentists," *Lancet* (1982): 1147–50; I. I. Shipp and I. Shapiro, "Mercury Poisoning in Dental Practice," *Compendium of Continuing Education* 4 (1983): 107–10.

The urinary mercury levels for 4,272 U.S. dentists who participated in the Health Assessment Programs at annual sessions of the American Dental Association during the years from 1975 to 1983 recorded a number of shocking findings. No matter how carefully they handle the metal, dentists themselves are being poisoned by methylmercury, mercury vapors, mercury particles, and other manipulative substances relating to this toxic material.

Although there is no safe or acceptable amount for mercury in the urine, 20 mcg per liter is considered to be on the high side of "normal." In studies conducted among participating dentists during the above recorded years of Health Assessment Programs[1]

- 19.1 percent were over the maximum "normal" level of mercury in urine;

- 10.9 percent were over the "maximum acceptable level" of 30 mcg of mercury per liter of urine, published by the Centers for Disease Control and Prevention (CDC);

- 4.9 percent were over 50 mcg of mercury per liter of urine, the level shown to induce potential tremors of the peripheral neuropathies;

- 1.3 percent recorded over 100 mcg of mercury per liter of urine, the level shown to bring on actual tremors.

Numerous situations and case studies have been published in the health professional journals that report on the personnel working in dentistry and industry who suffer from disease entities. The publications record high mercury measurements and associated polyneuropathies.[2]

---

1   C. Naleway and others, "Urinary Mercury Levels in U.S. Dentists 1975–1983: Review of Health Assessment," *Journal of the American Dental Association* 111 (1985): 37–42.

2   G. Macdonald, "Occupational Hazards in Dentistry," *Journal of the California Dental Association* 12 (1984): 17–19; P. Bloch and I. Shapiro, "Summary of the International Conference on Mercury Hazards in Dental Practice," *Journal of the American Dental Association* 104 (1982): 489–90; D. Mantyla and O. Wright, "Mercury Toxicity in the Dental Office: A Neglected Problem," *Journal of the American Dental Association* 92 (1976): 189– 94.

(Note: In the next chapter I will reveal the several motivations for dental professionals to ignore alarming sickness statistics at which they fixedly gaze but studiously disregard—even at the cost of their own safety and health.)

Assorted Disorders Caused by Mercury Amalgams

Gary A. Strong, D.D.S., of Billings, Montana, produced a short list of systemic pathologies from "silver" dental amalgam fillings. Dr. Strong, assisted by a variety of authoritative dental professional sources, offers the following number of assorted potential disorders caused by mercury amalgams:[1]

1. Tremors observed in fine voluntary muscle movements, such as in handwriting. The tremors eventually progress to convulsions

2. Inability to concentrate, including loss of memory

3. Sleep disorders with either insomnia or drowsiness

4. Gastrointestinal upset consisting of nausea and diarrhea

5. Loss of appetite

6. Birth defects in the newborn

7. Nephritis (symptomatic kidney disease)

8. Pneumonitis (lung inflammation)

9. Swollen neck glands and tongue

---

1   Council on Dental Materials, Instruments, and Equipment, "Recommendations on Dental Mercury Hygiene," *Journal of the American Dental Association* 109 (1984); 617–19; Council on Dental Materials, Instruments, and Equipment, "Mercury Hygiene Measures Recommended," *ADA News* (7 September 1981); ADA Mercury Testing Program, *Hg* (Chicago, Ill.: American Dental Association; no date), ADA pamphlet promoting in-office urine mercury testing program; P. Gronka and others, "Mercury Vapor Exposures in Dental Offices," *American Dental Association* 81 (1970): 923–25.

10. Ulceration of the oral mucosa

11. Dark pigmentation of the marginal gingiva

12. Loosening of the teeth

Our anonymous source, the wary New York dentist, confirms Dr. Strong's information. Then he cites a reference from the *Journal of the American Dental Association* that backs up his confirmation. This dentist, who feels uneasy with his ADA colleagues, states, "Amalgam fillings contain medically significant quantities of mercury. Published research has proven that the metal is not locked into the fillings, as some dentists erroneously claim. Dental mercury has been traced from the filling into the body tissues, including the brain, where it builds up over time. Brain and other nerve tissues are a key target for mercury toxicity, and human autopsy studies have demonstrated a direct correlation between the amount of mercury in brain tissue and the number of amalgam fillings present in teeth. My own professional society's literature says this.

"What can be done about the problem?" he asks. "Any new filling that you have placed in your mouth should not be mercury. If your dentist is insistent about putting mercury fillings in, find a new dentist. However, getting your amalgam fillings removed doesn't mean that any illness you have will be corrected. I don't tell people that they must have their amalgams removed. When asked, I do tell them, 'If I had any mercury in my mouth, I'd have it replaced immediately.' While, as a dentist, I cannot make statements about people's health regarding mercury, I will say that I have been removing mercury fillings for over fifteen years, and the health improvements I have seen in people have just been astonishing."

Seven

Documentation of Systemic Diseases Derived from Dental Amalgam Fillings

On August 14, 1992, retired California businessman William H. Tolhurst became the plaintiff in five separate legal actions he brought against particular supporters of dental amalgam filling material. Tolhurst sued those champions of amalgam he alleged caused him harm. The five defendants in the Superior Court of the State of California were

1. the American Dental Association (ADA), recognized as the authoritative health professional organization forcefully advocating installation of "silver" dental amalgams into people's decayed teeth;

2. Johnson & Johnson Consumer Products, Inc., manufacturers of amalgam formulations;

3. Englehard Corporation, packagers and wholesalers of advanced dispersion amalgam systems;

4. ABE Dental, Inc., distributors of amalgam supplies to dentists;

5. the plaintiff's former dentist, Thomas Fitzgerald, D.D.S., who had implanted amalgams into the man's teeth from which he experienced disease symptoms.

William Tolhurst charged that the defendants caused him personal injuries resulting from mercury toxicity through exposure to his mercury amalgam fillings. His first cause of action was for strict products liability against the dentist and various manufacturers. The second and third causes of action were against the same defendants for breach of warranty and negligence, respectively. The fifth cause of action was leveled only against the defendant dentist for negligence in dental treatment.

Most significant was the fourth cause of action, which was brought solely against the ADA. Mr. Tolhurst's complaint alleged that the American Dental Association was negligent in informing or failing to inform the public about the alleged dangers of mercury-containing amalgams. He pointed to the ADA as being liable for injuries to the public caused by products used by its members. He asked the court to formulate a new law that could impose liability on the ADA for every dental-related injury suffered by any person in the United States.

In a demurrer filed by attorney Robert S. Luft, the defendant responded, saying: "The ADA owes no legal duty of care to protect the public from allegedly dangerous products used by dentists. The ADA did not manufacture, design, supply, or install the mercury-containing amalgams. The ADA does not control those who do. The ADA's only alleged involvement in the product [amalgam] was to provide information regarding its use. Dissemination of information relating to the practice of dentistry does not create a duty of care to protect the public from potential injury."

Ruling on the demurrer, Judge Read Ambler dismissed the ADA from the case. William H. Tolhurst lost his legal action, and the American Dental Association bailed out on dental amalgam, leaving the product manufacturers, the distributors, all state boards of dental examiners, and all ADA and non-ADA dentists-users-members hanging.[1]

If you interpret the judge's decision, you will realize: the ADA, a dental trade union, escaped home free, but all American dentists who use the amalgam information disseminated by that union remain on the hook for damages they are doing to their patients by restoring teeth with mercury amalgam.

1   *W. H. Tolhurst v. Johnson & Johnson Consumer Products, Inc.; Engelhard Corp.; ABE Dental, Inc.; The American Dental Association, et. al.*, Calif. Superior Court, County of Santa Clara, Case No. 718228.

Potential Class Action Suits against Dentists and the ADA

The precedent-setting court decision had some chilling effects on the codefendants and all of dentistry. For instance, as a result of the ADA being let out of the case, Johnson & Johnson Consumer Products, Inc. discontinued manufacturing amalgam, and dentists must now turn for their metallic filling supplies to other sources such as Kerr Chemicals, Inc., Caulk Dentsply, and Silmet, Ltd.

Amalgam-using dentists who may give attention to their trade union's activities were unhappy about the ADA's setting them adrift, but the member-dentists continue to follow organized dentistry's party line. Such nonsensical thinking prevails today in the face of ever increasing scientific documentation casting doubt on the safety of dental amalgam. The only defense for its use has been the unwavering support of organized dentistry's mainstream members, and such support has functioned rather like a child's security blanket, offering assurance of protection that doesn't really exist.

The lawsuit revealed that the dentists' professional association washes its hands of legal responsibility for the potential adverse effects from its members' use of dental amalgam. Tolhurst offered as evidence that the ADA, in a February 19, 1985, letter from its executive director, J. M. Coady, D.D.S., had issued formal notification that , as a voluntary professional organization (a trade union), it has no legal authority to regulate the use of any dental materials. The ADA admitted then and accepts now that there is no scientific documentation establishing the safety of dental amalgam. It became apparent during Tolhurst's lawsuit that the defense of amalgam's safety is based only on the fact that it has been used for something like 160 years.[1]

The false hope by organized dentistry that use of dental amalgam can be defended on the basis of being a legally approved dental device, accepted and classified by the U.S. FDA, is delusional. Such acceptance and classification does not exist. Just like the big tobacco companies

---

1   ADA, Division of Scientific Affairs, "When Your Patients Ask about Mercury in Amalgam," *Journal of the American Dental Association* 120 (1990): 395–98.

and Dow Corning Corporation, manufacturer of silicone breast implants, the ADA and its members apparently are teetering at the edge of class-action suits as well.

On July 8, 1998, Dow Corning Corporation reached a payout settlement of $3.2 billion with tens of thousands of women who had brought upwards of 19,000 implant damage suits.

No doubt such legal actions eventually will be brought by eager attorneys leading groups of outraged consumers of dental care. Patients will likely want retribution for being implanted with toxic teeth by potentially death-dealing dentists. And these consumers will have a case that's probably bigger than any fought over silicone breast implants and cigarette smoking, combined. More consumers are wearing "silver" amalgam fillings in their teeth right now than ever have used silicone or tobacco.

Contrary to popular belief among dentists who mix and apply the mercurial compound, the FDA has *never* accepted and classified mixed dental amalgam. Instead, the FDA has accepted "dental mercury" and "amalgam alloy" individually as "safe and effective" dental devices—not mixed dental amalgam.[1]

In 1993, in a widely acknowledged Public Health Service (PHS) document on dental amalgam, the FDA admitted that it had never accepted and classified mixed dental amalgam.[2] And the ADA hasn't done so either.

Individually and as a group, the dentists seem unknowing about or disregarding of the fact that their own trade organization has refused to certify the safety of mixed dental amalgam. Still, these dentists persist in putting it into the mouths of their patients. Where is their conscience? What's happened to their ethics? Why do dental patients let them get away with it?

---

1   Food and Drug Administration, "Dental Devices: General Provisions and Classification of 110 Devices: Final Rule," *Federal Register* 52(155):30082-30106, 12 August 1987.

2   United States Public Health Service, "Dental Amalgam: A Scientific Review and Recommended Public Health Service Strategy for Research, Education, and Regulation," *Regulatory Work Report* (FDA) (Washington, D.C.: Committee to Coordinate Environmental Health and Related Programs, 1993), V1 2.

Self-Interest Conflicts of the FDA's/ADA's
Dr. John W. Stanford

The ADA certifies "dental mercury" and "amalgam alloy" separately, as I mentioned, not requiring biocompatibility testing for either product.[1] The fact that this mirrors the FDA position is no coincidence.

John W. Stanford, Ph.D., for two decades chairman of the FDA Dental Device Panel that recommended this single-certification policy for adoption by the FDA in 1980, was, at the same time, director of the ADA Council on Dental Materials, Instruments and Devices (CDMIE).[2]

During that period, Dr. Stanford wrote a letter stating that dental amalgam is a "reaction product" manufactured by the dentist in his or her office.[3] Therefore, while the dentists' trade union has not hesitated to certify other "reaction products," such as dental composites, cements, and impression materials, mixed dental amalgam cannot be certified by the ADA and is solely the responsibility of the individual attending dentist.

The FDA Dental Device Panel, under Dr. Stanford's chairmanship, also put nearly the same ADA wording on the record. Moreover, from the FDA's Office of Device Evaluation, Lillian Yin, Ph.D., director, Division of Ob-Gyn (obstetrics and gynecology), ENT (ear, nose, and throat), and Dental Devices, wrote such a letter too.[4]

If the ADA accepts no responsibility for the harm to human health that amalgam material causes, who does? The ADA's successful demurrer in the Tolhurst lawsuit says: "The ADA owes no legal duty

---

1   American Dental Association, ANSI/ADA Specification No. 1, "For Alloy for Dental Amalgam," 211 E. Chicago Avenue, Chicago, Illinois 60611; ANSI/ADA Specification No. 6, "For Dental Mercury," 211 E. Chicago Avenue, Chicago, Illinois 60611.

2   Food and Drug Administration, "Medical Device Classification Procedures," *Federal Register* 40(97):21848-21851, 19 May 1975.

3   ADA, letter from John W. Stanford, Ph.D., director, Council on Dental Materials, Instruments, and Equipment, 22 May 1986.

4   Food and Drug Administration, letter from Lillian Yin, Ph.D., director, Division of Ob-Gyn, ENT, and Dental Devices, Office of Device Evaluation, 1 April 1991.

of care to protect the public from allegedly dangerous products used by dentists." The court's ruling creates a couple of responsible parties: the practicing dentists themselves and the boards of dentistry of the states. Because of the state dental practice act in each state, this situation of responsibility has been established by law.

The consequence is that today amalgam-implanting dentists and their state boards of dental examiners are set to be the fall guys in any overall class action or individual legal action suits brought by patients who are showing immune suppression or autoimmune disease symptoms arising from their dental amalgams. Dr. Stanford's many years of FDA/ADA manipulations (certainly during the years 1975 to 1986) have kept his favorite ADA trade union out of the proverbial soup.

The conclusions are clear! If ever there is a legal liability for placing dental amalgam into humans, the practicing dentist and his or her state board of dentistry have been left holding the bag. No doubt financial payouts for legal defenses will be borne by the individual dentists sued. However, it will take state tax money to defend suits against state dental boards, so state residents will inevitably carry the burden. The potential for such lawsuits is compounded by the following:

The FDA has categorized mercury as a "drug" in its regulations for First Aid Materials. Since scientific documentation has clearly proven that mercury is released from *in vivo* (within a living organism) dental amalgam on a daily basis, and it does accumulate in human tissues over time, the placement of dental amalgam constitutes implantation of a time-released, highly poisonous drug into people. As a drug, mercury is more neurotoxic than lead, cadmium, or even arsenic.[1]

Being neurotoxic means that mercury escaping from dental amalgam fillings damages the dental patient's nerves. This neurotoxin is a poison that acts directly on the tissues of the central nervous system. Is it any wonder that there is potential for the development of

---

1   R. P. Sharma and E. J. Obersteiner, "Metals and Neurotoxic Effects," *Journal of Comparable Pathology* 91 (1981): 235–44.

Alzheimer's disease, multiple sclerosis, amyotrophic lateral sclerosis, or Parkinson's disease? Like the venom of certain snakes, amalgam mercury may move along the motor nerves to the brain. It is likely to be as poisonous as toxins made by certain bacteria or by the cell breakdown created by the botulism toxin of *Clostridium botulinum*.

Legal precedent has established that in any other medical circumstance, such implantation of a poison cannot be done without informed consent. When amalgam was placed into your teeth to turn them toxic, were you informed as to what it would do to your health? Did you give consent for such a sick effect? That's another possible issue to pursue in the courts.

Placement of Amalgam in the Mouth

You know that "silver" dental amalgam filling material usually contains not less than 50 percent mercury. As mentioned in chapter 6, the most popular brand of amalgam used in dentistry, the Nogama 2 Sabrablend from Silmet U.S.A. Corporation of Miami, Florida, contains a mercury to alloy ratio of 52 percent, or 1 part of advanced high-copper dispersion alloy (with silver, tin and zinc) to1.1 part of mercury. This ratio makes it easy for the dentist to work the amalgam into the patient's tooth, for the formulation offers high resistance to corrosion, convenient carving with no waiting time, and a smooth lustrous finish upon polishing. Working time for mixing Nogama 2 by the dentist is three to four minutes; carving time on the tooth allows the dentist eight to ten minutes; compressive strength occurs in one hour, with 22,000 pounds per square inch (PSI) of chewing allowed. In twenty-four hours the amalgam hardens so that its acceptance of chewing force increases to 65,000 PSI.[1]

Here is how the amalgam is worked for placement into the mouth: a capsule containing self-activating mercury stored inside is placed in a pestle. It gets released in small doses of minute atomized droplets

---

1   Silmet U.S.A. Corporation, "Nogama 2," package insert.

with every pestle impact during tituration by the dentist or dental assistant. This process ensures that all the mercury becomes diffused with the alloy at each stroke of the dentist's or technician's hand.

A competitive brand, Dispersalloy, a Fast Set Dispersed Phase Alloy, comprised of self-activating capsules, produced by Caulk Dentsply, a second amalgam manufacturer, publishes on its package insert that this product is "American Dental Association (ADA) Certified." Of course, this statement can't be true since, as indicated previously, the ADA has taken steps to stay out of legal entanglements by not certifying amalgam.[1]

Not to be outdone by a competitor, Silmet, Ltd. (the Silmet U.S.A. Corporation of Miami, Florida) stamps its package insert for Nogama 2 with the "Certified" logo of the Council on Dental Materials, Instruments, and Equipment of the ADA.[2] Considering the ADA's single-certification policy, it would seem that Silmet is making a fraudulent statement too.

There are other forms of mercury implantation materials in addition to amalgam capsules. There are pellets that break up rapidly into uniform microparticles, and the dentist can use mercury powder with or without zinc alloy that creates a formulation which carves especially well.

Unfortunately, no matter how carefully the dentist or assistant handles the admixture of mercury, some is destined to spill. And such spilling is a highly poisonous circumstance for the technician. The metal must be sponged away immediately and disposed of with great care; otherwise, the handler becomes poisoned.[3] That's a warning put out by the ADA. Can you imagine what physical and mental effects mercury amalgam must create when placed inside a patient's mouth?

---

1   Caulk Dentsply, "Dispersalloy 2 Spill Self-Activating Capsules, Fast Set 656-2862," package insert.

2   Silmet U.S.A. Corporation, "Dispersalloy 2."

3   R. Craig, W. O'Brien, and J. Powers, *Dental Materials: Properties and Manipulation* , 4th ed. (1987).

Some Adverse Physical Effects Created by Amalgam

Dentists usually do not consult patients to determine what materials to use for correction of dental carries. Most follow the ADA policy that dialogue with a patient on this issue is unnecessary and time consuming. However, some materials are hazardous to one's health under certain conditions, and mercury amalgam falls directly into that category. It creates some physical effects of which the patient is seldom informed. Backed by references from an exacting literature search conducted by the Australasian Society of Oral Medicine and Toxicology, the information that follows alerts you to numerous adverse physical effects created by the implantation of mercurial poison in your mouth.

Containing metallic substances consisting of 50 percent pure elemental mercury, 35 percent silver, 13 percent tin, 2 percent copper, and a trace of zinc,[1] amalgam leaches mercury continuously throughout the lifetime of the dental filling.[2] Mercury vapor is the main way that mercury comes out of amalgam, and this vapor is absorbed at a rate of 80 percent through the lungs into the arterial blood.[3] Mercury is more effective as a killer of cells (cytotoxicity) than many cancer chemotherapies. There is *no* harmless level of mercury vapor exposure.[4]

Amalgam mercury binds to sulphydryl (-SH) chemical groups, which exist in almost every enzymatic body process. Amalgam mercury will thus have the potential for disturbing

---

1   H. L. Queen, *Chronic Mercury Toxicity: New Hope against an Endemic Disease* (Colorado Springs, Colo.: Queen and Co. Health Communications, Inc. 1988), 15.

2   D. W. Jones, E. J. Sutton, and E. L. Milner, "Survey of Mercury Vapour in Dental Offices in Atlantic Canada," *Canadian Dental Association Journal* 4906 (1983): 378–95.

3   F. H. Langan, "The Use of Mercury in Dentistry: A Critical Review of the Literature," *Journal of the American Dental Association* 115 (December 1987): 867; F. Hanson, *Journal of Orthomolecular Psychiatry* 12 (1983): 144–201.

4   World Health Organization, "Environmental Health Criteria," *118: Inorganic Mercury* (Geneva, Switzerland: 1991).

all metabolic processes.[1] Mercury vapor is transported freely via the blood[2] and becomes absorbed directly into a dental patient's brain[3] by crossing the blood brain barrier. As shown in the prior chapter, mercury is implicated strongly in the pathogenesis of Alzheimer's disease.[4] Its easy blood transport results in a slow buildup of mercury in body tissues.[5]

Women of childbearing age with mercury amalgams in their teeth invariably poison their fetuses and infants, for mercury crosses the placenta.[6] In fact, the fetus stores up to eight times more mercury than lodges in the mother's tissues, although it does get stored and builds up in breast milk.[7] The metal in amalgam is likely responsible for infertility

1   C. Malmstrom, M. Hansson, and M. Nylander, paper presented at Conference on Trace Elements in Health and Disease, Stockholm, 25 May 1992; F. Goyer, "Toxic Effects of Metals," in *Casaret and Doull's Toxicology: The Basic Science of Poisons*, 3d ed. (New York: Macmillan Publishing, 1986), 582–609; V. Stejskal, *Memory Lymphocyte ImmunoStimulation Assay*, Sweden.

2   H. Matts, "Amalgam Hazards in Your Teeth," *Journal of Orthomolecular Psychiatry* 12, no. 3 (September 1983); P. Stortebecker, *Mercury Poisoning from Dental Amalgam: A Hazard to the Human Brain* (Stockholm, Sweden: Karolinska Institute, 1992); H. Huggins, "Observations from the Metabolic Fringe," paper presented at International Congress of Biological Medicine, Colorado Springs, Colorado, 1988.

3   Stortebecker, "Mercury Poisoning from Dental Amalgam"; P. Sheridan, "Amalgam Restorations and Mercury Toxicity," Master's thesis, University of Sydney, Sydney, Australia.

4   D. E. Vance, W. D. Ehmann, and W. R. Markesbery, "A Search for Longitudinal Variations in Trace Element Levels in Nails of Alzheimer's Disease Patients," *Biological Trace Element Research* 26/27 (July/December 1990): 461–70; Queen, *Chronic Mercury Toxicity*.

5   M. J. Vimy, Y. Takashashi, and F. L. Lorscheider, "Maternal-Fetal Distribution of Mercury Released from Dental Amalgam Fillings," Department of Medicine and Medical Physiology, Faculty of Medicine, University of Calgary, Calgary, Alberta, Canada, *FASEB*, 1990; F. L. Lorscheider and M. J. Vimy, *Lancet* 337 (4 May 1991); Stortebecker, "Mercury Poisoning from Dental Amalgam."

6   M. J. Vimy and others, "Maternal-Fetal Distribution of Mercury"; G. Drasch, "Public Announcement 25," *Bio Probe Newsletter*, January 1994.

7   M. J. Vimy and F. L. Lorscheider, "Intra-Oral Mercury Released from Dental Amalgams," *Journal of Dental Research* 64, no. 8 (1985): 1069–71; Matts, "Amalgam Hazards in Your Teeth"; Drasch, "Public Announcement 25."

in both men and women because it severely reduces the reproductive function.[1]

Amalgam mercury is probably the cause of numerous immune suppression diseases we are seeing today because it rapidly depletes the immune system. As shown by published medical journal studies, certainly it induces autoimmune diseases. It definitely increases the number and severity of allergies for people with amalgam fillings.[2]

---

1   EPA Office of Health and Environmental Assessment, *Mercury Health Effects Update Health Issue Assessment,* final report (1984); B. Gordon, "Pregnancy in Female Dentists: A Mercury Hazard," *Proceedings of the International Conference on Mercury Hazards in Dental Practice,* Glasgow, Scotland, 2 4 September 1981; L. P. Lee and A. Dixon, "Effects of Mercury on Spermatogenisis," *Journal of Pharmacology and Experimental Therapy* 194, no. 1 (1975): 171–81; Vimy and others, "Maternal-Fetal Distribution of Mercury"; P. Kuhnert, B. R. R. Kunhert, and P. Erkard, "Comparison of Mercury Levels in Maternal Blood, Fetal Chord Blood, and Placental Tissue," *American Journal of Obstetrics and Gynecology* 139 (1981): 209–12; J. B. Brodsky, "Occupational Exposure to Mercury in Dentistry and Pregnancy Outcome," *Journal of the American Dental Association* 111, No. 11 (1985): 779–80; V. Mohamed and others, "Laser Light Scattering Study of the Toxic effects of Methyl Mercury on Sperm Motility," *Journal of Andrology* 7, no. 1 (1986): 11–15; S. Jiff and M. Ziff, "Infertility and Birth Defects," *Bio Probe* (1987); M. Inouye, K. Murao, and Y. Kajiwara, "Behavioral and Neuropathological Effects of Prenatal Methyl Mercury Exposure in Mice," *Neurobehavior, Toxicology and Teratology* 7 (1985): 227–32; J. Koos and others, "Mercury Toxicity in Pregnant Women, Fetuses, and Newborn Infants," *American Journal of Obstetrics and Gynecology* 126 (1976): 390–409; Z. Khera and others, "Teratogenic and Genetic Effects of Mercury Toxicity. The Biochemistry of Mercury in the Environment," in J. O. Nriagu, ed. (Amsterdam, the Netherlands: Elsevier, 1979), 503–518; I. Mandel, "Amalgam Hazards: An Assessment of Research," *Journal of the American Dental Association* 122 (August 1991).

2   H. Matts, "Why Is Mercury Toxic? Basic Chemical and Biochemical Properties of Mercury/Amalgam in Relation to Biological Effects," paper presented at International Congress of Biological Medicine, Colorado Springs, Colorado, 1988; Stortebecker, "Mercury Poisoning from Dental Amalgam"; Huggins, "Observations from the Metabolic Fringe"; S. Babich and others, "A Survey of Metal-Induced Mutagenicity and Clastogenicity of Heavy Metals by Physiochemical Factors," *Environmental Research* 37 (1985): 253–86; K. Hansen and others, "A Survey of Metal-Induced Mutagenicity *In Vito* and *In Vivo*," *Journal of American College of Toxicology* 3 (1984): 381–430; L. Vercaeve and others, "Comparative *In Vitro* Cytogenetic Studies in Mercury Exposed Human Lymphocytes," *Mutation Research* 157 (1985): 221–26; L. Pelletier and others, "*In-Vivo* Self-Reactivity of Mononuclear Cells to T Cells and Macrophages Exposed to Hg C12," *European Journal of Immunology* (1985): 460–65; C. Veron, "Amalgam Dentaires et Allergies," *Journal of Biological Buccale* 14 (1986): 83–100; H. Huggins, *It's All in Your Head* (Garden City Park, N.Y.: Avery Publishing Group, 1990); Stejskal, *Memory Lymphocyte Immune Stimulation Assay*; S. Denton, *Proceedings of the First International Conference on Biocompatibility* (1988).

Mercury from amalgam is stored principally in the kidneys, liver, and brain, with kidney damage being a potential result. There will be a 50 percent reduction in kidney filtration as shown in a study of sheep after they underwent amalgam placement in their teeth.[1]

Mercury from amalgam is methylated in the mouth, and methyl mercury is more toxic than elemental mercury.[2] After chewing mercury vapor levels tend to remain raised for at least another 90 minutes, and during this time, immune suppression, brain cell damage, and other adverse health effects from the metallic poisoning is taking place. But amalgam mercury will also migrate through the tooth in which it's lodged.[3] This rate of migration is increased if a gold crown is placed over a tooth filled with amalgam (as had occurred with Dr. Jaro Pleva described in chapter five).[4]

Some uninformed consumers don't think of teeth as living tissue that are part of our bodies, but teeth have a massive communication with the physiology via blood, lymph and nerves. Because of this communicative network, amalgam mercury is absorbed into the body, according to the 1991 World Health Organization criteria, at a rate of 3 to 17 micrograms per day (mcg/day).[5] Additional to that rate, mercury release is elevated by increases in environmental

1   Denton, *Proceedings*; N. D. Boyd, H. Benediktsson, M. J. Vimy, D. E. Hooper, and F. L. Lorscheider, "Mercury from Dental 'Silver' Tooth Fillings Impairs Sheep Kidney Function," *American Journal of Physiology* 261 (1991): 30.

2   E. Heintz, V. Edwardson, S. Derand, and U. Birkhead, "Methylation of Mercury from Dental Amalgam and Mercuric Chloride by Oral Streptococci," *Scandinavian Journal of Dental Research* 91 (1983): 150–52; F. Rowland, P. Grasso, and B. Davies, "The Methylation of Mercuric Chloride by Human Intestinal Bacteria," *Experientia* 31 (1975): 1064–65; T. Yamada, "Formation of Methyl Mercury Compounds from Inorganic Mercury by *Clostridium Cochlearium*," *Journal of Fermentation Technology* 50 (1972): 159–66

3   C. W. Svare and others, "The Effects of Dental Amalgam on Mercury Levels in Expired Air," *Journal of Dental Research* 60, no. 9 (1981): 1668–71; K. Ott and others, "Mercury Burden Due to Amalgam Fillings," *Deutsch. Zahnarztl Z* 39, no. 9 (1984): 199–205; Vimy and Lorscheider, "Intro-Oral Mercury Released from Dental Amalgam."

4   Malmstrom and others, conference paper; Matts, "Why Is Mercury Toxic"; W. Till and others, *Welt/reform* 87 (1978): 1130–34.

5   Stortebecker, "Mercury Poisoning from Dental Amalgam."

temperature, friction (chewing and tooth brushing), and electrical currents (dissimilar metals in the mouth).[1]

So the poison implanted in your teeth will enter the body in a variety of ways: as elemental mercury, inorganic mercury, mercury vapor, charged mercury ions, and whole mercury particles that break from the filling. When the poison hits the brain, it gets stored preferentially in the hypothalamus and pituitary gland. The adverse effects are principally characterized by neurological symptoms manifested in the form of peripheral neuropathies, multiple sclerosis, Parkinson's disease, amyotrophic lateral sclerosis, and other pathologies. The damaging mercurial ions get transported along the axons of nerve fibers and become stored in most cells of the brain and body. Each area of tissue affected will produce its own set of symptoms.[2]

Another problem is that mercury binds to hemoglobin in the red blood cells, thus reducing oxygen-carrying capacity. There will also be blood vessel damage (micro-angiopathies) with a subsequent reduction in blood supply to the tissues.[3]

As for electrical currents created by dissimilar metals such as gold and amalgam in the mouth, they are definitely injurious to health. These currents are measurable in microamps, a higher electrical current than those operating in the brain and central nervous system. Rather, they operate in the very tiny range of nanoamps, which are 1,000 times less than microamps.[4]

1   A. R. Sheppard and M. Eisenbud, *Biological Effects of Electric and Magnetic Fields of Extremely Low Frequency* (New York: New York University Press, 1977); Langan, "The Use of Mercury in Dentistry"; R. Marxkors, "Korrosionserscheinungen an Amalgam-Fullungen und Deren Auswirkungen auf den Menschlichen Organismus," *Das Deutsche Zahn rztebl* 24 (1970): 53, 117, 170.

2   Vimy and others, "Maternal-Fetal Distribution of Mercury"; Goyer, "Toxic Effects of Metals"; Stortebecker, "Mercury Poisoning from Dental Amalgam"; W. Nylander and others, Fourth International Symposium of Epidemiology in Occupational Health, Como, Italy, September 1985.

3   Denton, *Proceedings*; Ott and others, "Mercury Burden Due to Amalgam Fillings"; J. Abraham, C. Svare, and C. Frank, "The Effects of Dental Amalgam Restorations on Blood Mercury Levels," *Journal of Dental Research* 63, no. 1 (1984): 71–73; Goyer, "Toxic Effects of Metals"; Lorscheider and Vimy, *Lancet*; Huggins, "Observations from the Metabolic Fringe."

4   Sheppard and Eisenbud, *Biological Effects of Electric and Magnetic Fields*; Matts, "Amalgam Hazards in Your Teeth"; Till, *Welt/reform*.

From animal experiments, medical scientists know that mercury from amalgam induces antibiotic resistance. There also is mercury resistance in bacteria lodged in the mouth and gastrointestinal tract.[1]

As for the level of mercury settling into brain tissue, there is a direct linear proportion to the number of surfaces of amalgam fillings in the mouth.[2] The amount of mercury lodged in the brain tissue of a fetus, newborn, or young child is proportional to the number of amalgam fillings in the mother's mouth.[3]

Medical literature recognizes that mercury causes single-strand breaks in DNA.[4]

In addition to these many adverse physical effects created by the mercury in dental amalgam, mercury is responsible as well for the development of some dire mental effects, like the fate of "mad hatter" whose condition was caused by handling mercury in the hat-making industry. Every person carrying a dental amalgam filling in the mouth has the potential to go mad from its mental effects.

Some Adverse Mental Effects Created by Amalgam

Mercury levels in the body derived from dental amalgam fillings cannot be assessed by either blood or urine levels.[5] But such filling material is the single greatest source of dietary mercury for the general population of the world, says the 1991 WHO criteria report.[6]

---

1   A. O. Summers, J. Wireman, M. J. Vimy, F. L. Lorscheider, B. Marshal, S. B. Evy, S. Bennet, and L. Billard, *Journal of Antimicrobial Agents and Chemotherapy* 37, no. 4 (April 1993): 825–34.

2   Denton, *Proceedings*; Matts, "Amalgam Hazards in Your Teeth"; Malstrom and others, conference paper.

3   Drasch, "Public Announcement 25."

4   Khera and others, "Teratogenic and Genetic Effects of Mercury Toxicity"; Babich and others, "Mediation of Mutagenicity and Clastogenicity of Heavy Metals."

5   Lorscheider and Vimy, *Lancet*.

6   World Health Organization, *Criteria 118*.

A number of adverse mental and emotional effects are created in people by their being exposed to ongoing leaching of mercury into the tissues of their brains. Persuaded by his own findings as presented in chapter 6, Dr. Boyd Haley, professor of medical biochemistry at the University of Kentucky, says: "I would not want to make a statement that mercury causes Alzheimer's disease, but there is no doubt in my mind that low levels of mercury present in the brain cause neural cell death and that this could lead to dementia similar to Alzheimer's disease. To the best that we can determine, mercury is a time bomb in the brain waiting to have an effect. If it is not bothering someone when they are young, especially when they age, it can turn into something quite bad."

"Regarding differences between extra-oral and intra-oral mercury vapor exposure and measurement, although there would be no difference between mercury vapor measured inside the mouth and outside the mouth, the exposure potential of intra-oral mercury would be much greater than that of extra-oral mercury vapor, as mercury is toxic through the routes of absorption and ingestion as well as by inhalation," Gilbert J. Saulter of Dallas, regional administrator for the Occupational Safety and Health Administration (OSHA) of the U.S. Department of Labor, wrote on November 26, 1986, to Bill Wolfe, D.D.S., H.M.D., P.A., of Albuquerque, New Mexico.

The result of such intra-oral exposure to mercury was measured through a survey conducted by the Foundation for Toxic Free Dentistry (FTFD) of Orlando, Florida, among 762 dental patients. (Note: For supportive information of what you're about to read, please see appendix A for the address and telephone number of the FTFD and contact that organization.) The 762 patients were either about to have their amalgam fillings replaced or they actually had recently replaced them. The collected data on symptoms of illness were turned over to the FDA for evaluation as to the mental/emotional or physical dangers resulting from mercury present in dental materials.

Among these 762 people, a total of 440 different illnesses were reported with the average number of symptoms per patient numbering 4.9. A total of 534 women and 228 men reported; their average age was 45.5 years. Among the women, 220 were younger than 40; among the men, 80 were younger than 40. The women experienced 2,916 symptoms and the men recorded 876.

For *depression*, 181 (23.75 percent) reported experiencing the symptom, but 100 percent of these patients advised that they changed to feeling cured when their amalgams were removed.

For *fatigue*, 325 (42.65 percent) had this symptom, but 95 percent (310) found themselves cured when their amalgams were removed.

For *allergies*, 221 (29 percent) were troubled by this symptom, but 88.68 percent (196) had permanent release from their allergic discomforts by amalgam replacement.

For *headaches*, 233 (30.5 percent) of all the people participating in the survey experienced them, but 95 percent (196) of these reported being cured after substituting their filling material with something other than mercury amalgam.

For *memory loss*, 109 patients (14.3 percent) went through this experience regularly, but 93.5 percent (102) of these found themselves recovered completely after amalgam removal.

For *multiple sclerosis*, 42 people (5.5 percent) reported MS-like symptoms, but 78.5 percent (33) of these said they were better or cured after taking out amalgams. Their range of improvement for MS-like symptoms was from 10 percent to 100 percent.

These are only a few of the health difficulties that improve from having dental mercury amalgam fillings replaced with less toxic materials. The following is an additional listing of signs or symptoms relating to amalgams present in the mouth about which much could be commented:

anxiety	metallic taste
bad temper	muscle tremor
bloating	nervousness
blood pressure, high or low	lack of energy
chest pains	skin disturbances (eczema)
dizziness	sleeping excessively (narcolepsy)
gastrointestinal upset	sore throat
gum disease	tachycardia
insomnia	thyroid difficulties
irregular heartbeat	ulcers in the oral cavity

irritability	urinary tract problems
lack of concentration	vision problems
numbness anywhere on the body	

Dentists often observe signs or hear complaints from patients about these kinds of symptoms. However, almost all of them make no connection to the poisons they're putting into the mouths of people. That's probably because any dentist who prefers to avoid malpractice troubles with patients and licensure difficulties with the American Dental Association seldom mentions mercury amalgams as the potential source for what's causing such physical, mental, or emotional signs and symptoms.

Eight

Why Dentists Love Amalgams and Deny Their Toxicity

The chapter you're about to read is the pivot around which much of this book revolves. Because there is so much shocking but documented information about the American Dental Association's love affair with dental amalgams, chapter 8 focuses on dentistry's vested interests and ethical confusion.

Oral Health Professionals Discuss Dental Materials

Commenting from his office in the state of Washington, a biocompatible dentist declared that he is apprehensive about being identified with negative statements about the American Dental Association. His license to practice could then be in danger. Still, he did speak on the record about the many different materials installed in the mouth by dentists as long as I did not reveal his name.

(Note: For a full description of what each of the separate oral metals implanted by dentists do to a person's overall body and brain physiology, please see chapter 10.)

The Washington dentist, who is a leader in his field, told me:

> Numbers of dental crowns are made from certain nonprecious metals such as chromium, nickel, and stainless steel. The steel, of course, is changed to be stainless by the inclusion of nickel into its formulation. Nickel is toxic. When some nonbiological dentists report that they don't use nickel but do utilize stainless steel, they are then shocked to learn from an informed source that the stainless steel is, in large measure, comprised of nickel. Science knows that nickel binds with the body's proteins to act allergenically.

Then the allergens will bring on a cascade of events which adversely affect the patient's sense of general well-being.

It's important for dentists to acknowledge that the human immune system contains immunoglobulins which react to various substances entering one's body. A person's age, sex, predisposition to the environment, and other factors play roles in how somebody responds to those factors. Although we may be exposed to many similar substances, all of us do not react in the same way to such materials.

More now than ever before, my colleagues who are biological dentists take note of what our patients tell us. Although we may not find substantive clinical evidence of a health problem, it's exceedingly important to listen to the individual as one taps into the built-in physiological computer to explain what's believed to be the trouble. When somebody advises that he or she feels a decline in well-being from the placement of a particular dental material, attention must be paid to that advisory.

Personally, as a biological dentist, I am acutely aware that what I put in a patient's oral cavity has systemic effects on that person. The mouth is attached to the rest of the body, and anything we do to this portal of entry for the gastrointestinal tract affects the patient's systemic well-being.

From Ronald Dressler, D.D.S.

"There are a whole range of materials used in dentistry today which have the potential for creating an adverse systemic effect," states Ronald Dressler, D.D.S., of Atlanta, Georgia. "Probably the prime substance that nearly everyone is talking about in my profession is 'silver'-mercury amalgam; then there are other problematic materials such as nickel-based metals used for crowns. But mercury in amalgams is the main abuser. It causes a massive number of symptoms, including minor hypersensitivity reactions, frequent headaches, ringing in the ears, chronic eye inflammation, chronic fatigue, easy tiring, excessive sweating, cold hands and feet, slow healing, frequent urination, memory loss, insomnia, difficult decision making, neuromuscular troubles, and other major neurological health problems such as Alzheimer's disease, Parkinson's disease, Lou Gehrig's disease, and multiple sclerosis. There's no known direct relationship to any major disease—something like multiple sclerosis—but mercury certainly is a key element in its causation.

"During my thirty years of practice, I've observed several hundred people having trouble from their mercury amalgam fillings," adds Dr. Dressler. "And I can clinically confirm that there is a mercury relationship present because, prior to amalgam removal, patients were experiencing disease symptoms which tended to improve or even disappear after their amalgam replacement. Heavy metals in general can be problematic, and that goes for silver, beryllium, cobalt, chromium, and such other materials used in the mouth in one fashion or another. Troublesome substances make up such items as removable partial dentures, crowns, and other appliances.

"For example, a patient of mine wearing a nickel crown was discomforted by an eczematous rash on her leg. When I removed that nickel crown and replaced it with a plastic one, within two weeks the rash had disappeared and stayed away permanently. I have seen changes like this with skin disturbances happen many times now," affirms Dr. Dressler.

Dr. Ron Dressler gives a legal definition for the holistic (biological) dentistry he performs. When asked to describe his routine dental office procedures, this is what Dr. Dressler states: "The emphasis of my practice is on biocompatible, mercury-free dentistry with which I treat patients who have been compromised by dental materials."

From Kenneth A. Bock, M.D.

"Dentist-treated teeth—profound cases especially involving dental mercury amalgams—have been responsible for numbers of my patients consulting me for the alleviation of chronic fatigue syndrome, allergies, sinusitis, and other difficulties with their health. Their conditions come on from mercury toxicity," says Kenneth A. Bock, M.D., medical director of the Rhinebeck Medical Center in Rhinebeck, New York. Dr. Bock focuses on family practice medicine with specialties in the treatment of allergies and cardiovascular disease. His primary tools for healing involve the use of nutritional therapy, immunotherapy, preventive medicine, and chelation therapy.

"I approach the whole issue of amalgams in the teeth with the understanding that they are a main source of systemic disease. At first I was skeptical about the amalgam issue, but over the years I've seen so much illness arising from mercury-filled teeth that amalgam toxicity makes a lot more sense to me now. It shows up clinically," said Dr. Ken Bock. "The trouble starts with the mercury amalgam's effect on intracellular enzymes and their uncoupling of the patient's oxidative phosphoralization [a usual body function].

"Challenging toxic patients with the detoxificating agent known as DMSA [2,3-Dimercaptosuccinic Acid] was proof to me that such amalgam toxicity exists," said Dr. Bock. "DMSA is an orally administered mercury chelating agent. Also I help patients to get rid of their health problems by using numbers of intravenous drips with vitamin C and EDTA [ethylene diamine tetraacetic acid] chelation therapy."

(Note: To gain a full description of DMSA, DMPS, EDTA, and several other detoxification methods for heavy metal poisoning that arises from dentist-treated teeth, please see chapter 9.)

From Bill Wolfe, D.D.S., H.N.D.

Bill Wolfe, D.D.S., H.N.D., a holistic (biological) dental practitioner and homeopath, who renders mercury-free and biological dentistry in Albuquerque, New Mexico, told me the story of when, at age sixteen, he worked as a part-time dental assistant to Byron Smith, D.D.S., of Austin, Texas. After fifty years, Dr. Smith is still actively providing an attentive, conventional form of dentistry in Austin. A couple of years ago he took in an associate dentist to relieve the burdens of his overflowing practice.

As a sixteen-year-old who was then acting as a part-time dental assistant, while aspiring to one day become a licensed practicing dentist, this is what Dr. Wolfe had witnessed:

"Back then, in 1963, the assistant's usual procedure was to mix liquid metallic mercury by hand for the dentist," explains Dr. Wolfe. "That's what I did for Dr. Smith. When those shiny little balls of mercury spilled onto the counter I would play with them—push the mercury around—and upon seeing those balls stick together, I'd pull them apart. While I waited in the operatory for my boss to carve and shape the amalgam in his patient's mouth, I'd have great fun with the mercury.

"But there was one afternoon I'll never forget. As Dr. Smith was busy with filling the dental amalgam into a child's tooth, he saw me playing at rolling those liquid mercury balls back and forth.

"That's when he turned in my direction, gave me a stare, leaned over, and in a stage-whisper said sharply, 'Don't do that!'

"Puzzled, I looked up and asked, 'Why not?'

"'It's a poison,' declared Dr. Smith.

"'A poison?' I wondered aloud. 'Then why are you putting it in the kid's mouth?'

"Not hesitating a moment, this long-experienced and well-established dentist responded, 'That's different!'"

Why Dentists Love Amalgam and Deny It's a Poison

Each time any dentist in North America fills somebody's tooth with "silver" mercury amalgam, the American Dental Association most likely receives a royalty payment. Depending on the amalgam formula and according to the bulk quantity of amalgam mixture sold to dental supply house distributors, a commission (royalty) is paid to the ADA by the individual amalgam manufacturer.

The ADA, through its Chicago-based American Dental Association Health Foundation (the ADAHF), with research facilities lodged in the Paffenbarger Research Center at the National Institute of Standards and Technology in Washington, D. C., owns production patent rights to mercury-amalgam. This circumstance is recorded for anyone to access in the United States Patent Office, a discovery made near the end of 1997 by the Swedish biological dentist, Ulf Bengtsson, D.D.S. Dr. Bengtsson's surprise revelation came about while he assisted his country's legislators who had been investigating and then formulating laws for the elimination of mercury-amalgam from that nation's dental offices. As of New Year's Day 1999, mercury amalgam was no longer allowed as a therapeutic dental device in Dr. Bengtsson's country. Dental amalgam filling material has been banned from use anywhere in Sweden.

According to patent records, Richard M. Waterstrat of Gaithersburg,

Maryland, invented a certain formula for amalgam and filed his U.S. patent application number 713,849 on August 12, 1976. Being an employee of the ADAHF under a standard work-made-for-hire agreement, Waterstrat thereafter turned over ownership of two U.S. patents that were granted to him to the ADAHF. Additional amalgam formulations were investigated thereafter, for it's an ongoing ADAHF research enterprise. As amalgam substitutes, dental composite materials are being formulated and patented as well. Thus, an organization under full ADA control today owns patents for the production of dental amalgam and composites. Among them, the ADAHF's patent ownership includes United States Patent number 4,018,600 Waterstrat, dated April 19, 1977, and United States Patent number 4,078,921 Waterstrat, dated March 14, 1978.

Under such circumstances, and judging that the American Dental Association, in forcefully advocating the use of dental amalgam fillings could be laboring under a serious financial conflict of interest that harms people, I contacted the ADA offices in Chicago. Introducing myself as a medical journalist, there I spoke with John Malone, an executive in the ADA's Department of Scientific Affairs.

My opening statement was, "I am writing about dental amalgam, and I understand that the American Dental Association owns patent rights for amalgam."

Mr. Malone said, "That's not true! I don't know where that came from. But we, the ADA Health Foundation as part of the ADA, do not own patents to amalgams. It's not patentable. Companies which manufacture it will have patented formulations, but the ADA does not own amalgam. We do own composite resins."

I responded, "But I have patent numbers granted to Mr. Waterstrat in 1977."

"That's probably not amalgam but some other version. Does it contain mercury?"

"Yes!"

"Well, R. M. Waterstrat was a researcher at the ADA Health Foundation, and it [his invention] probably was some amalgam version used for research purposes rather than for funding source," John Malone said. "He was around for a long time and is probably retired now. But I don't have any specifics. You're asking for contractual information, and I don't have that."

"I am trying to learn who receives royalties from the manufacturers producing amalgam," I responded.

"Companies who make amalgam have their own patents," said Malone. "It is they who get the income. There is no single amalgam formulation as there is for some composite resins."

I persisted, "Yes, but does the ADA Health Foundation receive a royalty for amalgam manufacture?"

Malone answered, "I don't know that. You would have to call the ADA Health Foundation."

Located at a different telephone extension, the American Dental Association Health Foundation uses the same Chicago toll-free phone number. I called and again, identified myself as a medical journalist and spoke to Bob Zarnicke at the ADAHF, whom I asked, "Who owns amalgam and its patents?"

Zarnicke replied, "The best person to talk to is Fredrick Eichmiller, D.D.S., director of the ADA's Paffenbarger Research Center component in Maryland, near Washington, D.C. Dr. Eichmiller is a researcher and dentist who deals with all the licenses and patents held by the ADA and outside the ADA but related to dental practice."

After introducing myself as a medical journalist, my exchange with Dr. Eichmiller was friendly and open. It went like this:

"Could you tell me who owns the patents on amalgam?"

"Almost all the patents on amalgam have expired," stated Dr. Eichmiller. "Yes, Richard M. Waterstrat did hold patents on amalgam composition which had been assigned to the American Dental Association Health Foundation. We did own a patent on one composition of amalgam which was never manufactured. Whatever he invented while working here would have been assigned to us."

I then contacted Richard M. Waterstrat, which netted the following information:

"All of my various patents on amalgam became the property of the American Dental Association. They own all patent rights on amalgam formulas. Mine was work-made-for-hire, and that's normal procedure."

I asked, "Does the American Dental Association assign those rights to manfacturers?"

"Yes, the ADA assigns them. They are happy to do that and ask for royalties. The [amalgam] manufacturers pay royalties," said Dr. Waterstrat. "They are paid directly to the ADA Health Foundation."

My follow-up question was, "Are they receiving royalties?"

Dr. Waterstrat answered, "Yes, they are getting some royalties, but not on mine. But some of the others, yes, like patents on composite materials. They get quite a bit of royalties on that. As far as I know, the ADA is not receiving royalties on amalgam formulations that I invented. But they do get royalties on other amalgam because they own the patents on it. That's the way it works!"

Returning the next day to speak on the phone with John Malone at the ADA Department of Scientific Affairs, I reminded him of my query, and he clearly remembered. When I apprised him of Dr. R. M. Waterstrat's two patents, Malone quickly said, "Presumably the ADA has patents on amalgams and composites which they license. I must confess that yesterday I answered incorrectly. I apologize for bad information. I should have answered: if there's any legal, contractual, or financial arrangements with reception of funds, the American Dental Association Health Foundation should be able to answer that question."

H. L. Mencken observed at one time: "Conscience is the inner voice which warns us that someone may be looking." Because nobody has been looking, the American Dental Association has not felt conscience-stricken for more than one hundred and fifty years (see the ADA's brief history, which follows). Until today, no medically informed person in the United States has been privy to the knowledge that the ADA makes money from encouraging its members to harm people's health by implanting poisonous mercury into dental patients' mouths.

Ethical Considerations the ADA May Allow Dentists

The Division of Legal Affairs of the American Dental Association issued a document in December 1990 addressed to all ADA members. It related to the ordinary dentist's taking into account certain ethical considerations in regard to dental amalgam removal. The ADA said it has an "Advisory Opinion" as an addendum to its *Principles of Ethics and Code of Professional Conduct*. This advisory opinion states:

Based on available scientific data, the ADA has determined through the adoption of Resolution 42H-1986 (*Trans*.1986:536) that the removal of amalgam restorations from the non-allergic patient for the alleged purpose of removing toxic substances from the body, when such treatment is performed solely at the recommendation or suggestion of the dentist, is improper and unethical. . . . A dentist who represents that dental treatment recommended or performed by the dentist has the capacity to cure or alleviate diseases, infections or other conditions, when such representations are not based upon accepted scientific knowledge or research, is acting unethically.[1]

Thus, if the dentist draws upon his or her professional knowledge and informs the patient about the hazards to health from chewing on amalgam filling material installed in the teeth, that dentist is considered unethical by the ADA. The consequence for a dentist pursuing behavior that's judged by his peers as unethical conduct is loss of license. This has happened repeatedly in most of this nation's states where the ADA carries any kind of political clout.

Alternatively, the ADA answers the sticky ethical question in another way as well. If one of its dentist-members asks, "May I ethically remove dental amalgam upon request from my patient?" The ADA organizational leaders respond:

The dentist who removes amalgam based on a request from a patient or the patient's physician is not acting unethically. The dentist also is not acting unethically if he/she decides not to comply with the patient's request, assuming there is no valid medical reason for removal based on a sound physician referral.[2]

Thus the ADA has cited the particular reason the book you're reading needed to be published. A dental patient who is carrying

---

1   Connecticut State Dental Association, *Ethical Considerations: Removal of Dental Amalgam* (Division of Legal Affairs, American Dental Association, December 1990).

2   Ibid.

poison in the mouth must be educated about its hazards, and I've endeavored to do exactly that. When my reader—the potential dental patient—has access to appropriate information, he may seek amalgam removal, which could be allowed by ADA bureaucrats without the ordinary dentist getting into trouble with his or her state's dental licensing board. Also, such knowledge will help the patient hold back the dentist from perpetuating the dental malpractice that may be conducted in the modern era.

Dental Malpractice Remains Rampant from No Informed Consent

The Jesus metaphor that "It is easier for a camel to go through the eye of a needle than for a rich man to enter into the Kingdom of God" is applicable to unethical dentists making money from the creation of illnesses by their amalgam installations.[1] The drive for riches apparently causes some dentists to put ethics behind them and go for the easy buck using mercury amalgams.

Dentists are possibly performing malpractice, as well, when they ignore a patient's right to participate in the important decision-making process for such amalgam installations. Patients have a prerogative to know the dangers of allowing mercury to be placed in their mouths. For any such procedure, they must give "informed consent."

Put simply, informed consent (a legal principal) requires that before the dentist touches or treats any patient, he or she has provided an appropriate amount of understandable information regarding the proposed treatment. Also, having received the appropriate information, the patient must agree to receive the treatment.[2]

Originally, this legal principle was grounded in the theory that

---

1   G. I. Nierenberg, *What You Need to Succeed in Business and Life* (New York: Nierenberg & Zeif Publishers, 1987), 15.

2   "Making Health Care Decisions," *President's Commission for the Study of Ethical Problems on Medicare and Biomedical and Behavioral Research* 3, appendix L (1982).

any unauthorized health care touching (or other kind of touching) constituted a battery (any illegal touching).[1] Therefore, the issue was simply whether or not consent to treatment had been obtained.

In the face of failure by the dentist to obtain the informed consent, or the provision of treatment beyond the scope of that consent, this circumstance could then form the basis for a battery claim against the dentist.[2] But in modern times the courts have steadily moved away from this simplistic approach and now, rather than battery, they've adopted what's known as a "negligence" standard.[3]

When dentists fail to reveal to their patients full information about the hazards of having amalgam fillings installed in existing dental cavities, these dentists are likely to be considered negligent by the courts. A ruling of dental negligence is equivalent to malpractice.[4]

The California Court of Appeal described the health professional's duty to obtain an "informed consent" as follows:

> A physician [dentist] violates his duty to his patient and subjects himself to liability if he withholds any facts which are necessary to form the basis of an intelligent consent by the patient to the proposed treatment. Likewise the physician may not minimize the known dangers of a procedure or operation in order to induce his patient's consent.[5]

At this time, according to established policy of the ADA, no dentist is allowed to warn his or her patient about the dangers of dental amalgams before installing them or to recommend their removal unless such patient expressly asks for true information on that subject. The American Dental Association seems to disallow its members from telling the truth, and therefore tends to violate its

---

1   *Schloendorff v. Society of New York Hospitals*, 211 New York 125, 105 N.E., 133 New York State. 1143 (1914).

2   Ibid.

3   *Rubino v. DeFretias*, 638 F. Supp. 182 (D. Ariz. 1986).

4   *Salgo v. Leland Stanford Jr. University Board of Trustees*, 154 Cal. App. 2d 560, 317 P.2d 170 (1st Dist. 1957).

5   Ibid.

"fiduciary" obligation to all patients treated by its members in contradistinction to laws adopted by the several states.[1]

Founded on the doctrine of negligence, there are four basic elements of an informed consent lawsuit:

- The dentist must have given incorrect, inappropriate, or inadequate disclosures (as deemed so in the court's jurisdiction) about amalgam dental fillings.

- The patient must have consented to and undergone the treatment that was the subject of the dentist's inadequate disclosures.

- The patient must be injured in some manner by the mercury placed in his or her mouth by the dentist.

- The patient must show that he or she would *not* have agreed to the procedure if that patient had possessed all of the relevant and vital information.[2]

Brief History of the American Dental Association

Throughout their history, leaders of the ADA have been advocates of dental amalgam. This organization, in fact, was born out of the negative reports and bitter professional controversy surrounding the application of amalgam as a dental filling material. ADA members loved amalgam from the moment of their organization's 1830s tooth-related inception into the United States by two con men, the Crawcours brothers. Dental amalgam brought the brothers instant wealth, while dental patients received lasting damage.

The leading educated medical-dentists of the day opposed putting mercury mixed with silver into the human mouth because they knew this mixture was poisonous and so declared it to be. An opposing group, the uneducated craftsmen-dentists, loved amalgam

---

1   *Canterbury v. Spence*, 464 F.2d 772 (D.C. Cir. 1972), *cert. denied*, 409 U.S. 1064 (1972).

2   C. A. Harris, *The Principles and Practice of Dental Surgery*, 2d ed. (Philadelphia: Lindsay and Blakiston, 1845), 259 60.

because it was so easy to use. They paid no mind to its toxicity. But, in his textbook on dental surgery—the bible of every dentist who worked at his trade—Dr. Chapin Harris wrote: "The amalgam of mercury and silver . . . is decidedly the most pernicious material that has ever been employed for filling teeth."

Believing in educating all of their fellow dentists about human anatomy, metabolism, and physiology, the medical-dentists joined together to form dental schools. Preferring to learn by the trial-and-error method, craftsmen-dentists opposed going to any such school. Between the two groups, there were about fourteen hundred dental practitioners in the United States in the 1830s.

In 1840 the medical-dentists decided to form a dental society, the American Society of Dental Surgeons (ASDS), to which they invited the craftsmen-dentists as members. Almost all dentists joined together. There was friendship between the two groups for a few years, until 1843, when the more educated members of the ASDS—filled with a loathing for the harm that amalgam was bringing to patients—passed a controversial resolution. It stated that the use of amalgam filling material is considered to be malpractice, and amalgams must be banned from the legitimate practice of dentistry. Thereafter, ASDS members were required to sign a pledge that they would oppose amalgam usage.

This pledge split apart the two dental groups—the well-educated *medicalists* and the trial-and-error *craftsmen*. Those craftsmen-dentists who refused to sign the pledge were considered unethical and were expelled from the American Society of Dental Surgeons.

By 1856 so many amalgam-using dentists had withdrawn or been expelled for unethical conduct that lack of membership caused the ASDA to disband as a professional society. It had run out of funds to function. Three years later the *amalgamists* formed the American Dental Association (ADA), jokingly referred to among its craftsmen-dentist members as the "Amalgam Dental Association."[1] They had hardly any acquaintance with medical

---

1   M. D. K. Bremner, *The Story of Dentistry* (Brooklyn, N.Y.: Dental Items of Interest Publishing Co., Inc., 1939).

practices and instead focused on the mechanical aspects of dentistry. And that's the way it has remained to this day. The American Dental Association's underlying concept continues to be that the teeth are separate from the body and have no influence over what occurs anatomically, metabolically, or physiologically.[1]

Why the ADA Persists with Harmful Practices for Dental Patients

In their excellent book, *Surviving the Toxic Crisis: Understanding, Preventing and Treating the Root Causes of Chronic Illness* (see appendix B) William Randall Kellas, Ph.D., and Andrea Sharon Dworkin, N.D., reveal to readers why, despite all the evidence that mercury in amalgam is toxic, officials of the American Dental Association persist in demanding harmful practices for dental patients by their dues-paying members. Here are the reasons offered by Dr. Kellas and Dr. Dworkin:[2]

- Like any powerful, politically oriented union, the ADA is protecting its own financial interests by supporting its poorly performing members.

- If ADA leaders admit their policies have been mistaken for the past one hundred and sixty-seven years, the lawsuits leveled on them from dental consumers would bankrupt the organization.

- Officers of the ADA would be forced to perform extensive and expensive scientific testing on amalgams with nothing to gain from it. Rather, doing such tests would be giving more ammunition to attorneys representing dental consumers for use against the ADA or its members.

---

1   J. E. Hardy, *Mercury Free: The Wisdom behind the Global Consumer Movement to Ban "Silver" Dental Fillings* (Glassboro, N.J.: Gabriel Rose Press, Inc., 1996), 55.

2   W. R. Kellas and A. S. Dworkin, *Surviving the Toxic Crisis: Understanding, Preventing and Treating the Root Causes of Chronic Illness* (Olivenham, Calif.: Professional Preference, 1996), 195.

- If ADA members really believed amalgam is harmless, they would be anxious to prove it with appropriate testing. But secretly they acknowledge among themselves that amalgam implantation is hazardous to the patients' health, so they avoid any semblance of such testing. Why furnish patients and their attorneys with ammunition for legal claims?

- ADA officials are more anxious to justify their position than in finding the truth. The dental industry is following the example of obfuscation set by the tobacco industry.

- The ADA accredits dental schools, issues licensing examinations administered by state boards of dental examiners, and provides all information studied by dental students; consequently, ADA members start into their dental practices totally biased in favor of ADA policies, which are mostly against the welfare of patients.

- Because of ADA pressure, almost all state dental boards forbid dentists to tell their patients about the toxicity of mercury in amalgam fillings. If your dentist does explain the truth about amalgam toxicity, he or she is putting their state license to practice dentistry in jeopardy. Then this reputable dentist will lose the means of earning a living.

Nine

Detoxification Procedures before and after Removing Dental Amalgams

Are you anxious to preserve the health of your loved ones and yourself? Do you want to get rid of the poison in your mouth? If so, there are certain toxic waste removal procedures to follow before and after removing dental amalgams. They do work well as protection from damage from mercury discharging during amalgam eradication, and this chapter describes them in detail.

Five Techniques of Mercury Detoxification

It is absolutely essential that any individuals who wish to remove "silver" dental amalgams engage in a mercury detoxification program. As mentioned, the detoxifying procedure should be performed both before and after replacing the fillings in tooth cavities. If mercury is indeed causing disease symptoms, the additional mercury toxins that get added to the patients' body before and during amalgam replacement may be enough to push these unfortunate people over the edge into illness. This extra burden of mercury will worsen their pathologies in the extreme, rather than making them better physiologically.

Some techniques of body cleansing such as detox bathing can be done for oneself at home. But in particular, there are three general and two specific detoxification programs against mercury poisoning. Since certain protocols must be followed, four of the five purification methods cannot be self-administered but rather must be given by skilled medical personnel exclusively. Two of the effective methods involve receiving intravenous (IV) infusions to neutralize mercury toxins that are poisoning the body fluids and tissues. A third detox technique is an internal/external sweat-induction program derived from Scientology's antiaddiction method developed by L. Ron Hubbard, the religion's founder. Two other protocols require that certain chemicals with affinity for toxic heavy metals be used to pull out the amalgamated mercury that has accumulated throughout the body.

The amalgam-removal patient should choose at least one or two or undergo all five detoxifications before and after embarking on dental amalgam filling replacement. These can get rid of the poison in one's mouth and clean out mercury from the body tissues so that immune system vitality may be restored. Undergoing such detoxifications is the way to avoid degenerative diseases such as cancer, and can advance progress toward healing if illness has already struck.

The simplest method is the IV-vitamin C mercury detox program, as described in the book *Chronic Mercury Toxicity: New Hope Against an Endemic Disease*, by medical journalist H. L. Queen. This 1988 book is published by Queen and Company Health Communications, Inc. of Colorado Springs, Colorado, and is among the most complete texts ever written on chronic mercury poisoning from dental manipulations by allopathic-type dentists. (See appendix B for further publishing information.)[1]

The second method of blood vessel infusion detoxification entails undergoing a series of IV chelation therapies with ethylene diamine tetraacetic acid (EDTA), as described in four particular books I have authored or coauthored: *The Chelation Way*, by Morton Walker, D.P.M. (Avery Publishing Group);[2] *Everything You Should Know about Chelation Therapy* by Morton Walker, D.P.M., and Hitendrah Shah, M.D. (Keats Publishing, Inc.);[3] *Toxic Metal Syndrome*, by H. Richard Casdorph, M.D., Ph.D., and Morton Walker, D.P. M.

---

1   H. L. Queen, *Chronic Mercury Toxicity: New Hope against an Endemic Disease* (Colorado Springs, Colo.: Queen & Co. Health Communications, Inc., 1988).

2   M. Walker, *The Chelation Way: The Complete Book of Chelation Therapy* (Garden City Park, N.Y.: Avery Publishing Group, 1990).

3   M. Walker and H. Shah, *Everything You Should Know about Chelation Therapy* (New Canaan, Conn.: Keats Publishing, Inc. 1997).

(Avery Publishing Group);[1] and *The Healing Powers of Chelation Therapy*, by John Parks Trowbridge, M.D., and Morton Walker, D.P.M., (New Way of Life, Inc.).[2]

(For publishing information on these four books about chelation therapy that I have researched and written, see appendix B. To contact the medical/professional organization that offers additional in-depth information about certification as a chelation therapist, the American College for Advancement in Medicine, see appendix A.)

A third method for physical detoxification requires the use of a sauna for inducing severe body cleansing through the skin by means of sweating. Two of the three detoxification techniques are described here, beginning with the latter, L. Ron Hubbard's sweat-induction program.

Then, the fourth and fifth techniques for dealing with body burdens of mercury from amalgams are to take treatments that provide one or both of the experimental chemical agents: 2,3-dimercapto propane-1-sulfonate (DMPS)[3] and 2,3-dimercaptosuccinic acid (DMSA).[4]

The Hubbard Protocol of Body/Mind Purification

There are three criteria for any program that reduces contaminating stores of heavy toxic metals such as mercury or polluting fat soluble chemicals like DDT (dichlorodiphenyltrichloroethane, a toxic

---

1   H. R. Casdorph and M. Walker, *Toxic Metal Syndrome: How Metal Poisoning Affects Your Brain* (Garden City Park, N.Y.: Avery Publishing Group, 1995).

2   J. P. Trowbridge and M. Walker, *The Healing Powers of Chelation Therapy: Unclog Your Arteries, an Alternative to Bypass Surgery* (Stamford, Conn.: New Way of Life, Inc., 1998).

3   A. Wannag and J. Aaseth, "The Effect of Immediate and Delayed Treatment with 2,3-Dimercaptopropane-1-Sulfonate (DMPS) on the Distribution and Toxicity of Inorganic Mercury in Mice and in Foetal and Adult Rats," *Acta Pharmacol Et Toxicol* 46 (1980): 81–88.

4   P. J. Kostyniak, "Methylmercury Removal in the Dog During Infusion of 2,3-Demercaptosuccinic Acid (DMSA)," *Journal Toxicol. Environ. Health* 11 (1983): 947–57.

%-3chlorinated hydrocarbon pesticide now banned in the United States). For such a detoxifying program or method to work effectively:

1. It must be nontoxic itself.

2. It must decrease the overall body burden of toxic metal, carcinogen, atherogen, allergen, mutagen, teratogen, filth, or any other form of disease-producing pollution.

3. It must reduce or eliminate symptoms caused by such pollutants.

The deceased, world renowned science fiction writer, philosopher, and humanitarian, L. Ron Hubbard, developed the technique of achieving a reduction in the adverse effects of metallic poisons, drugs, and pollutants. In 1979 Hubbard's research culminated in the protocol that I will summarize here from a lecture offered by Megan Shields, M.D. Dr. Shields delivered her talk to the American College for Advancement in Medicine (ACAM) on November 6, 1994, in San Diego, California. I was in the audience taking notes.

The Hubbard Protocol of Body/Mind Purification safely reduces adipose tissue levels of toxic materials stored in the body, using natural methods and without the administration of pharmaceuticals. Since the protocol's public introduction by Scientologists, a minimum of one hundred and twenty thousand persons worldwide have undertaken L. Ron Hubbard's detoxification technique.

Administration of the Hubbard protocol begins with a thorough health history and physical examination performed by an individual's participating physician. "A patient can be moderately ill and still undergo the treatment," said Dr. Shields. "Using it, I have successfully treated over three thousand people from age three to eighty-seven, sometimes with spectacular results. It is possible to treat persons with diabetes, hypertension, multiple sclerosis (who are notoriously heat intolerant), arthritis, and a host of other ailments. In each case modifications and adjustments must be made to tailor the program to that person. Good kidney function is a must, however, and persons with a diagnosis of congestive heart failure or cardiomyopathy are not good candidates."

The Hubbard therapy may be self-administered, but I recommend that it be taken under a physician's supervision. Sweating from the application of dry heat and flushing from dosing with niacin in the manner described below is highly effective to pull out the body's accumulated mercury.

Once treatment has begun, a precisely determined dose of niacin (vitamin B3) is taken by the patient. Because time-release (sustained-release) niacin is associated with liver dysfunction, the dose starts at 100 mg of immediate-release and *not* sustained-release niacin. The purpose of niacin ingestion is to cause a breakup of fat tissues (lipolysis) and the deliberate liberation of fat-stored toxins. The dosage of niacin is gradually increased until single doses of up to 5000 mg are taken without any noticeable effect (which may otherwise show itself as marked skin flushing, heating, and tingling). Once the detoxifying person has ingested the niacin, he or she then engages in aerobic exercise for up to thirty minutes to enhance blood circulation of the niacin and to cause mobilized toxins to be excreted by the body. Running is preferred as an aerobic activity, but this may be altered by using steady rope skipping, active rebounding on a minitrampoline, vigorous basketball playing, fast racket ball playing, hard-driving bicycling for long distances up steep hills, and so forth.

Next, for up to five hours daily, sweating is forced by use of wet or dry intermittent sauna treatment. The sauna must be maintained at a temperature ranging between 140ºF and 180ºF. And the sauna facility has to be very well ventilated. No weight loss is permitted, however, and potassium and salt with purified water are replenished as indicated by a check of the patient's vital signs by a medical doctor. Of course, the patient is weighed each day before and after treatment to guard against dehydration.

At the same time sauna treatment is being received, various polyunsaturated, cold-pressed oils are applied to the patient topically to block bowel and liver (enterohepatic) recirculation of toxins that are being excreted through the skin. An all-blend combination of the polyunsaturates—safflower, soy, peanut, and walnut oils—are preferred for application. This oil blend prevents any deposition in the liver of toxins from the lipolyz-ing fat.[1]

The patient also takes increased quantities of supplemental nutri-ents because of the potential for reduced absorption of these important nutrients, which can result in increased toxicity of persistent heavy metals such as mercury, nickel, titanium, and others and polluting chemicals such as PBB and PCB. These nutrients do a great deal of good. In one study, for instance, the clinician's administering of ascorbic acid (vitamin C) during polychlorinated biphenyl (PCB) detoxification eliminated liver enzyme activity degradation and histologic changes that otherwise would normally have been observed.[2]

Elimination of Toxic Metals from the Body and Brain

The vitamins A, C, and E, *Lactobacillus acidophilus*, the mineral selenium, the sulfhydryl amino acids L-cysteine, cystine, and methionine, and the foodstuffs garlic, apple pectin, and fiber are the nutrients used for their oral chelating effect as well. Some medical scientists maintain that a special liquid preparation called *biocatalyst water* can help dramatically in the detoxification process.

The synthetic amino acid ethylene diamine tetraacetic acid (EDTA), along with the substances British Anti-Lewisite (B.A.L.), cuprimine, penicillamine, and lithium carbonate are among the therapeutic chemicals that can be used to cleanse the human physi-ology of heavy metals, toxic metals, and chemical pollutants (includ-ing agent orange and those several toxicants that cause the Gulf War syndrome).

Particular amino acids, antioxidants, coenzymes, and other nu-trients are able to extract complexed heavy metals and toxic metals from human tissues. These beneficial substances detoxify the body

---

1   L. R. Hubbard, *Clear Body, Clear Mind: The Effective Purification Program* (Copenhagen, Denmark: New Era Publications International ApS, 1990).

2   D. W. Schnare, B. Max, and M. G. Shields, "Body Burden Reductions of PCBs, PBBs and Chlorinated Pesticides in Human Subjects," *Ambio: Journal of the Human Environment* 8 (1984): 5–6.

and brain so that pathological symptoms are minimized or avoided. All of the stored heavy and light toxic metallic substances are removed by the use of chelation therapy, the most intensive form of detoxification known to the medical community.

Intravenous Chelation Therapy for Metallic Detoxification

Intravenous chelation therapy is a safe, effective, comfortable, and relatively inexpensive treatment to detoxify and restore blood flow for those people who have an overburden of toxic metals in their tissue cells and along the walls of their blood vessels. During the intravenous chelation process, the ions of minerals floating in the bloodstream or other tissue fluids are captured and bonded into ringed structures by the EDTA synthetic amino acid that you have taken into your systemic circulation. The ions and the injected chelating agent eventually leave your body and brain through the two usual waste disposal systems, the urinary tract's kidneys or the gastrointestinal tract's bowel.

Intravenous chelation therapy has been known, but not generally used, by organized North American medicine for over forty-five years. About 5 million Canadians and Americans have benefited from the treatment. Around the world, approximately 38 million chelation infusions have been administered by chelating physicians in (alphabetically listed): Australia, the Bahamas, Belgium, Brazil, Canada, the Cayman Islands, Colombia, Costa Rica, Denmark, the Dominican Republic, Ecuador, Egypt, England, France, Germany, Greece, Hong Kong, Hungary, India, Indonesia, Ireland, Israel, Italy, Malaysia, Mexico, the Netherlands, New Zealand, Norway, Pakistan, Panama, Paraguay, the Philippines, Poland, Puerto Rico, Saudi Arabia, Spain, Switzerland, the United States, Venezuela, and the West Indies (Jamaica). Chelating physicians who are members of ACAM are located in these countries.

EDTA intravenous infusions remove undesirable metals from the body and brain, such as lead, mercury, cadmium, iron, aluminum, and arsenic. All metals, even essential nutritional elements, are toxic in excess or when they are abnormally situated anatomically. The

IV EDTA normalizes the distribution of most metallic elements in the body and brain. It improves calcium and cholesterol metabolism by eliminating metallic catalysts that cause damage to cell membranes through their production of "oxygen free radicals." Free radical pathology is known to be an important contributing cause of many degenerative diseases such as atherosclerosis, cancer, diabetes, the deterioration of aging, and much more. Free radicals themselves are, in fact, the sources of tissue degenerations. The administration of IV EDTA helps to prevent the production of harmful free radicals.

Usually, in accordance with the recommended protocol of the American College for Advancement in Medicine, an intravenous infusion for chelation therapy is administered over a four-hour period twice weekly. The safety of chelation therapy is absolutely proven. When properly administered by a physician who is fully trained and competent in the treatment's use, few, if any, side effects occur. Of course, as with any drug therapy, mild adverse side effects are possible. Vein irritation, mild pain, headache, and fatigue may occur. Occasionally a mild, transient fever appears. These and other inconsequential side effects, if they happen, are easily controlled by adjusting the duration and frequency of treatment, or with the use of other simple measures. Side effects tend to diminish after the first few treatments. Most patients hardly ever experience them.

Patients taking the treatment to unburden themselves of toxic metals that are causing symptoms of illness routinely report that they experience a reduction or disappearance of their difficulties. They acquire an increasing sense of well-being. Family friends are often the first to notice and report improvement in the way a chelation patient looks, behaves, and performs. Comparison of pretherapy and posttherapy diagnostic tests can provide objective evidence of the chelation treatment's effectiveness.

Oral Chelation Therapy

Actually merely a term of reference long used and somewhat misnamed, oral chelation therapy consists of certain nutritional agents taken by mouth that act as cellular detoxifiers. They tend to clean out waste products, pollutants, heavy metals, foreign proteins, and other poisonous materials from the body's cells. Such agents do this by displacing toxic substances in the cells or by diluting the electromagnetic energy stored in destructive free radicals that have been created by combining reactions within the tissues. The so-called oral chelating agents may include antioxidant nutrients, pharmaceuticals, metabolic factors, food substances, dietary supplements, herbs, homeopathic remedies, nutritional formulations, specific exercises promoting a person's systemic chelation, and other such ingredients. Over one hundred oral chelation agents and formulas for home use are readily available without prescription and over the counter.

The book, *Everything You Should Know about Chelation Therapy* (see appendix B), contains a full chapter devoted to a formula for an excellent oral chelating agent. This oral chelation nutritional formula was created by certified clinical nutritionist and doctor of chiropractic Michael Jude Loquasto, C.C.N., D.C., of Marshall's Creek, Pennsylvania.[1] Dr. Loquasto, favored with the name "Dr. Mike," by his patients, has created another nutritional formula and the dental diet. Both Dr. Mike's Dental Diet and Dr. Mike's Teeth and Gums Support Pack are dedicated to supporting all tissues of the oral cavity. They are discussed at length in chapter 16.

Medical consumers are finding out about intravenous and oral chelation therapy as life-extending programs and want them badly. Victims of degenerative diseases are desperate for the IV treatment to save their lives or to preserve their blood vessels, hearts, internal organs, limbs, vision, memories, bones, joints, neurons, and other parts of their body and brain.

The intravenous and oral chelating methods control common degenerative diseases such as arthritis, cataracts, stroke, heart attacks, diabetes, cancer, kidney disease, atherosclerosis, arteriosclerosis, radiation toxicity, osteoporosis, high blood pressure,

---

1   Walker and Shah, *Everything You Should Known about Chelation Therapy.*

senility, cirrhosis, Alzheimer's disease, schizophrenia, gangrene, varicose veins, glaucoma, hypercalcemia, angina pectoris, heart arrhythmias, impotence, Raynaud's disease, multiple sclerosis, lupus erythematosus, diabetic retinopathy, macular degeneration, Parkinson's disease, Lou Gehrig's disease, digitalis intoxication, heavy metal poisoning, toxic metal syndrome, intermittent claudication, sickle cell anemia, high-serum cholesterolemia, and chronic fatigue and immune dysfunction syndrome. The toxicity arising from dental mercury amalgams responds exceedingly well to EDTA chelation therapy and its accompanying nutritional oral chelators.

When I Had My Own Amalgams Replaced

When I undertook to have my dental amalgam fillings replaced with composites or gold by Stanley Machenberg, D.D.S., of Stamford, Connecticut (to whom I have dedicated this book), I went through a series of six IV treatments with EDTA. Such treatment was absolutely mandatory because my friend, Dr. Machenberg, practiced dentistry only conventionally according to the dictates of the American Dental Association. He was not oriented to holistic/biological dentistry. The protocol for amalgam removal was not followed back then.

My amalgam removal took place sixteen years ago, before my friend or I knew anything about the poisoning effects of mercury vapors associated with amalgams. Directly after the replacements, I experienced symptoms related to mercury toxicity. By now I have received upwards of one hundred and six EDTA intravenous infusions to accomplish the life-preserving regimen of chelation therapy. And I have researched the subject of chelation therapy thoroughly. I have written twenty-three published clinical journal or magazine articles and eight trade books on the subject of chelation therapy alone. In all, I have produced 2,200 published articles and 73 consumer health books (including this one).

From my own experience, I know that if ever amalgams must be removed because a dental patient or the parent of a minor patient finally understands the dangers wrought by them, appropriate protocols have to be followed as enforced by any mercury-free dental members of the four professional organizations cited in appendix C.

Which Dentist for Removing Amalgam Fillings?

It is imperative to consult only a holistic-oriented biological dentist who knows how to remove a patient's dental amalgam material safely. The removal must be accomplished in accordance with established tried and proven methods of amalgam withdrawal. As I have emphasized, the memberships of those four dental organizations listed in appendix C are comprised of skilled dentists who have knowledge and have taken training in the appropriate procedure for mercury amalgam fillings removal. Never request amalgam removal from just *any* dentist who is not properly prepared.

A procedure that is extremely important to follow is that the amalgams must be removed in the correct sequence. Fillings hold onto charged electrical current, and those amalgam fillings possessed of negative electrical charges should be removed before those with positive current. If performed in the opposite order, there may not only be an immediate worsening of symptoms, but it is also possible the symptoms will never be eliminated.

Thus you should choose the dentist to remove "silver" dental amalgams very carefully. Whether he or she is your personal friend in whom you have confidence (as was my situation), or a person you know only as a professional, the dentist you choose must be trained in the specific technique of amalgam removal as taught by Hal A. Huggins, D.D.S., of Colorado Springs, Colorado. This is a procedure learned by dentists when they become oriented to mercury-free/biocompatible and holistic (biological) dentistry. Dentists trained in this biocompatible method also investigate the existence of electricity and radio frequencies in the mouth. If taught at all, oral electricity is something that's hardly touched on in dental school.

As far back as 1880 a dentist described how an electrical current is generated when saliva comes into contact with a filling. But it wasn't until 1979 that modern dentists learned that electrical currents of the mouth occur as two types: positive and negative. At first the meaning was elusive but after observing a few hundred patients, it became apparent that people with more severe problems of health had fillings that registered negative current on an *ammeter*, a device for measuring electrical current. Also, it's known that four kinds of oral galvanism exist.

Galvanism is generally defined as any form of medical treatment using electricity, but in dentistry the term means much more because of the chemical battery created in one's mouth that offers a unidirectional electric current.

The Four Kinds of Oral Galvanism

There definitely is such a thing as galvanism in the oral cavity, a condition in which burns and other soft tissue changes such as gingivitis and bleeding are caused by an electrical potential difference. It's created by dissimilar metals in the oral cavity, with saliva serving as the electrolyte. Amalgam alloys include those dissimilar metals.

A dentist may create one or more of four types of galvanism that are responsible for bringing on various kinds of illnesses in the mouth, many of which are life-threatening.

First, there is the classic example of dental galvanism in which the "silver" dental amalgam placed in opposition or adjacent to a tooth restored with gold sets up an electric cell. The dissimilar metals in conjunction with saliva and body fluids close the contact and the circuit created is shorted so that the flow of electrical current passes through the tooth's pulp and produces pain.

Second, the potential pathway for these currents may occur between teeth in the same dental arch but not in contact with one another. Pain will shoot that way.

Third, and most widely recognized as a form of electrolytic action causing pain, is the classic case of dissimilar metals coming into contact when the mandibular and maxillary teeth occlude.

Fourth, a galvanic situation occurs when two adjacent teeth are restored with dissimilar metals. The current flows from metal to metal through the dentin, bone, and tissue fluids of both teeth. Then pain and discomfort hit.[1]

Be aware that gold and amalgam placed in contact in the oral

---

1   R I. Holland, "Galvanic Currents between Gold and Amalgam," *Scandinavian Journal of Dental Restoration* 88 (1980): 269–72.

cavity will definitely cause galvanic currents and increase corrosion of the amalgam with the release of mercury metallic ions. This vapor shoots up to the brain and is the likely cause for the elevated incidence of Alzheimer's disease around the world but most especially in the United States.[1]

Mercury Fillings Contribute to Alzheimer's Disease

Research reported by Dr. Hal Huggins indicates that once even a minute amount of mercury enters the brain from amalgams, it seriously damages nerve cells and produces the physical and structural dysfunction of brain tissue now linked with Alzheimer's.

The biochemistry is complex, but mercury damages a key substance needed for the brain's energy processes called creatine kinase, an enzyme that speeds up chemical reactions involving energy release. Autopsies show that the brain of a healthy person contains 2300 percent more creatine kinase than the brain of a person with Alzheimer's disease, affirms Dr. Huggins.

The brain needs creatine kinase to make another molecule called adenosine triphosphate (ATP), which is central to all energy processes in the body. Autopsies also show that the Alzheimer brain has reduced ATP levels compared to healthy subjects. ATP in turn is needed to keep a sequence of chemical steps going that end with the production of tubulin, a protein substance that gives cells (including brain and nerve cells) their shape and physical integrity. "The amount of reduction of tubulin activity is directly related to the degree of Alzheimer's," Dr. Huggins says. "No other type of neural degeneration or any other autoimmune disease of the nervous system shows a reduction in tubulin activity."[2]

At a mere concentration of six micromoles of mercury in the brain, there is a 69 percent reduction in tubulin activity, and at

---

1   Casdorph and Walker, *Toxic Metal Syndrome*.

2   R. Leviton, "Can Mercury Fillings Contribute to Alzheimer's?" *Alternative Medicine* 25 (August/September 1998): 52.

eleven micromoles, the tubulin reduction can be 92 percent, Dr. Huggins says.

In a Canadian study, rats were made to inhale a small amount of mercury vapor for four hours each day. The amount was comparable to that emitted by dental fillings, over time, in a human mouth. After two weeks, the animals' brains had formed the neurofibrillary tangles and cellular plaques within their brains characteristic of a human Alzheimer's brain. "The result of this process is that you lose brain cells and brain function," states Dr. Huggins.

Knowing this, the maverick dentist reversed the Alzheimer's disease of a particular fifty-year-old woman who had three mercury fillings and carried a nickel hip replacement (prosthesis). At the time of treatment, she was completely incommunicative with the external world. Her mind was not functioning. "She could handle the fillings," Dr. Huggins explains. "She could handle the prosthesis, but she couldn't handle both. The two together pushed her over into Alzheimer's." When Dr. Huggins removed the mercury fillings and detoxified the patient's body of all residual mercury by methods being described in this chapter, her Alzheimer's disease receded and she resumed talking and living normally.[1]

Sequential Amalgam Removal Is Mandatory

Those dentists who believe in replacing amalgams with substitute materials found that when negative current fillings were removed first, the patient had excellent chances for recovery of health. If the positively charged fillings were removed first, leaving negative charges behind, the patients rarely improved. Nobody knows why this circumstance is true, but it is. Thus sequential removal of amalgams according to their negative or positive charges is mandatory.

In the mouth, usual bacteria such as *Streptococcus mutans* (see chapter 15 for the oral cavity bacteria) can chemically change mercury vapor coming off the filling and cause it to become deadly

---

1   Ibid.

methylmercury, a chemical one hundred times more toxic than plain liquid mercury. (And mercury alone is the most toxic metal known to man.) It's possible that the chemical composition of saliva secreted immediately over a filling with negative electrical current would contain slightly less oxygen, making it more conducive to production of deadly methylmercury.

Another procedure to follow before removing dental amalgams is that there must be biochemical coverage with certain vitamin and mineral supplements before, during, and several months after the filling replacements. These nutritional supplements condition the cell membrane to enable the stored mercury to be excreted from the cells and to allow an increased amount of oxygen to get into the cells. There is a basic supplementation regimen to follow, which will be known by those trained as holistic (biological) dentists and ignored by any of the ordinary conventionally practicing, allopathic-type dentists who follow the American Dental Association party line. To become informed about appropriate nutritional supplementation for a healthy oral cavity, please see chapters 15 and 16.

Michael Gerber, M.D., Uses DMPS for Amalgam Detoxification

DMPS, the sodium salt of 2,3-Dimercapto propane-1-sulfonic acid, is the fourth amalgam detoxifier that's applied by some biological dentists and many holistic physicians who treat patients with complementary and alternative methods (CAM).

Showing an extraordinarily high affinity for grasping many different heavy metals, lifting them from the tissues, and taking them out of the body, DMPS is a chelating agent from the chemical group of vicinal dithiols that forms stable chemical complexes with those toxic and nontoxic metals. To remove patients' poisonous metallic substances, especially lead and mercury, DMPS may be administered by health professionals who are licensed to do so. These include medical doctors, naturopathic physicians, or osteopathic physicians. DMPS is given either orally or by injection.

Absorption of orally administered DMPS takes place rapidly, and a parenteral (intermuscular or intravenous) injection of the substance acts even faster. This substance brings about no mutagenic or teratogenic side effects; rather, DMPS is an effective antidote for heavy metal intoxications.[1]

A correctly performed treatment with DMPS not only unburdens a dental amalgam patient of mercury poisoning, it also acts simultaneously to provide the attending physician and dentist with diagnostic information.[2] toxifies almost all of the metals frequently employed by dentists, including cadmium, selenium, manganese, beryllium, nickel, chromium, vanadium, tin, silicon, mercury, rubidium, platinum, lithium, and more.[3]

Particularly with mercury toxins lodged in the body, DMPS forms stable, water-soluble complexes of Hg2 + ions[4] and methylmercury CH3Hg,[5] which go into solution and leave the body together as a waste product. For chronic mercury poisoning from amalgam

1   J. Aaseth, D. Jacobsen, O. Andersen, and E. Wickstrom, "Treatment of Mercury and Lead Poisonings with Dimercaptosuccinic Acid and Sodium Dimercapto-propanesulfonate. A Review," *Human Analyst* 120, no. 3 (1995): 853–54.

2   H. V. Aposhian, D. Gonzalez-Ramirez, R. M. Maiorino, M. Zuniga-Charles, K. M. Hurlbut, and R. C. Dart, "DMPS (Dimaval) as a Challenge Test to Assess the Mercury and Arsenic Body/Kidney Load in Humans and as a Treatment of Mercury Toxicity," paper presented at the Pacific Basin Conference on Hazardous Waste, Malaysia, 1996.

3   H. Zumkley and H. P. Bertram, "Spurenelemente-Klinische Bedeutung nach Heutigem Kenntnisstand. 2 Kadmium, Selen., Mangan, Beryllium, Nickel, Chrom., Vanadium, Silizium, Quecksilber, Rubidium, Platn., Lithium," *Much. Med. Wochenschr* 124, nos. 32, 33 (1982): 709–11.

4   H. V. Aposhian, "Development of New Methods for Dithiol Analysis and Urinary Excretion of DMPS and DMSA," progress report for May 1984 to June 1986, The Heyltex Corporation, Houston, Texas 77042, January 1997; L. A. Volf, "The Use of Unithiol as a Masking Reagent in the Complexometric Determination of Calcium and Magnesium," *Independent Laboratory USSR* 25, no. 12 (1959): 1507–08; D. B. Wildenauer, H. Reuther and N. Weber, "Interactions of the Chelating Agent 2,3-Dimercapto propane-1-Sulfonate with Red Blood Cells In Vitro. 1 Evidence for Carrier Mediated Transport," *Chem. Biol. Interact* 42, no. 2 (1982): 165–77.

5   A. P. Arnold, A. J. Canty, P. W. Moors, and G. B. Deacon, "Chelation Therapy for Methylmercury (II) Poisoning. Synthesis and Determination of Solubility Properties of MeHg (II) Complexes of Thiol and Dithiol Antidotes," *Journal of Inorganic Biochemistry* 19, no. 4 (1983): 319–27; R. M. Smith and A. E. Martell, *Critical Stability Constants*, vol. 6, second supplement (New York: Plenum Press, 1992).

fillings, oral dosage forms of DMPS are preferred because of the simpler procedure for long-term therapy. Generally, the preparation is given at a dose of 100 mg three times a day.[1] For small children with poisoning from dental amalgams, the oral DMPS dose is 50 mg three times a day.[2] The longest period of treatment recorded for amalgam mercury removal lasted for four-and-a-half years.[3]

"I am performing a two-hour urine collection taken from my numerous amalgam-poisoned patients after they've gone through the DMPS intravenous challenge test," says orthomolecular medicine physician Michael L. Gerber, M.D., of Reno, Nevada. "Often I find that a huge amount of mercury comes out of these poisoned people within just the first two hours. With a two-hour collection, the quantity of mercury content is much more impressive than the concentrations seen following a full twenty-four-hour urine collection.

"With dentists putting about one hundred tons of mercury into the mouths of perhaps 100 million Americans every year, we are facing a national tragedy in this country. It's only by good luck that we have DMPS available to pull out the metal from these people's bodies," Dr. Gerber told me. "Documenting mercury toxicity in someone was exceedingly difficult prior to our having DMPS, because the amalgamated mercury binds tightly onto connective tissue. It hardly shows in the urine without DMPS unless the patient has just eaten a mercury-filled thermometer or the equivalent. Then the doctor might find some indication of mercury concentrated in that patient."

DMPS is not an approved drug in the United States. In Europe, it is marketed by the Heyl Coeerzalle Company, under the brand name Dimaval at a recommended dosage of one tablet, three times

1   N. Neuburger, "Monographie: Dimercaptopropansulfonsaure," *Budesanzeiger* 13 (1994): 10.

2   F. H. Kemper, F. W. Jekat, H. P. Bertram, and R. Eckard, in *Basic Science in Toxicology; Proceedings of the Fifth International Congress of Toxicology*, eds. G. N. Volans, J. Sims, F. M. Sullivan, and P. Turner (London: Taylor & Francis Publishers, Ltd., 1990), 523–46.

3   C. E. Ashton, I. House, and G. Volans, "A Case of Severe Intravenous Metallic Poisoning Managed Successfully with Prolonged Dimercapto-1-Propanesulphonate Therapy," paper presented at the annual meeting of the European Association of Toxicology and Poison Control Centers, Istanbul, 1992.

a day. In the United States, Heyl Coeerzalle's name is Americanized to Heyltex Corporation. To acquire more information about the detoxification attributes of DMPS or to actually receive quantities of the product, contact the Heyltex Corporation. (See its officer, location, and telephone in appendix B.)

In addition to using DMPS for purposes of detoxification when he sees that his patients are overburdened by mercury, Dr. Gerber also administers IV EDTA chelation therapy or DMSA, another chelating substance for toxic metals.

What Is DMSA and What Does It Do?

Holistic and alternative medicine physician Michael B. Schachter, M.D., medical director of the Schachter Center for Complementary Medicine in Suffern, New York, applies DMSA for the elimination of mercury burdens from the body. Dr. Schachter also uses the product as a testing material to determine whether an individual's mercury levels may be the cause of a patient's health problem. He works with biological dentists toward ridding his patients of metallic poisons in their mouths.

DMSA, an abbreviation for 2,3-DiMercaptosuccinic Acid, is marketed under the trade name "Chemet" and the generic name "succimer." DMSA is approved by the FDA for treatment of lead toxicity in children, and it's also an excellent oral chelating agent for removing mercury from the adult body. It crosses the blood-brain barrier and pulls out toxic mercury from the brain and other body tissues.

"The active portion of the DMSA molecule, which binds mercury and other toxic metals, consists of two sulfur atoms next to each other. Frequently, the heavy metals are removed sequentially," explains Dr. Schachter. "For example, the treatment may first remove lead with only small amounts of mercury. Later, after much of the lead is removed, the mercury may begin to be chelated out in larger quantities."

A provocative dose of DMSA is provided by a laboratory asked to conduct a urine mercury test. The lab furnishes a container to hold urine collected by the patient over six hours. When the analysis of the urine indicates significant levels of mercury are present, it is a signal that the body tissue levels are high. That being the situation, Dr. Schachter prescribes DMSA for the removal of mercury and other toxic metals, such as lead, cadmium, arsenic, and nickel. This is done in conjunction with the removal of the source of the toxic metal contamination.

The dosage of DMSA generally prescribed at the Schachter Center is between 100 and 500 mg, taken on an empty stomach, three times a week, for five weeks. None is then taken for two weeks. The process is again repeated for five weeks. The test is then repeated. This cycle is repeated as often as necessary to reduce the metallic mercury load in the body.

If amalgams are not removed or removal is postponed, "it is predictable that tissue levels of mercury in the body will build up again as mercury is constantly released from the teeth," says Dr. Schachter. "In such cases, periodically repeating urine mercury testing and a course of DMSA chelation therapy is recommended."

Steven Bock, M.D., Uses DMSA for Detoxifying Mercury

Like DMPS, DMSA (legally used in the United States) is quite effective in removing mercury from the body after the individual has undergone prolonged exposure to the toxic metal from dental amalgam fillings. DMSA is the fifth program provided in this chapter for detoxifying the body after prolonged exposure to amalgamated mercury. The research of Joseph H. Graziano, Ph.D., a pharmacologist performing research at the Columbia University College of Physicians and Surgeons, indicates that DMSA has definite value against leaching mercury connected with amalgam removal.

"Working by the system that a patient is having symptoms of illness because of cumulative abuses, my brother [see chapter 7's interview with Kenneth A. Bock, M.D.] and I don't treat just one causative trigger. We look at the total sources of environmental factors, many of them related to oral ill health that comes from amalgam fillings, root canals, cavitations, fluoride in the drinking water, peridontal disease, and so forth," says medical doctor, certified acupuncturist, and chelation therapist Steven Bock, M.D., who practices medicine in Rhinebeck and Albany, New York. "I estimate that pathology of the teeth, in particular mercury amalgam toxicity, makes up from 40 to 50 percent of all of my patients' health problems. I've concluded that there is no normal level of mercury allowable in the body.

"Amalgams in teeth impair a person's enzyme systems. The mercury causes symptoms in someone whose reserve is low in the particular group of enzymes. That's where mercury toxicity shows up from our giving the patient a DMSA challenge test," Dr. Steve Bock explains. "Before the challenge, however, we acquire the patient's six-hour urine collection to achieve a baseline for how much undisturbed mercury is present compared to what the challenge pulls out.

"Then, my brother or I initially administer to this patient 500 mg of DMSA by mouth three times a week for a month. We take our patient off of the oral DMSA for a week and then perform another urine collection to see what the mercury burden has become," says Dr. Bock. "Next, we elevate the oral dosage of DMSA to 1000 mg three times weekly. Finally, just before the patient has amalgams removed, we drop the detoxifying DMSA dosage to 500 mg three times weekly. Immediately following the patient's amalgam removal, when mercury vapor has escaped from the mouth into the blood and brain, the DMSA dose must go up to 500 mg per day to pull the poison out of the body and brain. This higher DMSA dosage is accompanied by an intravenous infusion of free radical-quenching vitamin C. I also combine homeopathic kidney drainage remedies, because mercury has an affinity for the kidneys. I want my patient to have the kidneys in an elimination mode. There you have a part of the Bock brothers' technique of amalgam detoxification."

There are few, if any, side effects to DMSA at the recommended dose. There may be some detoxification symptoms from residual mercury buried in the patient's tissues, however. If this is the case, the temporary ill effects of such symptoms are far less of a problem than the permanent ill effect of high levels of mercury remaining in the body. In fact, the most common treatment of removing mercury from the system causes people to notice improvement in their short-term memory, sharper concentration, and a decrease in "foggy" thinking.

In addition to the five cited detoxification programs for neutralizing mercury poisoning, listed here with references for obtaining further information are some more detoxifiers provided by the medical research writer, H. L. Queen, from his textbook, *Chronic Mercury Toxicity*.[1] The additional mercury amalgam detoxifiers are:

N-Acetyl-D, L-penicillamine or NADP, which is newly available to medical doctors, osteopathic physicians, naturopaths, and dentists in North America.[2]

N,N'-di-phenyl-p-phenylenediamine or DPPD[3]

Polymercaptal Microspheres[4]

Thiol Antidote[5]

Methicillin[6]

Hemoperfusion[7]

---

1   Queen, *Chronic Mercury Toxicity*, 278.

2   H. V. Aposhian and M. M. Aposhian, "N-Acetyl-DL-Penicillamine, a New Oral Protective Agent against the Lethal Effects of Mercuric Chloride," *Journal of Pharmacology and Experimental Therapy* 126 (1959): 131–35; D. O. Hryhorczuk and others, "Treatment of Mercury Intoxication in a Dentist with N-Acetyl-D, L-Penicillamine," *Journal of Toxicology and Clinical Toxicology* 19, no. 4 (1982): 401–08.

3   S. O. Welsh, "The Protective Effect of Vitamin E and N,N'-Di-Phenyl-P-Phenylenediamine (DPPD) against Methyl Mercury Toxicity in the Rat," *Journal of Nutrition* 109 (1979): 1673–81.

4   S. Margel and J. Hirsh, "Chelation of Mercury by Polymercaptal Microspheres: New Potential Antidote for Mercury Poisoning," *Journal of Pharmaceutical Sciences* 71, no. 9 (September 1982): 1030–34.

5   E. Giroux and P. J. Lachmann, "Thiol Antidote to Inorganic Mercury Toxicity with an Uncharacteristic Mechanism," *Toxicology and Applied Pharmacology* 67 (1983): 178–83.

6   K. Twardowska-Saucha, "Evaluation of the Chelating Action of Methicillin in Prolonged Experimental Metallic Mercury Poisoning," *British Journal of Industrial Medicine* 43 (1986): 611–14.

7   T. J. Pellinen and others, "Letter to the Editor: Hemoperfusion in Mercury Poisoning," *Journal of Toxicology and Clinical Toxicology* 20, no. 2 (1983): 187–89.

Neonatal Extracorporeal Hemodialysis removes 6 percent of the body burden of methylmercury, compared to 1 percent through normal excretory pathways.[1]

Self-Detoxification at Home with Cleansing Baths

While some of the techniques of detoxification may seem overly sophisticated, medically expensive, or just too much trouble, certainly you can do something useful for yourself that doesn't require any more effort than bathing. Taking certain kinds of cleansing baths offers some excellent self-treatment methods of detoxification at home. They are recommended by mercury-free dentist Bill Wolfe, D.D.S., H.N.D., of Albuquerque, New Mexico. What follows are four types of bathing that work well to accomplish external and some internal detoxification:

Clorox Brand Bleach Bath: To detoxify mercury from the body as a result of leaching from dental amalgam fillings, prepare bath water with one-half to one cup of liquid Clorox brand bleach in a medium-hot bath. Soak in this solution for twenty to thirty minutes. Then rinse off with cool water.

Epsom Salt Bath: To detoxify mercury from the body as a result of dental amalgam fillings, prepare bath water with an average dosage of four pounds of Epsom salts. Spend from twelve to fifteen minutes in the tub (but not longer). Then rinse off with cool water. The Epsom salt may be absorbed so much through the

---

1   P. J. Kostyniak and others, "An Extracorporeal Complexing Hemodialysis System for the Treatment of Methylmercury Poisoning. 1 *In Vitro* Studies of the Effects of Four Complexing Agents on the Distribution of Dialyzability of Methylmercury in Human Blood," *Journal of Pharmacology and Experimental Therapy* 192 (1975): 260–69; M. E. Lund and others, "Treatment of Acute Methylmercury Ingestion by Hemodialysis with N-Acetylcysteine (Mucomyst) and Infusion 2,3-Dimercapto propane Sulfonate," *Journal of Toxicology and Clinical Toxicology* 22 (1984): 31–49; S. B. Elhassani and others, "Exchange Transfusion Treatment of Methylmercury-Poisoned Children," *Environmental Science Health* 13 (1978): 63–80.

skin that you'll experience diarrhea for a short time. (You may recall that drinking Epsom salts has a laxative effect.)

Apple Cider Vinegar Bath: To detoxify mercury from the body as a result of dental amalgam fillings, prepare bath water containing one quart of apple cider vinegar. Soak in the tub for thirty minutes using hot water, and rinse off with tepid water.

Seasalt and Baking Soda Bath: To detoxify radiation particles from the body as a result of overexposure to your computer or some other source or from mercury toxicity as a result of dental amalgam fillings, prepare bath water using a combination of one pound each of seasalt and baking soda. Soak for twenty to thirty minutes (average time is twenty-five minutes). Then rinse off with cool water.

The Safe Way for Your Dentist to Remove Your Amalgam Fillings

It's not my intention to have the newly enlightened and conscientious allopathic dentist use the section of information that follows as an instruction tool for amalgam removal. He or she should take such instruction from one of the membership organizations dedicated to holistic, biological, biocompatible, mercury-free dentistry. Instead, this section is offering the 220 million or more dental consumers in the United States with amalgam still in their mouths general information about the safe way to have dentists remove amalgam fillings without causing extra health difficulties.

Here is a summary of procedures for the reputable dentist to follow in order to accomplish safe dental amalgam removal:[1]

---

1   W. R. Kellas and A. S. Dworkin, *Surviving the Toxic Crisis: Understanding, Preventing and Treating the Root Causes of Chronic Illness* (Olivenhain, Calif.: Professional Preference, 1996), 201, 202.

- Use a rubber latex sheet called "dental dam" in the mouth to prevent the patient from swallowing mercury particles.

- Use a high speed vacuum to remove drilled-out bits of amalgam filling material and the mercury vapor accompanying it.

- Use drapes over the patient so that no mercury chips are carried home to members of the patient's family or absorbed through the patient's exposed skin.

- Have inhalation oxygen or clean air attached to the patient through a nosepiece rather than allowing that person to inhale mercury vapor-laden air through the mouth or nose.

- Use a lighted magnifying instrument to see and remove every bit of amalgam removed from the patient's mouth.

- Using a special blue light, check teeth for cracks, which are common with mercury fillings.

- Repair dental cracks to stabilize the patient's tooth structure before crowns are required.

- Indicate you take mercury toxicity seriously by wearing protective gloves and mask.

- Cut up the filling to remove it in sections rather than drilling or grinding it out of the patient's teeth; this technique avoids the inhaling or ingesting of fine mercury mist by the patient.

- Use an air filtering system in the dental office to protect not only patients waiting for service but also the dental office personnel.

- Perform biocompatible testing for any replacement materials, adhesives, anesthetics, or other chemicals to be applied to the dental patient.

A Typical Dental Appointment Plan for Amalgam Removal

Below is a procedural program followed by Mark S. Hulet, D.D.S., director of the Dental Mercury Treatment Center in Victorville, California. Dr. Hulet is a practitioner of preventive biological dentistry who almost exclusively engages in the removal and replacement of mercury amalgam dental fillings with more patient compatible materials. He has published the schedule for anyone to read and act on:

First Appointment:

1. Orientation, health history, complete oral examination, mercury vapor test, electrical test, evaluation and screening.

2. Counseling in diet modification and mineral supplementation; this counseling is required before the doctor begins mercury elimination from the teeth.

3. After evaluation of the patient's mouth, the following tests or recordings may be recommended:

biocompatibility testing	pulses, temperature,
blood chemistry	blood pressure, and so forth
lymphocyte viability testing	trace element analysis
complete blood count	urine mercury screening

Blood, hair, and urine are required from the patient in order to examine these specimens and determine the severity and effects of mercury on the patient's nutritional deficiency status. Results take approximately three weeks to come back from the laboratories

4. Within one week after the initial examination, a diagnosis and proposed treatment plan are reviewed with the patient by telephone. In addition to mercury and other metallic problems, this information includes all dental conditions discovered, such as periodontal difficulties.

Second Appointment:

1. Dental treatment consisting of mercury removal and replacement with bonded composite. The treatment usually is accomplished in one day.

2. More complicated dental treatments requiring crowns, bridges, reconstruction, and temporomandibular joint (TMJ) correctionusually are done in all-day appointments and in as few visits as possible.

3. Dental reconstruction and temporomandibular joint dysfunction requirements are evaluated and treated separately.

Third Appointment:

Post treatment evaluation takes place, which includes a urine mercury test at the third week. When indicated, laboratory tests at three-month intervals to monitor improvement are carried out. There are tests composed of blood chemistry, complete blood count, urine mercury excretion, and so forth.

A Final Note on Detoxification

Dietrich Klinghardt, M.D., of Seattle, Washington, who is considered by his colleagues to be the holistic doctors' doctor and teacher, has described a typical patient who is mercury intoxicated and additionally suffers from mercury sensitivity.

Lecturing at the Enderlein Enterprises Isopathic/Homeopathic Seminar on biological dentistry, Dr. Klinghardt told his colleagues: "If a dental patient is tested and shows he or she is allergic to mercury but still requires detoxification from being poisoned by amalgam fillings, the known detoxification procedures [as stated in this chapter] must be carried out again and again. Because of repeated mercury buildup, detoxification is required about every six weeks. Furthermore, there are effective detoxifying nutrient substances such as chlorella and other green foods, which when given on a continuous basis, seem to take on an appearance to the patient's physiology that basis, seem to take on an appearance to the patient's physiology that looks like mercury itself. In the same way that Pavlov's dogs displayed operant conditioned reflex, the mercury-sensitive patient becomes conditioned to chlorella."

To break this immune system response, whether it be to neutralize the allergens of mercury, chlorella, or anything else related to dental metal toxicity, Dr. Klinghardt advises that the medical doctor or dentist should create an antidote. This type of antidotal therapy may be accomplished by using some of the techniques espoused by clinical ecologists. In brief, they consist of creating homeopathic dosage remedies that are administered sublingually. For further information about the correct clinical ecological methods required, please contact the American Academy of Environmental Medicine (AAEM). You will find the AAEM address and telephone number in appendix A.

Ten

The Good and Bad of Substitutes for Dental Amalgam Fillings

The commonly implanted dental amalgam filling lasts for an average of eight years, often to be replaced with more silver/mercury amalgamated material. If you suffer with amalgam-associated symptoms of illness such as fibromyalgia, chronic fatigue syndrome, lupus erythematosis, rheumatoid arthritis, or another form of immune system suppression, instead of putting a fresh supply of toxic metal into the dental cavity, why not ask your dentist to substitute another, less toxic or nontoxic substance?

No artificial product will be as good as natural teeth, but any of the dental materials described below will be better than dental amalgam as the means of avoiding illnesses. While there are good and bad aspects to all of them, a substitute could be any of the following:

1. One of the white composite resin filling materials (for a description, see the next section in this chapter)

2. Some of the gold filling materials

3. Gold crowns

4. Porcelain

5. A porcelain fused to gold crowns

6. Porcelain fused to nontoxic metal crowns

7. Plastic

Anyway you do it, your treatment for mercury hypersensitivity or mercury toxicity from dental amalgam really starts with getting rid of the mercury still present in your mouth. Substitution for these toxic amalgam fillings usually leads to an immediate improvement in chronic fatigue syndrome, lupus erythematosis, parasite overgrowth, candidiasis, fibromyalgia, rheumatoid arthritis, mental confusion, impotency, unexplained fevers, sore throats, nausea, problems with falling asleep, depression, low motivation, low blood pressure, decreased libido, constipation, inappropriate weight gain, dry skin or hair, elevated cholesterol, glucose intolerance, allergies, cold intolerance, slow wound healing, anxiety attacks, tinnitus, joint pains, muscular aches, severe menstrual cramps, or almost one hundred other immune system suppression symptoms of disease.[1]

Substitute Alternatives for Mercury Amalgam

There's a better procedure to follow than waiting for dental filling corrosion to force you into amalgam replacement. That improvement has been recommended for inclusion here by Edward Arana, D.D.S., of Carmel Valley, California, president of the American Academy of Biological Dentistry. It involves allotting yourself the time and setting aside the money to take out every bit of mercury amalgam material in your dental cavities. Dr. Arana suggests that you consider replacing this highly poisonous metal with other, less toxic materials, such as dental gold alloy (gold mixed with palladium, copper, or cobalt). More sophisticated substitutes, preferred by some dental specialists, are enamel and dentin bonding composites. They are electric insulators and avoid electrolytic corrosion problems with metallic restorations in the same mouth. Additionally, composites are thermally insulated and protect the tooth's pulp against temperature changes.

You might ask, "What are the best alternative materials, other than gold, for replacing mercury amalgam? To answer this question,

---

1   P. Yutsis and M. Walker, *The Downhill Syndrome* (Garden City Park, N.Y.: Avery Publishing Group, 1997), 138, 139.

I quizzed six dentists who practice using methods advocated by Dr. Arana's American Academy of Biological Dentistry. Answers varied considerably, from glass ionomers to the Class 2 (plastic) resins to mercury-free amalgam to silver to porcelain. The most popular technique of refilling a decayed caries hole in the tooth were the Class 2 resins. The brand most often preferred for aesthetic reasons, ease of placement, lack of toxicity, low cost, and good wear was a resin called *Herculite*.

The resin composite, Herculite XR/XRV Enamel Paste, consists of the following molecular components with the addition of the dental profession's idiomatic abbreviations (acronyms):

- Bis-phenol-A-bis-(2-hydroxy-3-methacryloxypropyl) ether or BISGMA

- Triethyleneglycoldimethacrylate or TEGDM

- Ethoxylated bis-phenol-Apdimethacrylate or EBADM

- 2-Hydroxy-4-methoxybenzophenone or UV-9

- 2,6-Di-(tert-butyl)-4-methylphenol or BHT

- 1,7,7-Trimethylbicyclo-[2.2.1]-hepta-2,3-dione or CQ

- 10-Methoxy-1-sulfostilbene-3-triazolonapthalene, sodium salt or TINOPAL

- 2-(Ethylhexyl)-4-(dimethylamino)benzoate or ODMAB

- Fumed silicon dioxide or TS530

- Zinc oxide or OX-50

- *gamma*-Methacryloxypropyltrimethoxysilane or A174

- Barium aluminoborosilicate or SP345

- Titanium dioxide or TiO_2

- Pigments

Advantages of Substituting Composite for Amalgam

Enamel and dentin bonding composites contain no mercury or other toxic heavy metals. They are electric insulators and don't create electrolytic corrosion problems with metallic restorations in the same mouth. Additionally, composites are thermally insulating to protect the tooth's pulp against temperature changes, and their full strength is attained quickly to reduce early failure. Finishing and polishing of the composite is done during one placement appointment. Tooth structure bonding is effective, with little mechanical retention necessary. Better yet, no corrosion products are created by composites as with amalgams.

Of the composites, the 3M Corporation's self-cured restorative, P-10, is the most wear-resistant and strongest posterior resin bonded ceramic available. A relatively new 3M product called P-30 has good tensile and compression strength. Fillings made from P-30 are safe to put in your mouth, but the pain that comes on postoperatively, along with potential sensitivity and possible allergy may be complicating factors. Some people feel temperature sensitivity unless certain calcium hydroxide products and glass ionomer cements are placed as a base over the exposed dentin. Brushing with desensitizing tooth pastes helps to overcome some of the discomforting feelings of sensitivity. (But, as discussed in the coming chapter 14, avoid fluoride in toothpaste).

Contrasted with other amalgam substitutes, the following listing indicates that composites offer particular advantages. Composite materials used for filling dental cavities will

1. contain no mercury;

2. last almost as long as amalgam fillings;

3. be white, esthetically pleasing, and appear like natural teeth to another person;

4. *not* generate electrical currents in your head so that no radio waves are broadcast;

5. *not* produce any of the four types of galvanism in the mouth that occur from the placement of dissimilar oral metals;

6. *not* corrode;

7. *not* demand as much loss of tooth structure as with drilling for placement of amalgam fillings;

8. be thermally insulating so that no feelings of hot and cold discomforts present themselves;

9. be actually restorative and increase the strength of teeth into which they are placed (unlike amalgams, which don't restore anything but rather are entirely destructive).

Possible Sensitivity to Composite Materials

Composites are comprised of filling materials made out of ground glass powder mixed with a plastic binder. Implanting them requires more time from the dentist, so their application will probably cost more than amalgam fillings. There are light-cure composites and chemical-cure composites. In using the light-cured material, the dentist places the composite into a tooth in plastic form and concentrates a special light on the substance that causes it to harden in place. The chemical-cured fillings require two pastes that, when mixed together, set up a chemical reaction that hardens the composite in place.

Composite filling materials such as these are only partially safe, because about 50 percent of dental patients will likely experience some minor immune system reaction from them. A few immuno-reactive chemicals in these composites may produce more serious reactions, and then no form of composite may be employed as a substitute filling material. To ensure that you are not one of those who is highly sensitive to composite, the dentist should conduct serum compatibility testing.

"This [testing] is especially critical," warns author Tom Warren in his book, *Beating Alzheimer's*, "since many composites contain aluminum or tin. Both of these materials are heavy metal contaminants and may be harmful." Incidentally, Tom Warren rid himself of Alzheimer's disease by eliminating dental amalgam fillings from his oral cavity. (See Tom Warren's book listed in appendix B.).[1]

---

1   T. Warren, *Beating Alzheimer's: A Step towards Unlocking the Mysteries of Brain Diseases* (Garden City Park, N.Y.: Avery Publishing Group, 1991), 171.

(Read in this book's chapter 9 how Hal A. Huggins, D.D.S., reversed Alzheimer's disease for a patient of his by eliminating three mercury amalgam fillings from her mouth.)

In passing, I should mention that allergic people do tend to tolerate the light-cured composite materials better than they take to the chemical-cured materials. Dr. Hal Huggins has revealed this in his many writings.[1]

The glass ionomer materials are favored mostly by those dentists whose patients have encountered postoperative sensitivity to plastic resins. A few dentists have turned to implanting the nearly pure silver fillings, but most fear that the patient could risk toxicity to silver. One dentist from California, Joyal Taylor, D.D.S., president of the Environmental Dental Association (a holistic group of mercury-free dentists listed in appendix C), favors using solid porcelain. "There is no electrical conduction with porcelain as seen in gold alloy and other metals," states Dr. Taylor, "and it doesn't vaporize as do some composites. Cost is porcelain's only negative."

It's expensive. Overall, Dr. Joyal Taylor believes that porcelain is an excellent material for the highly sensitive or allergic patient.

Sensitivity to Every Form of Dental Substance

Scott R. McAdoo, D.D.S., biological dentist and former associate of Dr. Huggins, (who no longer practices dentistry at his own Huggins Diagnostic Center in Colorado Springs, Colorado), reports that allergenic-type reactivity to nearly every dental material occurs in 50 percent of his dental patients. In good conscience, consequently, Dr. McAdoo admits there is no dental material that shows up safe enough to beat the "toss of the coin" system of choosing an amalgam substitute. All materials placed

---

1   H. A. Huggins, *It's All in Your Head: The Link between Mercury Amalgams and Illness* (Garden City Park, N.Y.: Avery Publishing Group, 1993), 78, 79.

into the mouth by dentists have some form of sensitivity connected to them.

Dr. McAdoo recommends that the dentist should undertake a biocompatibility study beforehand to determine which materials to use and which to avoid. To learn more about such a study, you may wish to contact Dr. McAdoo at the Huggins Diagnostic Center (see the address listing in appendix D). Perhaps you'll be fortunate to reach that master dentist and holistic dental pioneer, Hal Huggins.

For reasons similar to those given by Dr. McAdoo, Walter Jess Clifford, M.S., R.M. (AAM), director of Clifford Consulting and Research, recommends that you read his report, *Materials Reactivity Testing*, before even thinking about removing the dental amalgam fillings in your mouth. The testing procedures required offer you an immunological determination of systemic sensitization to components that emanate from oral cavity biomaterials. You can contact Walter Jess Clifford about the evaluation techniques for sensitivity or receive his mailed report by paying US$15 to Clifford Consulting and Research. (See his laboratory's address listing in appendix D).

Amalgam Substitutes Are Mandatory

If a pregnant woman has dental amalgam fillings in her mouth, chances are high that her embryo or later the fetus (each appearing, in turn, during the developing baby's first trimester) is being poisoned by absorbing mercury through the placenta. The mercury is leaching from the fillings into the pregnant woman's blood stream. This poisonous ingredient then becomes part of the (mal)nourishment she is sending to her newly developing baby.

This theoretical statement was proven to be true in a 1994 medical investigation. Mercury concentrations were measured in various tissues of fetuses. The tissues were obtained from fetuses taken as a result of medically necessary abortions. Additionally, newborn babies who died mainly from sudden infant death syndrome were studied for mercury content of their tissues. The concentration of mercury in the kidneys and liver of fetuses and in the kidney and cerebral cortex of infants correlated significantly with the number of dental amalgam fillings in the mouths of the tested mothers.[1]

Commenting on this pathology study, Alan R. Gaby, M.D., of Seattle, Washington, who is medical editor of the *Townsend Letter for Doctors and Patients*, stipulated why amalgam substitutes are mandatory. Dr. Gaby wrote in his monthly column: "Mercury is one of the most toxic elements on earth. Small amounts of mercury vapor leach continually from dental amalgams and the potential dangers of this constant exposure have been debated vigorously. The present study suggests that fetal tissues accumulate mercury that leaches from the mother's dental amalgam. The possible adverse effects of dental amalgams on fetal growth and development warrant further investigation."[2]

Teeth Affect the Health and Function of Internal Organs

That mercury amalgam fillings, root canals (dead teeth with nerves removed—see chapter 12), cavitations (infection within the jawbone—see chapter 13), and periodontal disease (infections under the gums—see chapter 15) can affect the health and function of internal organs, including those of an unborn child, is a clinical reality that Thomas Rau, M.D., deals with every day. Dr. Rau is medical director of the Paracelsus Clinic in Lustmuhle, Switzerland, and he always looks for dental problems in his patients when he's assessing their cases.

Until now, among nearly all conventionally practicing physicians and for too large a number of alternative medicine professionals, the role of the teeth in overall health—that they influence and even disturb the individual's internal organs—is still a neglected, underresearched

---

1   G. Drasch and others, "Mercury Burden of Human Fetal and Infant Tissues," *European Journal of Pediatrics* 153 (1994): 607–10.

2   A. R. Gaby, "Literature Review and Commentary. Mothers' Amalgam-Mercury Accumulates in Fetus," *Townsend Letter for Doctors and Patients* 147 (October 1995), 19.

topic. But an open-minded approach to medical practice has led Dr. Rau to discover some surprising connections. The prerequisite for successful, long-term holistic care, he says, is the recognition of the importance of a patient's teeth in their overall health picture.

Dr. Rau practices medicine in a holistic or biological manner. "Biological medicine observes a person as one whole, functional biological unit. If one part of the body is sick, this will make other parts of the body sick also. One of the essentials to rebalancing the body's internal environment is paying attention to the teeth," Dr. Rau explains. "It is my philosophy that to practice with a high level of success it is of utmost importance to incorporate holistic dentistry.

"So many of the body's mechanisms of regulation, regeneration, adaptation, and self-healing are blocked due to dental problems, usually from a 'dental focus' (such as an infection under a tooth) or toxic metal load from mercury fillings or the palladium in gold fillings. The electrical charge (galvanicity) released from dental materials also creates trouble."

At his Swiss Paracelsus Clinic, the Center of Holistic Medicine and Dentistry, Dr. Rau employs five dentists as part of his clinical staff to treat the dental problems that would otherwise block healing. They rely on a variety of innovative techniques and instruments to gather precise medical information about the dental status of each patient. "It is necessary to first diagnose the burden to the body of the toxic dental materials," Dr. Rau says, "and we do this with DMPS. It flushes mercury out of the tissues and into the urine, which we then collect for analysis." (DMPS was discussed in chapter 9.)

Founded in 1990, the Paracelsus Clinic is the only outpatient health facility in Switzerland that combines "holistic, biological medicine with conventional and modern methods of regulation therapy and holistic dentistry," comments Dr. Rau. "This allows us to treat people in cases of acute or chronic disease which, many times, originate in the jaws and/or teeth, the connections of which are unknown to conventional doctors."[1]

---

1   R. Leviton, "Cancer, Miscarriage, and Your Teeth," *Alternative Medicine* 24 (July 1998): 56–62.

Biohazards in the Oral Cavity

"The oral cavity is a challenging environment," advises Dr. Hal A. Huggins, former director of his world-renowned multi-medical-discipline clinic but now director of its laboratory. The clinic is functioning without Dr. Huggins. It combines the disciplines of dentistry, medicine, nutrition, psychology, and other healing arts—all dedicated to the treatment of autoimmune diseases, especially those brought on by the dental amalgam disease syndrome. Chronic fatigue of the type related to chronic fatigue syndrome is the most common condition that brings patients to the Huggins diagnostic center. Dr. Huggins has shown in his journal writings and lectures to health professionals that any metallic amalgams must be replaced with safer materials. As a result of his observations on literally thousands of patients, and research that he has carried out, he wrote the explicit and well-documented 1993 consumer book, *It's All in Your Head: The Link Between Mercury Amalgams and Illness*. (See its listing in appendix B).

"The presence of heat, cold, pressure, and bone flexion make the strength of dental replacements critical if they are to be serviceable. Unfortunately, the materials which possess the best properties of strength are those that have a high degree of toxicity," Dr. Huggins warns. "Nickel, beryllium, copper, cobalt, and chromium are popular materials used for large dental replacements such as crowns, bridges, and removable prostheses. Small fillings (commonly called 'silver fillings') are composed of silver, copper, zinc, [sometimes tin or nickel] and large amounts of mercury (generally more than 50 percent). All of these materials have one other asset which makes them popular. They are inexpensive.

"Over the years, these dental materials have been contrasted with gold which enjoys the overall best properties, but has a greater cost," adds Dr. Huggins. "[Lower] cost has generally won out in the competition; however, neither the public, nor the doctors have been given any information about biocompatibility. Whether or not the material is a biohazard has not been a factor of concern, but the time has now come to recognize biohazards and their consequences."[1]

---

1   H. A. Huggins, "Autoimmune and Carcinogenic Responses to Dental Materials: Diagnosis and Treatment," *Explore More* 6, no. 3: 64, 65.

The Six Biohazard Metals Implanted in Your Mouth

Mercury is the greatest biohazard of all the toxic dental materials; but it oxidizes within the human body to an even more poisonous ingredient, methylmercury (MeHg). Organic MeHg is approximately one hundred times more toxic than the inorganic form. Mercury becomes methylated in the mouth, the stomach, the small and large intestine, and by the intestinal mucosa. It is easy to point out the autoimmune component in the diseases that MeHg produces for knowledgeable medical scientists to understand, since it brings about physiological destruction through commonly recognized mechanisms of destruction.

Amazing as it may seem, we are faced with the fact that the six potential constituents of dental amalgam—silver, copper, tin, zinc, nickel, and especially mercury—not only are pathogenic, but they are monitored under federal regulatory agencies. This monitoring takes place in most areas of human exposure such as in the work place, during leisure activities, in toys, as part of household cleaners, and for other places and uses. The one area of human exposure for which these six toxic heavy metals are excluded from federal regulation is in the dentists' placement of them into the human oral cavity.[1]

Yes, there is no governmental regulation of poisonous dental metals that are intimately implanted into your body. My suggestion is that you ask yourself the following questions:

Don't you have cause to wonder about this ludicrous set of U.S. government nonregulations?

Why has an exception been made for the dental profession?

Do you have these unregulated biohazardous substances implanted into your mouth as dental fillings or root canals?

Do you suffer from energy reduction and chronic fatigue related to the poison in your mouth?

Have you been aware that you are facing elements of dental danger?

---

1   Yutsis and Walker, *The Downhill Syndrome.*

Why Immune Suppression Arises from Dental Amalgams

There are two primary reasons for chronic fatigue, fibromyalgia, the yeast syndrome, or other immune suppression-type diseases to arise from carrying dental amalgam fillings in the teeth. A main reason is the electromagnetic transfer of ionic current from one type of metal bound to another, which was discussed in chapter 9. The other reason is its biochemical/medical association, which I will discuss now.

The biochemical/medical cause of immune system suppression coming from dental amalgam fillings is connected to the vapors of mercury and other heavy metals interfering in the formation of the blood element, heme.

Heme is the colored, nonprotein part of the hemoglobin molecule in the blood that contains iron. Heme carries oxygen in the red blood cells, releasing it to tissues such as the porphyrins, which give off excess amounts of carbon dioxide. (Porphyrins are pigments that bind [chelate] with iron, magnesium, zinc, nickel, copper, and cobalt and that are important in many oxidation/reduction reactions.)

When an interference from the six commonly used dental metals or other toxic metals occurs in the chemical transformation of the body's porphyrin series, including 8-carboxy porphyrin (uroporphyrin), through the other types of porphyrin such as the porphyrins-7-carboxy, 6-carboxy, 5-carboxy, and so forth—down to the final product "heme," porphyrins spill from the blood into the urine. Then porphyrins and heme are excreted out of the body as if they are waste products. This loss of potential hemoglobin as well as the associated loss of adenosine triphosphate (ATP), the body's stored energy, formed through heme reactions in the cytochrome series, is the largest contributing factor to reduction of energy for the body's metabolic events.

Any person with insufficient heme carrying oxygen to the body cells and tissues is destined to be fatigued no matter what mental, emotional, or physical stimulant might be taken. This explains our present epidemic of chronic fatigue syndrome and associated immune system suppression diseases.

Dental amalgams are leaching the porphyrines out of human metabolism and draining these mercury-poisoned people of their energy-supplying ATP, according to information provided by Dr. Hal Huggins and his associates.

Additionally, heavy metals in dental amalgams interrupt the distribution of erythrocytes and leucocytes throughout the bloodstream. In contrast, when dental toxic materials are removed from the mouth following a specific protocol that had been created by Dr. Huggins and is followed faithfully by his holistic dental disciples, a highly predictable improvement occurs in the differential distribution of red blood cells and white blood cells throughout the blood system. The occurrence of this improvement in physiological functions proves that an involved patient's immune responses are influenced by his or her dental amalgam fillings. It is to everyone's advantage (except perhaps for the dentist's disadvantaged time allotment) when safer substitutes are selected as replacements for the heavy metals of toxic dental amalgams.

Nonalloyed Gold Is the Best Replacement for Amalgam

As is obvious, when dental amalgams are removed from the mouth, they must be replaced with some other material or else the patient will be left with a hole in each tooth that held the amalgam. Such a hole may produce pain and other complications. While it has some small toxicity problems too, gold probably is the best substitute for dental amalgam. Still, gold filling material is most expensive. This noble metal has been used in dentistry longer than amalgam and is relatively biocompatible and nontoxic; therefore, it's a desirable alternative except for those few people who are reactive to gold in their mouths.

Dental gold is an alloy (gold mixed with palladium, copper, or cobalt). Problems of sensitivity reactions arise for a patient mostly when base metals are mixed with the gold. Then the ill person could have near-similar symptoms of the chronic fatigue and immune dysfunction syndrome that he or she is just getting over. Consequently, any dental patient should insist that the dentist use the best materials with a higher amount of gold. While it should be as high as possible, the dental gold percentages may vary in the replacement alloy from 2 percent to 92 percent.

In his book, *How to Save Your Teeth: Toxic-Free Preventive Dentistry* (see the book's listing in appendix B), biological dentist David Kennedy, D.D.S., of San Diego, California, wrote:

> The metals that the fewest people react to are gold and platinum. You can make good dental crowns with these metals. Titanium is popular at the moment, but I do not feel we know enough about the long-term biocompatibility of this material. By far the most common metal used in over 70 percent of dental castings today is nickel. Some dentists call nickel-containing stainless steel crowns "white metal." The question you should ask is, "What are the exact percentages of each metal in the crown?" I do not recommend any non-precious metal, for example, nickel, steel, or copper, be used in the mouth. These are long-term restorations and prolonged contact can cause sensitization.
>
> Many women cannot wear stainless steel pierced earrings due to systemic reactions to the nickel. If a nickel crown is placed on the tooth of a sensitive individual, the gums can deteriorate rapidly and become inflamed . Even if this does not occur, you are swallowing the dissolved nickel. I can assure you that few health-conscious physicians would recommend you swallow a daily dose of nickel, no matter how small, if you can avoid it.[1]

Unfortunately, a lot of dentists do add copper to gold alloys. Many people react adversely to copper. Unlike mercury, small amounts of zinc and copper are essential for life. They often are taken as nutritional supplements. But too much of these trace minerals can make people ill, and allergic reactions may develop from them. It's much better for your health to forbid your dentist from using any form of copper alloy when making a gold partial or crown.[2]

---

1   D. Kennedy, *How to Save Your Teeth: Toxic-Free Preventive Dentistry* (Delaware, Ohio: Health Action Press, 1993), 88, 89.

2   J. Leirskar, "On the Mechanism of Cytotoxicity of Silver and Copper Amalgams in a Cell Culture System," *Scandinavian Journal of Dental Research* 84 (1974): 74–81.

If you are not allergic to gold and can afford the cost, it is ultimately among the best of filling materials says pedodontist Flora Parsa Stay, D.D.S., of Oxnard, California in her book, *The Complete Book of Dental Remedies.*[1]

1   F. P. Stay, *The Complete Book of Dental Remedies* (Garden City Park, N.Y.: Avery Publishing Group, 1996), 175.

Eleven

Tissue Toxicity from the Heavy Metals Implanted by Dentists

You may know that Napoleon Bonaparte died a prisoner in 1821. In 1961 a group of university historians pressured the government of France to dig up Napoleon's body in order to finally determine the cause of the former emperor's death. This was done, and a mineral analysis of the corpse's hair was performed. The analysis found that his hair contained one hundred times the normal level of the heavy toxic metal arsenic. Such a finding suggested that "the little corporal" probably had been poisoned.[1]

Yet the poisoning was not necessarily carried out by Napoleon's political enemies, but rather it could have come from any number of unsuspected but potential sources on the Island of St. Helena, where he was imprisoned. Poisoning may have come from Napoleon's eating contaminated seafood, drinking impure well water, burning coal, or consuming polluted poultry. He may have succumbed from arsenic in livestock feed additives, wood preservatives, wine, wallpaper dye, colored chalk, or any number of other chemical pollutants of that time.

Because they bring about so many disease symptoms, including the one nearest to our topic of interest, the toxicology of metals used in dentistry has attracted some notice from consumers as well as the scientific/holistic dental community. Metallic pollutants of all varieties have been infused into the planetary ecosystem at an ever increasing

---

1   G. McDonald, "Arsenic in Napoleon's Hair," *Nature* 4798 (1961): 103.

rate in the twentieth century with its technological explosion, and polluting metals will show themselves to be much worse in the new millennium. Unquestionably, toxic metals are hazardous to human existence and certainly should not be implanted into the mouth as is done by the multitudes of mechanically minded, allopathic-practicing dentists.

The Extent of Human Metallic Toxicity

Toxic metals are loosely defined as those elements whose presence at certain concentrations are known to interfere with normal metabolic functions, usually at the level of the enzymes put out by human cells. Several of the more poisonous metals, such as lead, mercury, cadmium, and aluminum, have no known biological role in the human or animal body. Others, such as nickel, arsenic, and copper are thought to be essential at lower concentrations, but are poisonous at high levels. Some metals are especially predisposed to producing immune system suppression when they are placed in close proximity to human tissues as are the dental restorative materials. As stated in chapter 3 by holistic oncologist Vincent J. Speckhart, M.D., of Norfolk, Virginia, "There is no place for metal in the mouth."

But in actuality, toxic heavy metals are overrunning our bodies, according to Garry F. Gordon, M.D., of Payson, Arizona, former president of the American College for Advancement in Medicine, now founder and president of the International College of Advanced Longevity Medicine, located in Chicago, Illinois. Dr. Gordon told me, "Because of modern industrial technology, each person living in Western countries today is known to be at least a thousand times more polluted with toxic metals and/or heavy metals than was anyone who lived when Christ walked the earth."

Contamination of the human body with various toxic heavy metals besides mercury is common. Metallic poisoning is likely a main contributing factor for the occurrence of illnesses in many Western industrialized peoples. There are, in fact, twenty-two damaging toxic and heavy metals, but in addition to mercury, only five others are entering our environment in ever increasing amounts: cadmium, lead, aluminum, arsenic, and nickel. These metals and mercury are indestructible, recycled, and poison both internal and external body processes. While the toxic metals may be polluting a man or a woman's physiology as the result of occupational exposure or generalized ecological contamination, other metals are actually implanted into individuals by health professionals such as dentists and orthopedic surgeons.

As for dentistry, in addition to mercury, dentists implant other more subtle but less recognized metallic poisons such as copper, palladium, tin, titanium, aluminum (as salts), cadmium, cobalt, nickel, silver, and zinc. (More metals are named below.) At one time, those modern day party-line followers of the American Dental Association used to implant lead into the mouth, too, and created their share of lead poisoning.

If it can be avoided, under no circumstance should anyone allow himself or herself to remain in prolonged intimate contact with toxic heavy metals or even toxic light metals such as aluminum. Otherwise, your risk of experiencing symptoms of Alzheimer's disease, immune system suppression, or even a full immunological collapse are exceedingly high. If any of these health difficulties happen, not only are you predisposed to loss of mental capacity or infections of all types, you are likely to die quickly.[1]

Dental Patient Health Hazards Not Arising from Mercury

Because of the introduction of new nonprecious dental metal alloys, dental technology has become hazardous for those persons who open their mouths for dentists to work inside them. Such usage brings patients into contact with a variety of potentially dangerous materials such as nickel, gold, chromium, cobalt, beryllium, molybdenum, gallium, copper, tin, zinc, palladium, titanium, and other metals. In the subsection that follows, I will describe some of the

---

1   H. R. Casdorph and M. Walker, *Toxic Metal Syndrome: How Metal Poisonings Can Affect Your Brain* (Garden City Park: N.Y.: Avery Publishing Group, 1995).

discomforts or outright diseases that occur from allowing any of these metals to be implanted into your mouth.

My information on health hazards *not* arising from mercury but rather from other dental metals comes from the research efforts of Howard G. Hindin, D.D.S., of Suffern, New York, who for more than thirty years has practiced holistic (biological) dentistry. Dr. Hindin furnished me with documentation on the hazardous dental alloys described below but in no particular order. All of them are dangerous to your health and life when implanted in your mouth. The metals become most hazardous to one's health when allowed to remain for several years or longer, leaching their metallic poisons. Provided by Dr. Hindin, here is the shocking report on a few of the individual toxic heavy metals that dentists implant in their patients' mouths:

Poisoning from Dental Nickel

Nickel (*niccolum,* chemical symbol *Ni*) is among the most dangerous and greatest illness-producing of dental materials. Periodically, nickel implantation causes the dental patient to experience various sicknesses such as nervous headaches with associated tiredness of the eyes, dimness of vision, dizziness, and slight nausea. Symptoms of nickel poisoning also include weak digestion, general dyspepsia, constipation, and catarrh. Frequently a cracking sound is heard in the cervical vertebrae when the head is moved, and the crown of the head will hurt as if it's being hammered with a nail. The upper lip will twitch, there will be violent sneezing, and the nose will feel stopped up.

Someone looking at a person poisoned by nickel will see signs of redness and swelling at the tip of their nose and the victim will suffer acute pain that extends to the head's vertex and through the temples.

Sore throat strikes from nickel toxicity and causes great tenderness along the right side of the throat, which is sore to the touch. There will be a loss of appetite, with acute pain in the stomach, which extends upward to the shoulder. There will be intense thirst and hiccuping. A sour, fetid secretion oozes from the patient's molar teeth. Hoarseness and a dry, hacking cough are present. Stitches in the chest get so bad that the person is obliged to sit up and hold his or her chest and head to relieve the pain. The patient will itch all over, which is worse on the neck and which cannot be relieved by scratching. Young women will have scanty and late menses, accompanied by pain.[1]

Toxicity from Dental Tin

The chief poisoning symptoms of tin (*stannum*) center on the nervous system and respiratory organs. Tin toxicity causes emotional upset with a sense of sadness, anxiety, and the dread of seeing people. The dental patient's head aches in the temples and forehead, with motion causing the pain to worsen. The pain gradually increases and decreases as if the head is constricted by a band. The forehead feels pressed inwards and ulcerations of the earring holes (if present) in the lobes of the ears occur. The patient poisoned by dental tin alloys experiences obstinate and acute coughing fits.

Dental tin is truly discomforting. In the throat, for instance, tin toxicity produces much adhesive mucus that's difficult to detach. The smell of cooking causes the patient to vomit; thus, there is a perpetual sensation of emptiness in the stomach. A cramp-like colic is present around the navel, which is relieved only when hard pressure is placed against the abdomen.

The woman who has tin poisoning will feel a bearing down sensation with a weak, sinking feeling in the stomach. Menses come early and are profuse. There will be both pain in the vagina that extends upward and backward to the spine and a white vaginal discharge.

The voice is hoarse from tin toxicity; a dry cough is part of the symptom complex, with mucus forming that must be expelled by forcible and violent coughing. In tin poisoning, the patient's cough is excited by laughing, singing, and talking, and it worsens when lying on the right side. During the day the patient expectorates a copious green, sweetish mucus. The poisoned person's chest feels so sore and weak that the individual can hardly talk at all.

---

1   O. Boericke, *Materia Medica with Repertory*, 9th ed. (San Francisco: Miller, June 1927), 468, 469.

Sleep is managed only with one leg drawn up and the other stretched out in a characteristic "tin toxicity position." The extremities undergo a paralytic weakness. Fatigue invariably is chronic and tiredness becomes so extreme that the patients have difficulty holding onto objects; they begin to drop things. The ankles swell and limbs give out suddenly when the tin-poisoned person is attempting to sit down. Spasmodic twitching of the muscles of the forearm and hand shows up. Fingers jerk when holding a pen.

With poisoning from tin in the mouth, fever forms and higher body heat comes on in the evening; exhausting night sweats develop, especially toward morning. Perspiration accumulates in copious amounts on all skin surfaces but principally on the forehead and nape of the neck. The sweat of an individual with dental tin toxicity is smelly and musty—really offensive to someone standing nearby.[1]

Necessary Zinc but Not as a Dental Implant

Zinc (*zincum metallicum*) forces the tissues all over the body to feel as if they were worn out; yet the sensation gives rise to somnambulism. Zinc toxicity also is the source of screaming out at night during sleep without the patient being aware of it. There will be varicose veins, especially of the lower extremities and a sense that bugs are crawling over the skin, a sensation that by itself prevents sleep.

Itching is present in the thighs and in the hollow of the knees. And zinc poisoning brings on a number of neurological discomforts such as frequent high fevers with shivering down the back, night sweats, profuse sweat on the feet, and cold extremities.[2]

Traces of Copper are Needed but Not as Dental Implants

Copper (*cuprum metallicum*) causes spasmodic muscles, cramps, convulsions and, beginning in the fingers and toes, a violent contractive and intermitting pain. Copper causes the worst nausea of all metallic toxins.

---

1   Ibid., 605, 606.

2   Ibid., 683 86.

This sense of digestive illness is usually accompanied by excessive vomiting, stupor, convulsions and pain, all of which increase when the patient experiences any kind of movement and touch.

Dental copper toxicity brings about some mental quirks such as the victim having fixed ideas that are malicious and morose. The poisoned patient uses unintended words and is fearful. Purple and red swellings of the head develop, which are associated with convulsions. An odd sensation comes over the individual as if water were being poured down and along the sides of the head in a stream. Also, giddiness accompanies this patient's many ailments.

Aching forms over the eyebrows, and the patient shows a fixed, staring, sunken, glistening set to the eyes, which are turned upward, crossed, or experience quick rolling movements of the eyeballs; or there may be constantly closed eyes. The face of the person poisoned with copper is distorted and pale bluish in tone with blue lips, contraction of the jaws, and foam at the mouth.

The person's nose will be congested with blood from the toxic metal being incorporated into his or her tissues. And the patient is likely to complain of a strong metallic, slimy taste in the mouth with a flow of saliva dripping from the lips. The unfortunate person with copper poisoning exhibits constant protrusion and retraction of the tongue, like a snake.

The gastrointestinal tract exhibits various symptoms from copper toxicity. For instance, there will be hiccuping preceding stomach spasms. Vomiting is relieved by drinking cold water, and the fluid is heard descending through the esophagus into the stomach with a gurgling sound. The abdomen is tense, hot, and tender to the touch. The stools are black, painful, bloody, and a weakness with ineffective spasms of the rectum is experienced.

For a woman, the menses appear too late in the cycle, and they are protracted. Cramps from the abdomen are so severe they extend into the chest before, during, or after suppression of the menses.[1]

---

1   Ibid., 246, 247.

Symptoms Coming from the Silver
in "Silver" Fillings

Silver (*argentum metallicum*) poisoning arising from dental use chiefly centers on the joints (articulations) and their component elements such as the bones, cartilages, and ligaments. The small blood vessels close up or wither and carious affections such as decay or tooth breakdown result.

Silver toxicity will result in a dull paroxysmal neuralgia over the left side of the head, gradually increasing and then ceasing suddenly. The scalp will feel tender to the touch.

Dizziness with an intoxicated feeling will come over the patient, especially when he or she looks at running water. The head will feel empty and hollow, and the eyelids will redden and thicken. There will be an exhausting inflammation of the mucous membranes of the nose (rhinitis) with a nasal discharge and frequent sneezing. Pain will appear in the facial bones and between the left eye and frontal eminence. The patient will have a sense of melancholy and hurriedness, yet time will seem to be passing slowly.

Dental silver toxicity takes a toll on the throat, with raw, hawking, gray, jellylike mucus forming. The throat will get sore from coughing, and there will be a profuse and easy morning expectoration. Professional singers will sometimes totally lose their voices, since the larynx will feel sore and raw with a red area seen near the supra sternal fossa. The soreness will worsen from use of the voice. Laughing will cause coughing. Reading aloud will result in hemming and hawking of phlegm. A great weakness of the chest will take place that's worse on the left side. There will be an alteration in the timbre of the voice and pain in the left lower ribs. For voice improvement, silver must be removed from the mouth.

Silver poisoning will cause severe backache, which will result in bent-over walking with oppression of the chest. Urination will be profuse, with urine that is turbid and that has a sweet odor.

Men will be struck with a feeling of crushing pain in the testicles, and there will be seminal emissions without sexual excitement. Urination burns.

Women's ovaries will feel too large when palpitated by an examiner and there will be a painful sense of bearing down. There may be prolapse of the uterus, an eroded spongy cervix, a foul-smelling, excoriating white discharge from the vagina (leukorrhea), pain in the left ovary, or a sore feeling throughout the woman's abdomen, which is worsened by jarring.[1]

Cobalt Intoxication

Cobalt (*kobalt*, chemical symbol Co) produces a sensitivity dermatitits and hypersenitivity of the lungs characterized by asthmatic symptoms, including cough and shortness of breath. Chronic exposure to cobalt is a generalized intoxication syndrome, which can produce a progressive respiratory disease termed *hard metal disease*.[2]

Suicidal Tendencies from Beryllium Toxicity

Beryllium (*glucinum*, chemical symbol Be) is a dentist killer. Of all potentially hazardous substances used by dentists or dental technicians, beryllium probably presents the greatest health risk to them in particular. This circumstance is especially true if beryllium is combined with mercury, which also stimulates the compulsion to suicide. Indeed, combined in mercury amalgam dental fillings, beryllium is the likely reason dentists suffer the highest rate of suicide among all the health professionals. Often 2 percent beryllium by weight is added to nonprecious alloys to lend strength and improve casting characteristics.

For the dental patient, this metal leads to a lung impairment called berylliosis, characterized principally by progressive shortness of breath and chest pain. Even very brief exposure can result in eye, nose, and throat irritation. Approximately 17 percent of acute poisonings can be expected to progress to the chronic, generally progressive, and debilitating disease that involves other organs such as the liver, skin, lymph nodes, and spleen. There is no question that

---

1   Ibid., 71, 72.

2   J. S. Lee, A. C. Kimball, and W. N. Rom, "Dental Laboratory Health Hazards," *Dental Laboratory Review* (November 1983): 22–26.

beryllium produces lung cancer in animals and is probably a human carcinogen.[1]

Skin Disease from Gallium

Gallium (*gallia,* chemical symbol *Ga*) occasionally causes mild dermatitis, a skin disease resembling eczema. Gallium antigens cause an antibody response that manifests itself externally as an epidermal eruption.

Nearly all of these dental metals, when combined into alloys, especially mercury, nickel, and beryllium, are toxic to genetic material within human cells (These dental metals are genotoxic.) They change the genetic code within the cellular molecules of deoxyribonucleic acid or DNA. (They're mutagenic.) Such mutations can be a main source of birth defects in newborns. No woman contemplating pregnancy should allow any of these toxic metals to remain in her mouth.

Non-Implanted Toxic Metals

The ingestion of toxic metals destroys the brain tissues and nerve cells by increasing cellular membrane permeability, allowing for the leakage of nutrients out of the cells, and inhibiting enzyme production, which, in turn, depresses the body's chemical reactions. There will be lowered energy in all physiological parameters so that chronic fatigue syndrome becomes inevitable.

Toxic heavy metals are the great destroyers when penetrating within the human body and brain. They are the prime sources of dementia of the Alzheimer's type. The toxic metals are discussed in the broadly circulated 1995 consumer book, *Toxic Metal Syndrome,* coauthored by H. Richard Casdorph, M.D., Ph.D., and Morton Walker, D.P.M.[2] Toxic metals encourage the transmutation of

---

1   Ibid.

2   Casdorph and Walker, *Toxic Metal Syndrome,* 143–52.

other elements into themselves and thereby increase the level of toxicity of those elements.[1]

Tables 11-1, 11-2, and 11-3, which follow, list a few of the heavy toxic metals, and aluminum, which isn't classified by chemists and physicists as being "heavy" because it has a specific gravity of less than five. However, aluminum definitely is toxic, especially to the brain. Listed within the tables are the sources, occupational exposures, and complex of signs and symptoms exhibited by the poisoning that comes from prolonged exposure to the dentists' implantation of metals in their patients' mouths. The really deadly dental metals I've selected to discuss are mercury, aluminum, cadmium, and lead.

Mercury Toxicity

In the modern era, thousands of people in hazardous situations are exposed to mercury daily. Of course, dentists, their assistants, dental hygienists, and dental laboratory workers are more exposed to the inhalation or skin contact with this deadliest of metals known to mankind. It is a scientific and sociological truth that suicide among dentists is the highest of any learned profession. Thus this profession's exposure to the toxic mercuric metal accounts for their high incidence of chronic marriage disruption, divorce, death by suicide, and psychiatric involvement.

---

1   H. R. Alseben and W. E. Shute, *How to Survive the New Health Catastrophes* (Anaheim, Calif.: Survival Publications, 1973), 2.

Table 11-1

Occupational Exposures to Mercury, in Addition to Dentistry:

artificial flower workers

cap loaders

cartridge makers

chemical workers

cosmetic workers

dental laboratory workers

dental technicians

detonator cleaners and fillers

dry battery makers

dye makers

electroplaters

embalmers

embalming fluid makers

engravers

felt hat makers

file makers

fulminate amalgam workers

fur handlers

gold refiners

hair workers

incandescent lamp workers

ink makers

motion picture machine operator

lead platers

lithographers

manometer makers

mercury boiler workers

mercury bronzers

mercury miners

mercury salt workers

mercury solder workers

mercury switch makers

mercury vapor lamp makers

metal refiners

mirror silverers

painters and point makers

pharmaceutical workers

physicians

pottery decorators

printers

radio tube makers

storage battery makers

thermometer makers

welders

wood preservers

zinc electrode makers

Signs and Symptoms of Mercury Toxicity:

Mental Illnesses Arising from Mercury

depression and anxiety	irritability
fearfulness	loss of memory
frequent bouts of anger	metallic taste
hallucinations	persecution complex
inability to accept criticism	weight loss
inability to concentrate	indecision
slight tremors of hands, head, lips, tongue, or eyelid	

Mental/Physical Illnesses Arising from Mercury

anorexia	headache
chronic low body temperature	hypersensitive reflexes
constricted visual field	insomnia
drowsiness	loss of energy
excitability	sensitive tongue

Physical Illnesses Coming from Mercury

anemia	gingivitis	numbness
bad breath	high blood pressure	nutritional defects
bleeding gums	irregular gait	paralysis
bronchitis	joint pains	shaking
chills	loose teeth	sore throat
colitis	lost appetite	stomach pain
coughing	low blood sugar	trembling
fatigue	mouth sores	urinary frequency
fever	nausea	visual changes
flu-like discomforts	nervousness	vomiting

Aluminum Toxicity

The use of aluminum (*alumen,* chemical symbol *Al*) and its numerous products is ubiquitous throughout the societies of all the industrialized nations and most third world countries. Additionally, *Al* makes up 8 percent of the Earth's crust; consequently, prolonged exposure to this nonheavy toxic metal is all too common and a source of many diseases. In particular it causes dementia of the Alzheimer's type.

Table 11-2

Sources of Aluminum, Other Than Dentistry

cooking utensils	deodorants and antiperspirants
baking powder	McIntyre powder
antacids	building construction materials
aluminum cans	packaging materials such as foil
insulated cables	alum in drinking water
insulated wiring	coal burning
soil	beer
maraschino cherries	pickles
milk products	aluminum nicotinate
nasal sprays	toothpaste
ceramics	cigarette filters
automotive exhausts	tobacco smoke
pesticides	animal feeds
FD and C color additives	vanilla powder
bleached flour	table salt and seasonings
American cheese	fumigant residues
arthritis treatments	feldspar and mica
dust from industrial manufacturing	sutures with wound-healing coatings

aluminum chelates of polysaccharide-sulfuric acid

dermatitis, burn, and wound remedies

Kaopectate and other such medications containing Kaolin, an aluminum

Occupational Exposures to Aluminum:

metal powders

bauxite ore production

aluminum products

paper industry

textile industry

glass industry

synthetic leather manufacturing

welding

explosives manufacturing

porcelain industry

pyrotechnical devices manufacturing

manufacturing aluminum abrasives manufacturing

Signs and Symptoms of Aluminum Toxicity:

aluminum pneumoconiosis (inhalation of aluminum dust)
—pneumothorax
—pulmonary fibrosis with emphysema
—dyspnea
—right-sided cardiac hypertrophy
—lacelike shadowing on lung X-ray films
—Shaver's disease: cough, substernal pain, weakness, fatigue

phosphate and aluminum binding in the gastrointestinal tract
—aching muscles
—rickets
—osteoporosis

skin reactions and miliaria
(acute inflammation of sweat glands)
encephalopathy
Alzheimer's disease
childhood hyperactivity

gastrointestinal distress
>—stomach inflammation and colitis
>—flatulence and acid eructation (belching)

nephritis
liver dysfunction
childhood psychosis

Cadmium Toxicity

Cadmium (*cadmia*) is poisonous to every human body system, whether dentally installed, orally consumed, sublingually ingested, injected, or inhaled. Cadmium tends to accumulate in body tissues; therefore, increasing the uptake of environmental cadmium is hazardous to human health under any circumstances. Inhaled cadmium (as from cigarette smoking) is better absorbed into the tissues than ingested cadmium. Once absorbed, the elimination rate for cadmium is quite slow so that low-grade toxicity with the patients' subclinical symptomatology is common, especially among those people whose cadmium sources are occupational.

Table 11-3

Sources of Cadmium Toxicity, in Addition to Dental Implantation:

drinking water	black polythylene and rubber
evaporated milk	plastic tapes
processed foods	refined wheat flour
soil	oysters, kidney, and liver foods
cigarette smoke	other forms of tobacco
ceramics	superphosphate fertilizers
alloys	paint pigments
electroplating	cadmium vapor lamps
rustproofed tools	marine hardware

Elements of Danger

welding metal

solders

fungicides

pesticides

copper refineries

rubber tires

soft drinks from vending machines with cadmium piping

urban street dust

silver polish

polyvinyl plastics

sewage sludge and effluents

rubber carpet backing

burning motor oil

soft water running in galvanized pipes

Occupational Exposures to Cadmium:

polymetallic ore smelting

electroplating

painting with cadmium pigments

cadmium alloy manufacturing

cadmium vapor lamp manufacturing

fungicide manufacturing

tetraethyl lead manufacturing

rustproofing tools, hardware, and so forth

zinc ore smelting

paint manufacturing

jewelry making

ceramic making

nickel-cadmium battery manufacturing

process engraving

soldering

Signs and Symptoms of Cadmium Toxicity:

chronic fatigue

hypertension from cadmium in kidneys

slight liver damage

hypercalcuria

yellow coloring of teeth

emphysema

pain in sternum

iron-deficiency anemia

kidney calcium stones (nephrocalcinosis)

loss of sense of smell (anosmia)

pain in lower back and legs

reduced birth weight in newborns

hypophosphatemia

decreased lung function

decreased vitamin D production

proteinuria

aminoaciduria

carcinogenesis

milkman's syndrome
(pseudofracture lines in the
scapula, femur, or ileum)

glucosuria

prostate cancer

increased mortality

itai-itai (osteomalacia in
middle-aged women with dietary
deficiencies)

Twelve

Death Stalks Your Gums from Root Canals

Our anonymous dental source from upstate New York named this chapter for me from his dental professional beliefs.

"We're faced with a situation in which many of you reading this may have what can become a major problem. If you possess any teeth with root canals, or have had teeth extracted without the surrounding membrane being removed with the tooth (and the odds are that it wasn't), right now thousands of ugly, disgusting, toxin-forming bacteria are ravaging your body systems. They're trying to destroy vital organs as fast as possible," he said.

"I would suggest you finish reading this information quickly," concludes the dispirited dentist. His implication is that you do something about ridding yourself of dental root canals.

The Dangers and Avoidance of Dental Root Canal

In the early part of the twentieth century, when one or more of a person's teeth became diseased or the dental pulp sustained injury, the accepted treatment was to remove such a dysfunctional calcified structure. Beginning in the late 1950s, however, these same types of pathological teeth were no longer always being extracted because of a complete alteration in the practice of conventional dental therapeutics and surgery. Thus modern endodontic dentistry was born.

Today, diseased teeth are successfully saved by the dental health professional, using a specialty procedure referred to as *root canal therapy* or *endodontics*. To the public's long-term detriment, unfortunately, acceptance of endodontic treatment has steadily been on the rise. For example, in 1969 six million root canal fillings were done and the number is increasing annually. Root canal installations rose in 1996 to more than 25 million, and for the year 2000 it's estimated by dentists belonging to the American Association of Endodontists that over 30 million such procedures will be performed each year thereafter.

These dental root canal fillings hold concealed life-threatening dangers for anyone who allows them to remain in place without taking precautionary measures. Really, as our source has warned, death does stalk your gums. This chapter is about the hazards of root canal therapy and how to neutralize such dangers if endodontic treatment becomes mandatory for somebody who must undergo it or who already has root canaled teeth installed.

The Troubles Arising from Root Canals

Most often, pockets of infection exist under those teeth that undergo root canal fillings even after endodontic therapy. This happens because regular general dentists or even the endodontists trained in this treatment seldom, if ever, eliminate all the bacteria and toxins from the diseased dental roots. Invariably, pockets of infection remain under the teeth that are undetectable on usual X-ray examination by even the most astute dental professional. Pathogenic microorganisms are allowed to remain, which in the long-term can bring on well-established disease and even death. I will tell you why.

Pathogenic bacteria lodged in root canals persist for years without the patient's knowledge and, as a result, disseminate their infectious processes throughout the body. Most likely, the tooth was removed originally because it was infected, and those infectious bacteria remain no matter how much sterilizing irrigation is performed. This circumstance has been proven innumerable times by investigating dental surgeons.

When foci of infection are present, toxins leak from these bacterial pockets—whether in teeth or anywhere else in the body—and depress the function of one's immune system, leading to degenerative diseases. Foci of infection are especially predominant in root canal fillings, and these bring on chronic disorders of a degenerative nature. Examples of such chronic illnesses connected to prolonged dental infections are systemic lupus erythematosis (SLE), multiple sclerosis (MS), parkinsonism, various cardiac manifestations, infectious arthritis, liver or kidney troubles, and much more—even malignant tumors.

Oncologist Josef Issels, M.D., Says Dental Foci Cause Tumors

In his highly praised and valuable book, *Cancer: A Second Opinion*, the respected and world renowned German cancer specialist Josef Issels, M.D., took a stand against saving a devitalized tooth at all costs. Dr. Issels died of pneumonia on February 11, 1998, a few weeks after his ninetieth birthday, in California. He was among the first to maintain that cancer is, in all its stages, a disease of the entire person, arising from the combined effects of manifold endogenous and exogenous mentally and physically harmful factors. Impaired teeth are definitely part of those factors producing malignant tumors. The oncologist repeated this admonition in nearly all his books, essays, and lectures to both colleagues and consumers. He was opposed to root canal work implanted by endodontists. Only recently have his findings become acknowledged by holistic (biological) dentists but not yet by orthodox practicing dentists.

Dr. Issels's book, cited here, explains that a tooth is no isolated lifeless thing uninvolved in the body's processes. Rather, Dr. Issels assures us:

> There is a lively metabolic interchange between the interior and exterior milieu of the tooth. And this two-way process takes place along many thousands of hyperfine, capillary canals joining the pulp cavity to the exterior surface of the tooth.
>
> Foci of infection lie quiet but active within devitalized teeth. The dentinal canals and dental capillaries contain large microbial colonies. The toxins produced by these microbes in a tooth with a root filling can no longer be evacuated into the mouth, but must be drained away through the cross-connections and unsealed branches of the dentinal and capillary canals into the marrow of

the jawbone. From there, they are conveyed to the tonsils, and thus the flow systems of the body. In fact, the conservation treatment [root canal] literally converts a tooth into a toxin-producing "factory."

When inflammation spreads to the marrow of the tooth socket, it causes osteomyelitis. Toxins will be able to advance unhindered into the marrow spaces, the tonsils, and into the body. In my cancer patients, I have found that such non-encapsulated foci were particularly common, as one would expect from people whose body resistance had been lowered. My clinical experience has produced evidence of a causal connection between foci and [malignant] tumour development.

If total treatment [of cancer] is to be performed, it is necessary to remove not only any devitalized teeth but also any hidden dental foci remaining in the jaw.

Further, total removal of devitalized teeth and their roots must not be the end of the dentist's activities. Each alveolus—the tooth's socket in the jaw—should be radically cleared down to the healthy bone. In that way the development of a residual ostitis or of a cystoma may be prevented. It is not only the tooth which may be a focus, but the adjacent tooth-fixing apparatus as well.[1]

It's been shown without doubt by practitioners of biological (holistic) dentistry and the medical doctors who support them that once an infection coming from teeth is cleared up, many of a patient's disease symptoms do disappear. The body's immune capability takes over and kills off or at least inhibits the overgrowth of infectious organisms.

Given the estimated three miles of microcanals within a single endodontured tooth, there can be considerable bacterial trouble engendered, according to George E. Meinig, D.D.S., author of *Root Canal Cover-Up*. If you are one of the unfortunate majority who have undergone root canal therapy, you are facing a serious potential health problem. Here are three sad facts with which you must cope:

---

1   J. Issels, *Cancer: A Second Opinion* (London: Hodder and Stoughton, 1975), 120–22.

1. From the pathogenic organisms lodged inside a root canal, bacterial toxins get into your bloodstream near the tip of the tooth root.

2. Minute amounts of these toxins, which Hal A. Huggins, D.D.S., of Colorado Springs, Colorado, declares are one thousand times more poisonous than botulism, circulate throughout the body, wreaking   biological havoc.

3. Immune suppression with the eventual appearance of one or more crippling degenerative diseases is among the results of root canals. [1]

Antibiotics Don't Work for Root Canal Infections

Antibiotics can't kill the bacteria, because the microbes aren't reachable with drugs once trapped inside the devitalized tooth. Antibiotic pharmaceuticals don't penetrate the tooth's dentin. Thus infection spreads from the dental root canal and moves through the bloodstream to an area of body weakness. "One third of all disease in the United States can be either directly or indirectly traced to dental infections," says Dr. Meinig, who is a founding member of the American Association of Endodontists and dentist for the Twentieth Century Fox Studio in Hollywood, California. Foci of infection remain to cause chronic depression of one's immunity. Dr. Meinig had practiced endodontics for over forty-eight years, and more recently he has studied the phenomenon of infectious foci from root canal fillings almost exclusively.

Dr. Meinig based his upsetting pronouncement initially on the twenty-five years of research conducted by Weston A. Price, D.D.S., M.S., who first published the results of his investigations in 1923. Meinig wrote that Dr. Price's research showed how 25 percent of patients whose family histories were free of degenerative diseases and who had topnotch immune systems "could expect to have and retain

---

1   G. E. Meinig, *Root Canal Cover-Up* (Ojai, Calif.: Bion Publishing, 1994).

root canal fillings and live without complications arising therefrom through old age." But the other 75 percent of patients were different. Root canals for them were significant and life-threatening sources of ill health.

Dr. Price, director of the Research Institute of the National Dental Association for fifteen years, demonstrated that dead teeth and root canals made people sick in the extreme. They produce scleroderma, rheumatoid arthritis, ankylosing spondilitis, cancer, many autoimmune diseases, and numerous other chronic health problems.

Cysts, Osteomyelitis, and Ostitis in the Jawbone

From their tendency to produce adverse immunomodulatory effects, dental root canal corrections are almost more dangerous than dental amalgam fillings. Root canal implants deteriorate under the dead teeth into focal bacterial infections that potentially bring on chronic fatigue syndrome and other such illnesses. Also, remote neural/fascial disturbances can come from inflammatory changes near the roots of teeth that barely show on radiographs (X-ray films). The bone inflammation arises from osteomyelitic foci created by displaced teeth, by teeth used as buttresses for bridgework and therefore subjected to excessive stress, and by radicular, paradental, or follicular cysts.[1]

In cysts, there is a constant decomposition of protein. This, together with the tendency of cysts to grow, is sufficient reason for their removal. The same reasoning applies to a variety of dental difficulties, including odontomas (tumors comprised of enamel, dentin, cementum, and pulp tissue that may be arranged in the form of a tooth), conglomerates of dental tissue, hypercementoses (excessive deposition of secondary cementum on the root of a tooth, which

---

1   W. J. Faber and M. Walker, *Pain, Pain Go Away* (Menlo Park, Calif.: Ishi Press International, 1996).

is caused by localized trauma or inflammation), and all sclerosing processes in the jawbones. Gingivitis (inflammation of the gums), stomatitis (inflammation of the mucous membrane of the mouth), and parodontoses (inflammation around the teeth) produce pockets, which become sources of chronic inflammation and irritation.

A stomatitis that occurred years ago in the dental patient with no visible changes at the time can have left behind a latent interference field with associated bacterial infection. It may become active at a later date by some second insulting trigger factor to the system.

The importance of ostitis in any search for an interference field is becoming more readily recognized by therapists who administer treatment for the vague, syndrome-like illnesses. *Ostitis* (also spelled *osteitis*) is inflammation of a bone, involving the haversian spaces, canals, and their branches, and generally the medullary cavity, and marked by enlargement of the bone, tenderness, and a dull, aching pain. Ostitis is one form of *osteomyelitis,* inflammation of bone caused by a pyogenic organism, which may remain localized or may spread through the bone to involve the bone marrow, cortex, cancellous tissue, and periosteum.

Formerly, the patient's defensive capability was sufficiently intact to enable the gums to heal by themselves after a dental extraction. Nowadays, environmental and internal pollution have reduced this immune defensive capability. It's a state made worse through the routine use of antibiotics as a main contributing factor to chronic, residual ostitis. What's seen by the therapist is a persistent chronic inflammatory condition sometimes with infection in the maxillary and mandibular bones of the patient's jaw. Their identification and evaluation need to be accomplished on viewing X-ray films by means of an oral panogram (a full circumventing view of all teeth and gum areas of the mouth).[1]

The dental surgeon must think more globally than merely as an extractionist of infected or impacted teeth. The dental surgeon has an important role with regard to the pathological processes taking place in

---

1   W. J. Faber and M. Walker, *Instant Pain Relief* (Milwaukee, Wis.: Biological Publications, 1991).

a person's body and not only in his or her mouth. Such an informed dentist can be an invaluable ally and not only a "narrow-gauge doctor." A partnership should be formed between the physician who attends to patients having dental difficulties and the dental surgeon fixing them. Such a partnership will be a genuine boon to those long-suffering patients who are victimized by foci of infection in the jaw directly related to the endodontics of root canal therapy.[1]

The Radiographic Panorex Key to Diagnosis

Spanish stomatologist Ernesto Adler, D.D.S., calls the wisdom teeth "teeth of misfortune," because almost all wisdom teeth, especially those out of alignment, have deep marginal pockets that promote chronic bacterial growth and inflammatory irritation. Dr. Adler observes that the real misfortune of wisdom teeth occurs after their extraction. Standard orthodox dental training teaches practitioners not to clean out (curette) the surrounding bone tissue, because this procedure is considered unnecessary. The result of this lack of cleansing is that bone heals over the surface of the now-vacant bone socket, but the infection remains. Often the unsuspecting patient experiences very little discomfort initially, when the ostitis (bone infection) remains in its chronic state. These areas generally escape detection if dentists employ the usual orthodox guidelines of X-ray diagnosis.

The key to diagnosis of ostitis is to carefully examine the patient's dental arch by means of the panorex or panoral radiographic exposure. The panoral X-ray technique uses a single radiograph of the entire mouth and both jaws. Often the changes seen on this film are not sharply defined and can generally be recognized by their blurred bone structure. Too bad that the panorex and its biological dentistry concept are not commonly used by the vast majority of dentists.

If there is one vital message this book provides, it is: the dental

---

1   P. Yutsis and M. Walker, *The Downhill Syndrome* (Garden City Park, N.Y.: Avery Publishing Group, 1997).

profession must become aware of the pivotal role its practicing members play in the overall health of their patients' body and mind. Dentists can help to wipe out the incidence of immune system suppression and its devastating more generalized, symptomatic, degenerative disease complications.

Prevent Immune Suppression from Root Canals

To prove how toxic removed endodontic material is, Dr. Weston Price sewed root-canaled teeth under the skin of laboratory rabbits. Within three days these rabbits were dead from the same condition that had sickened those human beings from whom the teeth were extracted. In fact, this bacterial dental material was so toxic that Dr. Price could produce the same results of disease and death in each of twenty-seven successive generations of rabbits, using the same infected tooth, even after autoclaving it at high temperatures for more than twenty-four hours.

There is a solution to the problem of root canals, of course. Extraction of the root canaled tooth, a thorough cleaning of the infected jawbone, and then sterilization of the entire area reverses these deadly conditions in a dramatically short time, usually in a few days. When the tooth with an endodontic filling is removed, the periodontal ligament that attaches this tooth to the underlying bone must also be removed, advises Dr. Hal Huggins. Otherwise, a pocket of infection remains. Full removal of the tooth, the periodontal ligament, and the surrounding areas of dead jawbone stimulates the old bone to produce new bone for healing.

The trouble with root canals is that conventionally practicing dentists doing endodontics fail to carry out the whole procedure to a full conclusion, and that is another main message that is specific to this chapter. In the sections that follow, I am informing medical/dental consumers how to take defensive actions against oral cavity abuse engineered by unskilled dentists who incorrectly install root canals. The procedure wouldn't be so dangerous to the patient's immune system if proper procedure and better root canal filling material were employed.

Morton Walker, D.P.M.

Use of a Root Canal Filling Material from Europe

For those root canal patients who don't want to lose any teeth, there is a truly effective alternative medical/dental procedure that works well to prevent immune system suppression. Informed prospective root canal patients can place demands on their endodontists to use the corrective medical/dental alternative. What does it entail? The dentist who is about to install a root canal must use a particular filling material that protects against underlying infectious microbes.

The patient must ask the dentist to use a dental protective preparation consisting of calcium oxide (CaO), zinc oxide (ZnO), and a special ethyl glycol/watery liquid. The combination—known as Biocalex—has been employed by European dentists for over two decades, but usually American endodontists don't apply these three highly compatible agents for their patients' prevention against foci of infection. This is the circumstance, even though the three agents are approved for U.S. import by the FDA. For strictly commercial reasons, endodontists of the ADA won't approve its members' use of the European product. This organized professional dental group of dental specialists, the American Association of Endodontists, offers no reason related to the technical excellence of Biocalex.

Here is how the Biocalex compound works. The calcium oxide has an affinity for endodontic liquids. This characteristic results in a volumetric expansion of Biocalex's healing components that penetrate the hundreds of tiny inaccessible canals or tubules that had brought nourishment to the formerly functioning tooth. The tubules do nothing more than act as shelters for expansion of bacterial growth and accumulation of their poisons. The poisons slowly leak out into the systemic fluid flow of one's body. By chemical conversion, calcium oxide changes to calcium hydroxide, which ultimately converts to calcium carbonate [$Ca(CO2)$], creating a wall of calcification, thereby sealing root apices and vital dentinal tubules.[1]

---

1   M. Georgopoulou and others, "*In Vitro* Evaluation of the Effectiveness of Calcium Hydroxide and Paramonochlorophenol on Anaerobic Bacteria from the Root Canal," *Endodontic Dental Traumatology* 9, no. 6 (December 1993): 249–53.

By application of Biocalex, anaerobic bacteria within the diseased root are killed. Calcium oxide is highly effective as an endodontic sterilization agent and also for decreasing the recovery time before final filling of the root canal. Studies show that CaO usage results in the absence of any germs (perfect asepsis) in root canals. No other root canal filling material used by American endodontists creates such a sterility effect.[1]

You Can Cure Root Canal Infection and Immune Suppression

For the first time ever, information I am presenting here furnishes all medical and dental consumers with the means of curing infections derived from their root canals. This may be carried out without removing the root canals themselves. Additionally, autoimmune disease and generalized immune system suppression arising from carelessly administered root canal therapy may be eliminated altogether, even without removing or correcting the existing root canal.

The cure comes from discoveries made during the period 1916 to 1925 by German Professor Guenther Enderlein, Ph.D. (1872-1968). A zoologist and bacteriologist by profession, Dr. Enderlein spent sixty years researching a series of medications eventually produced by Sanum-Kehlbeck GmbH and Co. KG of Hoya, Germany.

Prions Are the Likely Cause of Root Canal Infections

These remedies, introduced into the United States about five years ago as antipleomorphic therapies, were developed by Dr. Guenther Enderlein to inhibit bacterial growth and simultaneously neutralize the residual bacterial toxins in root canals. In actuality, many of them are true, minute homeopathic concentrations of live

---

1   A Cavalleri and others, "Comparison of Calcium Hydroxide and Calcium Oxide for Intercanal Medication," *G-Ital.-Endodonzia* 4, no. 3 (1990): 8–13.

microorganisms (and in appendix B are labeled with the designation of "Homeopathic/Isopathic Pleomorphic/Enderlein"). Dr. Enderlein's research includes two major breakthroughs:

1. An understanding of the life cycles and role of primordial parasitic microbes able to change shape, form, and character (known by scientists as *pleomorphism*)—discovered to be certain protein molecules referred to in modern medical science as *prions* (pronounced PREE-ahns)—a class of unusual virus-like infectious particles, and

2. A way of using the means of dismantling these microorganisms about which doctors are taught nothing in medical or dental school.[1]

Kurt Roessel, D.D.S., of Meisenheim-Glan, Germany, wrote to me: "I never use antibiotics or 'wonder' drugs in my dental medicine practice because they often choke off the immune system's response to an illness. In Germany and the United States, scores of medical doctors now enthusiastically use the Pleomorphic-Enderlein (the name in North America) or Sanum-Kehlbeck (the name in Europe) remedies to treat patients for specific illnesses."[2]

The Corrective Enderlein Root Canal Therapies

Remedies for neutralizing the pathogenicity of root canal poisons created by bacteria and other microbes inside the dentinal tubules consist of biological medications, some of which are homeopathically diluted to low concentrations, and suspensions of Mycobacteria or bacilli. These preparations work on the body as a whole (systemically), although their effectiveness can be enhanced

---

1   G. Kolata, "Viruses or Prions: An Old Medical Debate Still Rages," *New York Times*, 4 October 1994, section C, 1.

2   E. Enby, P Gosch, and M. Sheehan, *Hidden Killers: The Revolutionary Medical Discoveries of Professor Guenther Enderlein* (Hoya, Germany: Semmelweis-Institut, 1990), iv.

by local application. The biological medications contain benign protein particles or colloids, called *protits*, that fight disease-causing microorganisms. They assist antibodies produced by the immune system as well and stimulate the immune system response to disease.

Unlike antibiotics and other drugs that often require strong doses to kill pathogenic organisms, the medications developed by Dr. Enderlein work by changing the harmful microbes in the body fluids to nonaggressive forms, which permits gentle self-healing (isopathy). Harmful bacteria and their toxins are broken down and excreted through natural processes. Because these remedies promote healthy cell metabolism and hormonal balance, the body's internal environment experiences profound changes that benefit the entire systemic constitution.

To produce its biological medications, the manufacturer isolates beneficial protit forms from cultures of different molds and fungi during the spore-producing stage, a technique perfected by Dr. Enderlein. The protits, which act as bioregulators in the body, are then diluted and suspended in a specially prepared stabilizing solution.

"The Enderlein biological medications are ideal for changing the body's internal milieu and preventing or healing disease," says Karl-Andreas Guischard, M.D., of Hamburg, Germany. "Dr. Enderlein's preparations represent an important therapy against a wide range of chronic and acute diseases that I treat in my daily practice. The therapy is a basic and effective approach to fighting the causes of illness, and does not merely treat symptoms. As more medical doctors and dentists learn to use these medications in the future they will surely experience many therapy successes that can be documented and passed on to other health professionals."[1]

These remedies developed by Dr. Enderlein are the definitive answer to threats against the health of all people from root canal fillings.

---

1   *Sanum Post*, 1988, 4:5–9.

What Root Canal Therapy Is Not Supposed to Be

Within each natural tooth there is a formation of soft tissue, the dental pulp, which contains nerves, arteries, veins, and lymph vessels, all surrounded by bone-like tissue called *dentin*. The dentin supports the enamel on the tooth's exterior surface to make up the entire dental structure. The dentin also contains dental pulp tissue extending from a pulp chamber in the tooth's crown down to the root's tip, and these are held in the root canal.

When the pulp is damaged by trauma or some other cause, it attempts to heal itself. If it cannot, bacteria invade and cause an infection, which tends to abscess and bring death to the pulp. Root canal therapy attempts to clean the pulp chamber and seal it to prevent recontamination of the root canal system. Cleaning and sealing do often occur from the dentist's ministrations, but leaving behind a nonsterile root canal is the source of health-imperiling and even life-threatening danger for an unknowing patient. Immediately below is a description of one such brief but illustrative situation of effects from nonsterile root canal therapy:

Results of research by Professor Boyd Haley, the University of Kentucky Medical Center biochemist, confirmed that a significant percentage of root canal teeth contain high enough levels of toxins to adversely affect human health. As reported by *The International DAMS Newsletter,* Dr. Haley tested forty teeth containing root canal fillings that he received from five different dentists nationwide. Fewer than 22.5 percent of these root-canaled teeth showed little, if any toxicity; however, another 47.5 percent of them contained moderate levels of deadly poisons. These poisoned teeth caused the dental patients to suffer from symptoms of many types of degenerative diseases. And another 22.5 percent of root-canaled teeth indicated that they contained even higher dangerous levels of toxicity. The poisons present were actually manufactured inside foci of infection floating around the canals of supposedly cleaned teeth roots. The poisons had been spreading throughout the blood streams and lymphatic vessels of those immune-suppressed patients manifesting degenerative diseases. These sick people had undergone root canal therapy, the apparent source of their immune suppression.

Ordinarily the poisons pooled at the bottom of root canals slowly leach into the individual's blood stream to produce a subclinical condition of disease. Symptoms of illness may be subtle or not show themselves. The immune system is becoming suppressed continuously, however, and such suppression leaves that person open to opportunistic infections such as herpes, colds, flu, pneumonia, human immunodeficiency virus (HIV), fungal invasion, parasitic infestation, and more.

As part of the University of Kentucky study, toxins were extracted from the root-canaled teeth by the simple process of placing each tooth in 1 milliliter (ml) of distilled water for twenty minutes. Dr. Haley says more poison was released in the extract when the periodontal ligament surrounding the tooth was scraped before processing. This was a highly significant investigation performed by a biochemist who is strictly objective and oriented to science—completely neutral.

Dr. Haley's Daughter Becomes Well Once Again

Dr. Haley, who does not render health care of any type but rather is a laboratory investigator, was impressed enough by what he found that he convinced his twenty-six-year-old daughter to have her two root-canaled teeth extracted. The young woman, who had been diagnosed with chronic fatigue syndrome and suffered almost continuously from severe migraine headaches, overcame her symptoms of illness almost immediately. The migraines that had been part of her everyday existence for more than three years simply disappeared. Now Dr. Haley's daughter no longer suffers from chronic fatigue syndrome either. In fact, she exhibits more energy than when she was a teenager, he says. Root canal toxins were the sources of the young woman's health difficulties.[1]

Dr. Haley has joined with a colleague, Dr. Curt Pendergrass, at the University of Kentucky Medical Center, to develop an externally applied root canal test. It determines whether root canal teeth

---

1   B. Haley, "Root Canal Teeth Contain Toxins According to New and Old Research," *International DAMS Newsletter* 6, no. 4 (Fall, 1996): 1–3.

already present in a patient's mouth are the reason that person is chronically ill as the result of immune suppression. The Haley/Pendergrass test is a remarkable diagnostic breakthrough furnished to dentists by Dr. Haley's company, Affinity Labeling Technologies, Inc., located at the Advanced Science and Technology Commercialization Center, University of Kentucky in Lexington, Kentucky. (See appendix D for location details.)

Energetic Relationships between Teeth and the Whole Body

The human body's systems, organs, tissues, cell structures, and even the organelles inside each cell respond favorably or adversely to foreign substances coming in contact with any physiological part. The teeth being among those body parts, when something from the outside becomes incorporated within them (such as endodontic [root-canaled] materials), an energetic interrelationship begins and carries on to either a desirable or an antagonistic end. Most of the time, root canal fillings produce a chronically negative physiological response that results in subtle symptoms of illness.

To illustrate my point, the following is an investigation by the Laboratory for Biocompatibility Research on Implant Materials conducted at the Istituti Ortopedici Rizzoli in Bologna, Italy. Six Italian medical scientists—one with the double degrees of physician and dentist—experimented at this Istituti Ortopedici Rizzoli with endodontic cements usually used for filling root canals. The investigators' goal was to learn if any of the cement materials affected the cellular cycle of human bone-growing cells (osteoblasts).

Cultured on petri dishes (*in vitro*), three groups of endodontic compounds were tested. Group I encompassed three zinc oxide and eugenol-based cements (under the brand names Tubliseal, Argoseal, and N2). Group II consisted of three cements with a phenol group other than eugenol (AH26, Forfenan, and Methode R/R). Group III included two calcium hydroxide ($CaOH$)-based cements, which are applied by dentists almost exclusively in Europe (Biocalex and Endocalex). The study showed that all of the standard endodontic cements used in the United States altered the cell cycle of *in vitro* cultured osteoblasts. But Biocalex, which is not approved by the American Dental Association and not employed by endodontists or other American dentists, didn't bring about any negative osteoblastic changes in the test tube.[1]

Those broadly applied American endotontic cements definitely did cause adverse systemic inhibition of cell proliferation, which does tend to suppress the human immune system. Furthermore, locally they are responsible for the failed healing of the slowly expanding, spherical aggregation of mononuclear inflammatory cells (the apex granuloma) that forms within the root canal. This bloody tumor remains as an ever present source of infection for the root-canaled patient. Bacterial toxins then spread throughout the body to bring on a vast variety of degenerative diseases.

The energetic interrelations between the teeth and other body systems include the endocrine glands; the sensory organs; the paranasal sinuses; the joints between bones; segments of the spinal marrow and skin; the vertebrae; the internal organs such as the stomach, large intestine, gall bladder, urinary bladder, and small intestine; the central nervous system and limbic system; and the mammary glands (causing breast cancer). Dysfunctioning root canals bring about an immense amount of damage to a person's physiology. Along with dental amalgam fillings and fluoridation, this is the likely underlying reason for so many autoimmune illnesses being experienced currently among the North American and European populations. Realizing that autoimmune diseases most likely are dentally caused, medical/dental scientists could eliminate them.

The Occurrence of Cavitations at Extraction Sites

In the early 1950s, some European physicians and dentists noticed that certain old dental extraction sites in their patients had

---

1   D. Granchi, Su. Stea, G. Ciapetti, D. Cavedagna, St. Stea, and A. Pizzoferrato, "Endodontic Cements Induce Alterations in the Cell Cycle of *In Vitro* Cultured Osteoblasts," *Oral Surgery, Oral Medicine, Oral Pathology, Oral Radiology Endodontics* 79 (1995): 359–66.

sealed over the top, leaving behind holes where the teeth's roots used to be. Thereafter, European and North American clinical journal articles began appearing that described the condition they called "alveolar cavitational osteopathosis," or ACOs, frequently referred to by dentists as *cavitations*. (Note: see the next chapter on cavitations in which ACOs are currently identified and explained as NICOs.)

These cavitations actually were appearing as holes in the patients' jawbones as a result of lack of healing at those sites where the lining of dental sockets had not been removed. Lack of such removal probably is nothing more than the performance of careless dental surgery, for almost every dental student learns that removal of the lining of a tooth's socket is necessary after the pulling of teeth.

Between the tooth and the bone lies a layer of connective tissue called the *periodontal ligament* (*perio* is Greek for "around," and *dontal* refers to the tooth). When a tooth is removed, the ligament most often remains behind. If not taken out at the time of surgery, this ligament stops the bone from regenerating in order to fill the space that's left. Consequently, the socket heals over with a thin layer of bone and new gum tissue; the socket never fills in with good solid bone. As a result, this void stays as a hole or cavitation in the bone that fills with microbial toxins. Toxic products floating in the body's fluids become perpetual sources of stress to the immune system. It's another reason for immune suppression to develop and degenerative disease to set in.

Looking through the microscope, two main types of cells will be identified lining the cavitations. First there are the pathological organisms, streptococci, which unquestionably produce infection. Second are monocytes, the particular form of white blood cell invariably present in one hundred different kinds of arthritis, especially osteoarthritis, rheumatoid arthritis, ankylosing spondilitis, scleroderma, systemic lupus erythematosis, and many more joint disorders. The high incidence of arthritides among populations of Western industrialized countries most often results from the presence of cavitations in people's mouths, which stimulate the formation of large numbers of monocytes.

The immunologic challenge is intensified for a person with cavitations. When tissue biopsies are performed on bone immediately adjacent to a root canal-filled tooth, lymphocytic cells of chronic long-term immune abuse are found in profusion. This shows an ongoing nidus of autoimmune disease.

The Dental Solution to Cavitations

What's the solution to cavitations? Although I go into detail about this subject in the next chapter, here is a smattering of information that hints at the condition's correction. At least one milliimeter of bone around the extraction site must be the surgically removed. That's the well-proven answer to preventing holes (cavitational ostitis) in the jawbone.[1]

It's the careless or unskillful dentist who brings on this life-threatening, doctor-caused (iatrogenic) problem of cavitations. In contrast, the prevention of cavitations is simple, fast, and painless.

How does someone about to undergo dental surgery ensure cavitations are prevented? I advise readers with the potential of having holes created in their jawbones to emphasize to their treating dentists to merely take an additional minute after an extraction to clean out the socket with a slow-speed drill and rinse the space properly. Make this statement before treatment ever begins. When this is done, the healing proceeds much more rapidly with less bleeding and little or no pain. If the dental surgeon objects to being told what to do so that you may avoid cavitations, find another dentist. You need such a cavitation like you need another hole in your head.

The Definite Dangers of Dental Root Canals

Five years ago, thirty-four-year-old Mrs. Margaret Blackstone of Milwaukee, Wisconsin, underwent a root canal procedure on her front

---

1   H. A. Huggins, "Cavitations" in *Position Papers: Amalgam Issue, Root Canals, Cavitations* (Colorado Springs, Colo.: Huggins Diagnostic, Inc., 1991), 23, 24.

tooth—number eight—one of the incisors, which caused miserable problems. The woman described how it had pained her terribly. Almost every other day for two months she was forced to return to her dentist, who worked on the root canal to make the pain bearable. The dentist finally managed to achieve some desensitization for Blackstone.

Nine months later, however, a series of health problems started for the piano teacher and homemaker who was attempting to become pregnant with her first child. "I went through a hysterectomy because of excessive vaginal bleeding," she said. "The surgeon also took my left ovary. I was devastated by realizing that I would never mother my own children. A short time after leaving the hospital, I started to experience ongoing troubles with my gastrointestinal tract. For one thing, I was always constipated, which had never been the case before. I didn't feel well at all, but repeated enemas finally gave me some relief.

"Next I developed sinus problems, and they brought on severe headaches," Blackstone continued. "The doctor tried to treat me with antibiotics for a long time before discovering that all my sinus cavities were filled with polyps. He referred me for surgery to remove them. Even so, I still had sinus pressure and very thick drainage.

"Then I began to feel burning sensations in my esophagus and stomach, which went on for two months and slowly faded away. I developed severe burning in my vulva after this which kept up for two years while I consulted numerous gynecologists to find out what was causing the sensation. No one discovered the reason for such burning nor did any doctor help me get rid of it," she wrote in a letter to George Meinig, D.D.S. "It just continued on and on. Then, three months ago I woke up to severe pain in my right side. I couldn't even stand up because of the pain. In the hospital emergency room, diagnostic ultrasound showed that there was a large mass growing off of my remaining ovary. It was part cystic and part solid and required emergency surgery.

"The surgeons told me that the mass was full of infection and blood and that my ovary was twisted. They cut it out. Now I have no more ovaries or uterus at age thirty-four. I'm just an empty shell who can't procreate. The doctors had no idea why the ovary was so abnormally twisted," Blackstone confided to Dr. Meinig. (Dr. George Meinig furnished this letter for my use in this publication.)

"But my problems seemed to be solved, including the burning vulva and discharging sinuses by my having that front root canal pulled out along with the correction of a cavitation discovered by my biological dentist. He cleaned out the root canal and the hole in my jawbone and used several of those unusual American Pleomorphic/Enderlein, homeopathic/isopathic remedies as part of his usual therapeutic procedure. No more health problems have appeared for me, and it's five months since the root canal has been removed. I'm so happy to feel like a well person once again. I should have had the root canal removed a long time ago."

The High Price of Root Canals

The price of root canal fillings is an expensive one to pay, much more than money, for it entails a variety of health problems that could lead to a series of serious illnesses and even bring death. Dr. Hal A. Huggins states, "I have found nothing more vicious than the reactions people have to root canals."[1]

In his 1925 article published in the *Journal of the American Medical Association*, Dr. Weston A. Price reported that a large variety of degenerative diseases arise from root canal therapy. Among them are endocarditis and other heart troubles, kidney and bladder disorders, arthritis of all types, rheumatism, mental illness, lung problems, pregnancy complications, crippling degenerative diseases that don't respond to treatment, and most kinds of bacterial infections.

As I described earlier, Dr. Price discovered that these same health problems are transferable to rabbits when root-canaled teeth are taken from people who suffer with the diseases. If the teeth are implanted under the skin of these rabbits, usually the laboratory animals die from the same disease affecting the human victims.

---

1   H. A. Huggins, *It's All in Your Head* (Garden City Park, N.Y.: Avery Publishing Group, 1993), 83.

Meanwhile, those particular persons giving up the root-canaled teeth get rid of their illnesses.[1]

Toxicity Testing of Root-Canaled and Cavitational Teeth

It would be a good thing to know if your immune system is functioning appropriately and, if not, to take measures to correct it. Don't you wish that you could determine the status of your immunity? Of course, the medical profession makes that possible to do by undertaking certain laboratory examinations of your body fluids—urine, blood, sputum, and other secretions. However, today you can have your oral areas of cavitation and those teeth containing root canals tested to determine if they are hazardous to your health.

As mentioned earlier in this chapter, the laboratory test of one's oral cavity was developed by Dr. Boyd E. Haley and James Pendergrass, Ph.D., Affinity Labeling Technologies expert. They have perfected a technique for detecting the toxicants (poisons) in the tooth extracts and cavitational material taken from patients who are happy to give up their root canal fillings. The two researchers have perfected technology used worldwide for elegant biochemistry studies on the structure and function of proteins and enzymes. This same technology has been adapted by them for dental diagnostics. They test the discarded teeth taken from people who possess endodontic and cavitational faults.

Using their technique for the determination of dental difficulties, Drs. Haley and Pendergrass have published about 120 peer reviewed journal articles that explain its application to the testing of toxic materials. Their analysis for oral toxicants of root-canaled teeth and cavitations is sensitive, fast, easy and inexpensive for dentists employing the test and for patients desiring to have the test done. The Boyd/Pendergrass method and its advantage is offered for use by the informed medical/dental consumer as well as for dentists. A simple biological screening procedure is used to determine both the

---

1   W. A. Price, "Dental Infections and Related Degenerative Diseases," *The Journal of the American Medical Association* 84 (24 January 1925): 254–59.

level and type of poison to which the patient is being exposed so that decisions regarding further dental procedures may be made. To learn how you may gain access to their test, I suggest that you contact the two University of Kentucky scientists. (See appendix D.)[1]

Is Your Dentist Performing Root Canal Fillings Properly?

Dr. Meinig writes: "One can't study tooth decay without also giving thought to the problems of periodontal disease (pyorrhea). Those who have a marked tendency to develop dental caries are also prone to develop degenerative disease afflictions and, in addition, their ionic calcium levels are depressed. . . . It is time for dentists and patients to realize the decay of teeth is not just a local disturbance but is actually a systemic disease which involves the whole body."[2]

Performing root canal therapy requires removing infection from areas of dental decay. Many of the procedures performed in endodontics involve large sections of bone loss at the end of a root of the tooth. When the dentist does the root canal filling, one of the requirements is to see that bone fills in with new bone. To accomplish this for the patient, infection must be cleaned away entirely. The following summary is a brief description of the *proper* endodontic procedure that should be undertaken by a conscientious dentist:

After the extractionist or endodontic therapist removes the infected tooth, the dentist must also remove the periodontal ligament or membrane, which is a fibrous tissue that holds the tooth in its socket. This ligament keeps the tooth from falling out. Along with the dysfunctional tooth, it is usual for any periodontal ligament to become infected, and it is still attached securely to the surrounding bony socket even after the tooth is excised. The American Association of Endodontists recommends that the dentist go into the socket with a

---

1   B. Haley and J. Pendergrass, "Characterization and Identification of Chemical Toxicants Isolated from Cavitational Materials and Infected Root Canaled Teeth: *In Situ* Testing of Teeth for Toxicity and Infection," personal communication, 4 February 1997.

2   Meinig, *Root Canal Cover-Up*, 85, 88.

slow-moving drill and remove that periodontal membrane (ligament) and about 1 mm of the bony socket itself to prevent reinfection from occurring. Most dentists fail to either take out the periodontal ligament or do the bone removal. That's performing a mismanaged dental procedure, tantamount to medical/dental malpractice.

Another health professional, Robert C. Atkins, M.D., medical director of The Atkins Center in New York City and the author of six books, including *Dr. Atkins' New Diet Revolution* (M. Evans, 1992), is dead set against root canal therapy performed by standard practicing dentists in the conventional manner.

Dr. Atkins writes in his monthly newsletter: "Your dentist would like to sterilize that dead tooth, but because of the intricate system of dentin tubules that runs through it, the best he or she can do is to seal it up in a root canal. Unfortunately, that also seals in various bacteria that, deprived of oxygen, produce extremely toxic waste products called *thioethers*. These thioether toxins escape into your body through the junction of tooth and bone.

"There's nothing your immune system can do about it, because the immunoglobulin and white cells are too big to squeeze into the dentin tubules. Your tooth becomes a permanent and protected source of poison for the rest of your body, increasing your risk of such autommimmune conditions as arthritis, multiple sclerosis, lupus, suppression of bone marrow, and, most commonly, autoimmune thyroiditis (also known as Hashimoto's disease), which often leads to a subtle decrease in the functioning of the immune system," concludes Dr. Robert Atkins.[1]

Get Rid of Root Canals or Take Precautions against Them

Why are infections under root canal fillings stressful to the immune system? Because they are *focal infections*, meaning as I've defined, they linger, doing damage, and remain unrecognized as the

---

1   R. Atkins, "Is Other Dental Work Harmful," *Secrets of the Atkins Center*, monthly newsletter (September 1996), 11, 12.

source of difficulty. They're in a place where bacteria transfer their poisons to other tissues, glands, or organs, setting up entirely new infections. Some 95 percent of all focal infections start in root canals, other teeth, and the tonsils.

"If you are experiencing health problems after root canal fillings have been performed, no matter how long ago, you should suspect that infection is coming from the lateral canals of that root-filled tooth. These are accessory tubules that come out of the tooth root but that don't show up on X-ray films," advises former practicing endodontist Dr. George Meinig. "They are not easy to visualize, and it's impossible to treat them properly with ordinary methods available to conventionally practicing dentists. Endodontists today are assuring patients that there's nothing wrong with the treatment being offered, but they refuse to acknowledge that accessory tubules of the root canals can become infected."[1]

The way to know if your root canal is toxic is in two ways: (1) undergo a series of laboratory blood and urine tests to determine the viability of your immune system and, (2) undertake the root canal dental toxicity testing invented by Drs. Haley and Pendergrass that I have described. Knowing your immunological status and whether or not a root canal filling is producing poison are the two mandatory precautions required by anyone victimized by one of the chronic degenerative diseases or an autoimmune disease such as chronic fatigue syndrome. Then adopt some of the treatment options put forth in this chapter: have root-filling with Biocalex, use Dr. Guenther Enderlein's Homeopathic/Isopathic therapies, or participate in nutritional immune system boosting with diet and nutrients as is described in chapters 15 and 16.

Taking these precautionary measures and the therapies accompanying them is the least you can do to assure the restoration of good health for you or your loved ones.

---

1   L. Lee, "Laura Lee Interview with George Meinig, DDS & Dr. M. LaMarche: Cavitations & Root Canals," *Townsend Letter for Doctors and Patients* 157/158 (August/September 1996): 48–154.

Japanese Green Tea to Counteract Root Canal Infection

Antibacterial and bactericidal actions of four kinds of commercially obtained extracted Japanese green tea were tested against twenty-four bacterial strains isolated from infected root canals. The five Japanese investigators, all dentists, found that certain components in Japanese green tea provide good bacteria-killing properties when applied as a treatment measure for infected teeth, especially against those particular microorganisms commonly found in the mouth. The microbes against which the four Japanese green teas were tested and found effective included:

Streptococcus mutans	*Eubacteria lentun*
S. sanguis	*E. limosum*
S. intermedius	*Actinomyces israeli*
Staphylococcus aureus	*Lubteium rogosae*
S. epidermidis	*Propionibacterium acnes*
Actinomyces naeslundii	*Veillonella parva*
A. viscosus	*V. alcalescens*
Lactobacillus casei	*Fusobacterium nucleatum*
L. acidophillus	*Bacterides endodontalis*
Peptococcus mugnus	*B. intermedius*
P. niger	*Bifidobacterium bifidum*
P. coccus intermedius	*Fusobacterium nucleatum*

The dental researchers concluded their published report with a positive outlook. They wrote: "Japanese green teas do not have an irritating potential. The results [of this investigation] suggest that extracts of Japanese green tea may be useful as a medicament for treatment of infected root canals."[1]

---

1   N. Horba, Y. Maekawa, M. Ito, T. Matsumoto, and H. Nakamura, "A Pilot Study of Japanese Green Tea as a Medicament: Antibacterial and Bactericidal Effects," *Journal of Endodontics* 17, no. 3 (March 1991): 122–24.

Thirteen

Cavitational Causes of Jawbone Deterioration

In letters mailed to my source, the upstate New York dentist, a foot doctor documented his awful experience with oral cavity pathology. The upstate dentist provided me with the foot doctor's documents. This distressed dental patient wants his horror story told as a means of alerting others to the cavitational causes and cure of jawbone deterioration. His was a series of dentist-caused (iatrogenic) difficulties from which the now-fortunate man has recently recovered.

Having practiced podiatric medicine in St. Paul, Minnesota, for over four decades, during August 1998 seventy-two-year-old Allen J. Nordhelm (pseudonym) underwent six decavitational surgical operations on dental sockets. All six extractions involved root-canaled teeth. While this was a lot of tooth pulling to be done in a short time, the multiple procedures have considerably improved the podiatrist's physical, emotional, and mental health. What follows is Dr. Allen J. Nordhelm's factual narrative of his oral cavity consternation as told by him in three lengthy letters written, in turn, to George E. Meinig, D.D.S., F.A.C.D., of Ojai, California; Christopher J. Hussar, D.D.S., D.O., of Reno, Nevada; and the New York dentist who, in turn, furnished them to me.

The Cavitated Patient's Tale of Dismay with Dentistry

"When I was about age eight I fell down while skating and chipped off a small corner of the left central incisor (tooth number 9).

During my mid-teen years, this same chipped incisor became inflamed and developed an infection. Our family dentist offered my mother and me no choice except to perform a root canal procedure, and it was done," writes Dr. Nordhelm. "I didn't know about such things then, and neither did my mom, but this 'good guy' dentist failed to clean out the tooth's nerve socket and left in some root material. His poor dental technique was destined to be the beginning source of much illness for me.

"In my early twenties the root canaled incisor turned dark and another 'first-rate' dentist recommended extraction, advising that a dead tooth was not healthy to have in one's mouth. I believed him," Dr. Nordhelm affirms. "So, I allowed the extractionist to yank my tooth and install a bridge. Like the prior dentist, of course, this second fellow did not ream out the socket either and left behind the periodontal ligament, which we know now must not be allowed.

"It's my belief that all of my recent dental difficulties are founded on this inadequately removed root canal, because the poison left at its base spread through my jawbone. It affected my lower left molar (tooth number 19), which required a root canal be performed on November 3, 1988. And my upper right molar (tooth number 3) required another root canal on January 23, 1991," says the podiatrist. "Some time passed and then both of my lower left premolars abscessed. Consequently, two root canals had to be implanted on June 18, 1994. With more poison spreading along my jaw, both upper right premolars developed infections and two more root canals were put in on April 24, 1996. These many infections and the endodontics to correct them had me feeling absolute agony. The pain was tremendous and lasted excessively long.

"But then, approximately two months after the last root canal procedure, my real health problems began in earnest. First I was struck by a bilateral peripheral neuropathy [functional disturbance at the nerve endings] of the lower extremities. Then gradually other adverse symptoms started to appear. In turn, I was hit by marked bilateral occular [eye] headaches, trigeminal neuralgia [pain at the fifth cranial nerve] on both sides of the face, recurrent angina pectoris [heart pain], occasional acute attacks of left-sided pleurisy [lung inflammation], sporadic cardiac arrhythmias [irregular heart beats], and recurrent insomnia [chronic sleeplessness]," explains Dr. Nordhelm.

"From so much illness, I experienced a steady weight loss, dropping from 155 to 114 pounds. I looked like a strawless scarecrow. Then minor ongoing tinnitus struck my left ear, and acute rheumatism with severe sensations of coldness developed in both legs. The chilling rheumatism became so bad that to get any sleep, I was forced to wear thermal underwear bottoms at night and pack my limbs with hot water bottles," Dr. Nordhelm says. "Later I came down with general nervous irritability manifested physically by a tic of my left eyelid. Chronic fatigue syndrome hit so hard that I was forced to give up skiing, a sport I've enjoyed since being a little kid.

"In addition to the many serious physical impairments, I was additionally experiencing an ever increasing arterial hypertension [high blood pressure], which reached a peak on September 1, 1997, of 221/122. This elevated blood pressure continued despite my physician's prescription of 30 mg daily of Vasotec in a divided dose morning and evening," added the patient. "With my swallowing all of this high blood pressure medicine, fluid accumulated in my tissues, which necessitated the doctor prescribing diuretics for me to pop down each morning. Of course, I couldn't ever be far from a toilet, since about every half hour throughout each day I felt an urgency to urinate.

"Throbbing neuralgic pains from both sides of the jaw radiated up into both of my ears, temples, and eye orbits, which pains persisted for months. And, a fungus spread itchy dermatitis-like lesions, which ran up and down the anterior aspect of my right leg and eventually affected the same area of my left leg. Neither the bacterial antibiotic neopsorin, tea tree oil, dermatitis creams, an antifungal antibiotic, or anything else took away the fungal lesions. I itched and scratched much of the time.

"Eventually, with all my energy depleted for coping with these many adversities, I could no longer attend to my podiatry patients' needs. I had to close my office and quit working altogether. My enforced inactivity and big financial loss put my family and me in terrible circumstances," declares Dr. Nordhelm. "I remained a wreck in this way for another year until I read a book, *Root Canal Cover-Up*, written and self-published by George

E. Meinig.[1] In Dr. Meinig's book, I recognized myself. The same multiple symptoms associated with cavitations, which result from root canals or poorly excised teeth, had struck me. Thus, it was this book which alerted me to the dental dismay which lies as the underlying source of my massive number of afflictions."

As you'll learn later in this chapter, Dr. Allan Nordhelm has now had his cavitated difficulties solved. He consulted a holistic (biological) dentist who performed the kind of cavitational cleanout that should have been done initially, starting when the patient was a young boy.

Underlying Pathology Causing Cavitational Poisoning

During the period from May 1915 to November 1930, Weston A. Price, D.D.S., M.S., of Cleveland, Ohio, conducted laboratory and clinical research and published reports, some of which I mentioned in chapter 12. Dr. Price's research proved that root canals implanted daily by general dentists and endodontists into thousands of mouths worldwide by his fellow dentists are the underlying sources of massive numbers of physical afflictions. The profession of organized allopathic dentistry here and abroad has studiously ignored the Price research. Invariably, the endodontic procedures dentists perform bring about infection with subsequent immune suppression. The resulting disease symptoms are exemplified by what had happened to Allen J. Nordhelm, D.P.M., of St. Paul, Minnesota.

In a series of twenty-five published clinical journal articles and three dental books (most of them referenced in chronological order in footnotes on the following two pages), Dr. Weston Price documented "the effects of root-filled teeth on systemic diseases," says Dr. Price's admirer, Dr. Hal A. Huggins.[2]

---

1   G. E. Meinig, *Root Canal Cover-Up* (Ojai, Calif: Bion Publishing, 1994).

2   H. A Huggins, *The Price of Root Canals* (Colorado Springs, Colo.: Huggins Diagnostic Center, 1993), i.

For more than seventy-five years these Weston Price papers have been kept away from the consuming public by members of the American Dental Association, which wishes to avoid putting the endodontists out of business or causing their colleagues to be sued. Yet much of his investigations had been undertaken while Dr. Price worked as director of the Research Institute of the National Dental Association (NDA).

"Under the NDA auspices he conducted clinical studies on thousands of patients and tens of thousands of rabbits which gained him a position of high popularity as a speaker and publisher internationally," continues Dr. Huggins. "Of the over 220 papers and three major books that he authored during his lifetime, most of it [his experimentation] was conducted at the NDA Research Institute. And Dr. Price refused any salary for this dedicated service."[1]

So what did the Price experiments uncover about root canals that relate to poisoning from cavitations? It's all exposed in Dr. Price's papers, some of them published in the *Journal of the American Dental Association* along with other dental journals.[2]

---

1   Ibid.

2   W. A. Price, "A Report of the Progress of the Research Commission of the National Dental Association," *The Dental Review of the Illinois State Dental Society* (May 1915); W. A. Price, "The Prevention of Systemic Diseases Arising from Mouth Infections and the Purpose and Plan of the Research Institute of the National Dental Association," *Cleveland Medical Journal* 14 (October 1915): 657–68; W. A. Price, "The Pathology of Dental Infections and Its Relation to General Diseases," report of the Canadian Oral Prophylactic Association, February 1916; W. A Price, "The Present Status of Our Knowledge of the Relation of Mouth Infection to Systemic Disease," *Dental Review* 31, no. 4 (April 1917): 271–97; W. A. Price, "The Relative Efficiency of Medicaments for the Sterilization of Tooth Structures," read before the National Dental Association at its twenty-first annual session, 23 October 1917; W. A. Price, "The Relation of Dental Operations and Dental Lesions to Systemic Lesions," *Oral Health* 8, no. 4 (April 1918); W. A. Price, "Report of Laboratory Investigations on Root Filling Materials," *Journal of the National Dental Association* 5, no. 12 (December 1918); W. A. Price, "Address Delivered to a Mass Meeting of Toronto Dentists, in the Interests of the Canadian Dental Research Foundation," *Oral Health* 10, no. 11 (November 1920): 381–83; W. A. Price, *Dental Infections, Oral and Systemic*, vol. 1 (Cleveland, Ohio: Penton Publishing Col, 1923); W. A Price, *Dental Infections and Degenerative Diseases* (Cleveland, Ohio: Penton Publishing Co., 1923); W. A. Price, "Dental Infections, Oral and Systemic," *Oral Health* 13 (December 1923); W. A. Price, "Newer Data for Establishing a Basis for Judgment Regarding Focal Infection with Special Consideration for Child Welfare," report for the Northern Ohio

Explanations of the Price findings were given by Dr. George Meinig and biological dentist Michael LaMarche, D.D.S., of Lake Stevens, Washington, appearing together on the *Laura Lee Radio Show*, hosted by Laura Lee of Bellevue, Washington (telephone 800/243-1438 to receive the recording of their joint appearance). The Meinig/LaMarche radio interview is in the public domain, and it was republished in the August/September 1996 issue of the *Townsend Letter for Doctors and Patients*. During the course of that interview, a particular patient situation was given as an illustration.

"Dr. Price treated a man with kidney trouble who had a root-filled tooth," Dr. Meinig explained on the *Laura Lee Radio Show*. "He removed that patient's tooth and put it under the skin of a healthy rabbit; the rabbit got kidney trouble and died within a few days. Then Dr. Price took the tooth out of this dead rabbit, surgically of course, and washed it in soap and water, disinfected the root filled tooth with a disinfectant, and placed it under the skin of another rabbit. This second rabbit came down with kidney trouble and passed away too. He then took that same root-filled tooth out of the second rabbit, disinfected it, and for a third time placed it into a healthy rabbit,

---

Dental Association, June 1924; W. A. Price, "Focal Infection and Its Relation to Restorative Dentistry," *The Dental Outlook* 11, no. 9 (September 1924); W. A Price, "Dental Infections and Related Degenerative Diseases," *Journal of the American Medical Association* 84 (24 January 1925): 254–59; W. A. Price, "Fundamentals Suggested by Recent Researches for Diagnosis, Prognosis, and Treatment of Dental Focal Infections," *Journal of the American Dental Association* (June 1925): 1–26; W. A. Price, Affirmative of the Buckley-Price debate, "Resolved, That Practically All Infected Pulpless Teeth Should be Removed," *Journal of the American Dental Association* (December 1925): 1–38; W. A. Price, "The Responsibility of the Management for the Effect of Focal Infection (Especially Dental) on the Life, Health, and Efficiency of the Employee," *Dental Items of Interest* (December 1925); W. A. Price, "Some Systemic Expressions of Dental Infections," *Annals of Clinical Medicine* 4, no. 11 (May 1926): 943–74; W. A. Price, "Dental Infections: Their Dangers and Prevention," *Radiology* (May 1928): 3–20; W. A. Price, "New Fundamentals for the Treatment and Prevention of Dental Disease Based on Calcium Utilization and Disturbance, with Special Consideration of Factors Determining When an Infected Tooth Becomes a Liability," *Journal of the American Dental Association* (March 1929); W. A. Price, "Some Contributing Factors to the Degenerative Diseases, with Special Consideration of the Role of Dental Focal Infections," *Dental Cosmos* (October/November 1930).

which developed kidney trouble and died. Dr. Price repeated the same experiment thirty times.

"The reason he performed this laboratory experiment over and over again was that he wanted to prove to himself and to the world that infectious material [attached to root-canaled teeth] was able to be transferred [from living animal to living animal and from one location in the body to another]. The only way he knew how to show this was to do more animal experiments," Dr. Meinig said. "Now one of the things that happens with these root-filled teeth is that when they are removed it is very often the periodontal membrane [ligament] that is infected. The surrounding bony socket remains in the jaw and sometimes healing gets rid of the infection but many times it does not. What happens then is an infection occurs in the jawbone."

"And is that when this [new and unfamiliar] term, *cavitation*, comes in?" asked Laura Lee, in addressing her question to Dr. Michael LaMarche.

"Yes. A cavitation actually is a cavity within the bone, which was formerly occupied by a tooth. This cavity inside the jaw that is lined with dead bone causes pain," said Dr. LaMarche. "Dr. Jerry Bouquot, an oral pathologist, began researching this condition extensively in the early 1990s. He named such a jawbone cavity a *Neuralgia Inducing Cavitational Osteonecrosis*, but most dentists commonly use the acronym *NICO*."[1]

While NICO is the defining term for damage left behind by the application of poor dental technique for the implantation of root canals, other names that describe the resulting jawbone pathology include *chronic ostitis* or *osteitis, avascular necrosis, trigger point bone cavity, alveolar osteo pathosis, ischemic osteonecrosis, Ratner's bone cavity, aseptic osteonecrosis, alveolar cavitation pathosis, avascular necrosis, intraosseous ischemia, invisible osteomyelitis, Robert's bone cavity,* and *G. V. Black's forgotten disease.*[2]

---

1   L. Lee, "Cavitations and Root Canals," *Townsend Letter for Doctors and Patients* (August/September 1996): 48–55, 148–54.

2   S. Stockton, *Beyond Amalgam: The Hidden Health Hazard Posed by Jawbone Cavitations* (North Port, Fl.: Nature's Publishing, 1998), front cover.

Oral pathologist and clinical laboratory director Jerry E. Bouquot, D.D.S., M.S.D., of Head and Neck Diagnostics of America, a division of the Maxillofacial Center for Diagnostics and Research of Morgantown, West Virgina, performs tissue biopsies on extracted teeth. Upon request, Dr. Bouquot furnishes dentists and other health professionals reports on extracted teeth and additional specimens, including gross descriptions, microscopic descriptions, microscopic diagnoses, and clinical diagnoses. Much of the time he is kept busy evaluating specimens and responding with biopsy reports to dentists concerning their patients' pulled teeth. (See Dr. Bouquot's laboratory address in appendix A).

A textbook definition of the NICO cavitation has been offered by four dental/medical experts. They define this dentist-created pathology in the following manner: "Neuralgia-inducing cavitational osteonecrosis [NICO] is a low-grade, nonsuppurative, radiographically 'invisible' osteomyelits of the jaws diagnosed in some patients exhibiting atypical facial pain or trigeminal neuralgia. The intraosseous NICO lesion closely resembles ischemic or aseptic necrosis of the long bones in its histopathologic and clinical presentations and, therefore, may result from poor vascular circulation of the bone marrow of the jaws."[1]

Trigeminal neuralgia, also known as *tic douloureux*, is a disorder of the sensory nucleus of the trigeminal nerve, producing bouts of severe, seconds-long, lancinating pain along the distribution of one or more divisions of the trigeminal nerve. Most often the pain strikes within the mandibular or maxillary divisions of the nerve. It may or may not occur when cavitation or NICO is the underlying jawbone pathology.

---

1   "Neuralgia-Inducing, Cavitational Osteonecrosis," in *Oral & Maxillofacial Pathology* (Philadelphia: W. B. Saunders Publishers, 1995).

How to Recognize If You Have a Cavitation

NICO characteristically affects persons forty to sixty years old but has been diagnosed in patients ranging in age from eighteen to eighty-four. Women are affected twice as frequently as men. Any tooth socket site (alveolar process) along the upper or lower jawbone (mandible or maxilla) may be involved, but the third molar areas most often show the disease. Approximately one-third of NICO patients complain of more than one alveolar site of involvement, and 10 percent of the victims possess dead bone (osteonecrosis) lesions in all four quadrants of the jawbones. Dr. Bouquot explains that the average duration of neuralgia pain before a biological dentist diagnoses NICO's presence in the patient's jaws is six years, but the duration can range in length from a few months to more than twenty years.[1]

Cavitation, or NICO, is almost always identified in people with facial pain that mimics neuralgia, even to the point of occasionally possessing trigger points similar to those of trigeminal neuralgia. The involvement site is best identified by searching for a small zone of increased sensitivity or hyperesthesia or normal pain response in an area otherwise anesthetized by injection of a local anesthetic agent. (This examination, which uses procaine or some other local anesthetic, is known as the McMahon hyperesthesia/anesthesia test.)

Seldom are there visible alterations of the oral cavity's overlying mucous membrane (the mucosa). Also, the typical NICO lesion is not visualized well or perhaps not at all on panoramic radiographs, magnetic resonance imaging (MRI), computed tomography (CT), or any form of radioisotope bone scans, except technetium-99 scans. Many NICO lesions do present themselves as "hot spots" by application of the technetium-99 diagnosis technique. Unless he or she has a vast amount of experience in reading simple periapical X-ray films, a dentist won't see the subtle changes that distinguish NICO. When visible, however, NICO lesions usually present poorly demarcated, nonexpansile radiolucencies. Using technical dental language,

---

1   J. E. Bouquot, "In Review of NICOS, G. V. Black's Forgotten Disease," Edition 4.3, 1995.

Dr. Jerry Bouquot states that involved teeth appear "often with irregular vertical remnants of lamina dura associated with old extraction sites in the region."

The Cavitat, a sonogram diagnostic device for detecting NICO lesions, was recently invented by an engineer who was devastated by both cavitations and mercury amalgams. These toxic dental procedures performed on Robert Jones of Springfield, Virginia caused him to develop amyotrophic lateral sclerosis ,(ALS). When he eventually got rid of the poisonous conditions in his mouth, Bob Jones recovered from the ALS symptoms and is mobile once again.

As described by attendees of the second annual International Congress of Bioenergetic Medicine, the Jones Cavitat is an acoustic sound wave diagnostic instrument that provides a three-dimensional perspective image of the interior of the jawbone at suspected osteomyelitis sites. The Cavitat was designed by Mr. Jones for the needs of dental surgeons who require a more positive method to identify and accurately locate necrotic lesions. In clinical tests with over six hundred patients (and in followup studies of another four thousand dental patients), the Cavitat performed without a single false positive or negative and has indicated ischemic osteonecrosis in detail. Following the successful detection by the Cavitat, a significant number of patients have undergone the indicated surgery to remove NICO lesions.[1]

The way you can determine that you've been made the victim of either a poor root canal implantation technique or malpracticed extractionist dentistry is by the residual pathological effects of cavitation. Also, you may fit the profile of the typical cavitation patient.

First off, you're probably middle age or older, since the disease seldom occurs in people younger than thirty-five. It's well established but unexplained that the right side of the face is affected in more patients than the left by a ratio of 1.7 to 1. And the female-to-male sex distribution is 1.17 to 1. The pain of trigeminal neuralgia associated with cavitation is of a penetrating, searing, or lancinating type often set off by touching an oral trigger point or by chewing or

---

1   Stockton, *Beyond Amalgam*, 44.

brushing the teeth. And as mentioned, the interval between extraction and onset of pain ranges from months to many years later.[1]

How NICO or Cavitation Is Permanently Corrected

"Over the last ten years, I've verified a secret about chronic pain. It may be caused by previously unsuspected infections in the jaw and can be easily eliminated through simple surgical procedures," says dentist and osteopathic physician Christopher John Hussar, D.D.S., D.O., of Reno, Nevada. "I say 'verified' because, surprisingly, medical literature from the 1850s indicates that U.S. physicians were aware that chronic, untreated dental infections could produce serious symptoms elsewhere in the body. In fact, although this application has since been discredited, physicians once routinely recommended having teeth extracted as a cure for arthritis.

"The concept of chronic dental infections producing pain elsewhere in the body used to be more widely accepted in American medicine; these infections were known as a cause of 'focal disease.' Most American doctors and dentists seem to have forgotten this link but, since 1988, using an approach called *neural therapy*, I have performed thousands of dental procedures to remove chronically infected or dead bony tissue to relieve unexplained pain," Dr. Hussar states.[2]

In my coauthored book, *Instant Pain Relief,* William J. Faber, D.O., of Milwaukee, Wisconsin, and I describe neural therapy for providing instant pain relief for dental patients with disease symptoms far removed from their oral cavities. It's possible for the skilled injectionist to reverse chronic joint pain, headaches, blindness, hearing disorders, arthritic pain, rheumatoid problems, and all manner of other unexplained pain disorders. This neural therapy technique has given life back to people who were suicidal because of their ceaseless

---

1   R. P. Langlais, O. E. Langland, and C. J. Nortje, "Neuralgia-Inducing Cavitational Ostenoecrosis," in *Diagnostic Imaging of the Jaws* (Philadelphia: Williams & Wilkins Publishers, 1995).

2   C. Hussar, "No More Chronic Pain," *Alternative Medicine Digest* 15 (1996): 30–34.

pain and other body discomforts. Dr. Faber, Dr. Hussar, and dozens of other skilled health professionals who use local anesthetics are highly successful in removing disease symptoms permanently by the administration of neural therapy. (See appendix A to acquire more knowledge about the subject.)[1]

Here is how neural therapy treats cavitations: the procedure involves injecting a local anesthetic, such as Xylocaine, novocaine, procaine or lidocaine, into a scar, nerve ganglion, or an infected area of the jaw to numb, then block, the nerve flow—in this case, through a specific tooth or tooth site, which was found by use of the McMahon hyperesthesia/anesthesia test described above. If the pain is abolished with this injection, you can be certain that the dentist has found the primary problem site in the jaw.

"The dental sockets and ridges on the upper and lower jaws develop lesions or cavities as a result of chronic infections. The lesions are hollow, set inside the jawbone," continues Dr. Hussar. "When you open up these lesions and see the mush that comes out, you can understand why these infection sites will not heal on their own. I have opened up sections of jawbones and taken out decayed vegetable matter such as corn and carrots that had become locked within the original extraction site and were not reabsorbed by the body.

"Inside these jawbone cavities you may also encounter viruses, bacteria, yeasts, and parasites, all of which contribute to the harmful dental focal disturbance. The mouth is the filthiest place in the body," Dr. Hussar assures us. "Extraction of the root-canaled tooth and a thorough cleaning out of the infected jaw reverses these conditions in a dramatically short time, usually in a few days. . . . The bone cavitates, or forms a mushy depression (a cavity) subject to infection and the death of bone tissue. This results when the bone of the extraction site refuses to heal properly, literally leaving the root outlined.

"This situation leads to dead bone (osteonecrosis) that produces nerve pain (neuralgia), usually in the head, face, neck, or shoulders. But NICO can produce problems elsewhere in the body, such as heart

---

1   W. J. Faber and M. Walker, *Instant Pain Relief* (Milwaukee, Wis.: Biological Publications, June 1991).

disease, low back pain, intestinal disorders, pain in the groin or legs, all without accompanying facial pain," affirms Dr. Hussar. "I have treated many low back pain patients by removing infected bone in the third%-4 molar area. Chronic fatigue and arthritic pain disappear in many patients with these conditions after I've removed their dental infections."[1]

In the final analysis, treatment of the neuralgia-inducing cavitational osteonecrosis requires vigorous curettage of the bone cavities. And such cleaning should be repeated, if necessary. And there probably should be antibiotics or healing herbs such as olive leaf extract, oil of oregano, burdock root, and other natural antimicrobial agents administered to the dental patient. Agents like these induce healing and filling of cavities with new bone. Responses of patients to this treatment consist of significant-to-complete pain remission and systemic disease elimination.[2]

Once the jawbone defect is removed, the hole left by a cavitation heals from the bottom up. Intense facial pain subsides dramatically or disappears completely. I must include a disclaimer, however, which is offered by the textbook, *Oral & Maxillofacial Pathology*. The authors say, "One third of patients thus treated experience no pain relief. Also, the disease has a strong tendency to recur or develop in additional jawbone sites. Often, a repetition of the same surgical procedure is necessary. A 70 percent overall 'cure' rate (pain-free for an average of five years) has been reported, but additional studies are required for a corroboration of this figure."[3]

Returning to the Cavitational Case of Dr. Allen J. Nordhelm

"Having read Dr. George Meinig's book, my eyes were opened, and that's when I went hunting for an extractionist or other dentist who would clean out the cavitations that I knew were poisoning my

1   Hussar, "No More Chronic Pain."

2   Langlais, Langland, and Nortze, "Neuralgia-Inducing Cavitational Ostenoecrosis."

3   Neville and others.

blood stream. I contacted Dr. Meinig, who referred me to Dr. Christopher John Hussar, and I traveled from St. Paul to his Reno office for removal of my six root canaled teeth," writes podiatrist Allen J. Nordhelm, D.P.M.

"My general health has now improved considerably. The arterial hypertension has been reduced to an acceptable level. My rheumatism stopped; the fungus has disappeared on its own; and every other symptom of discomfort has left me. I'm free from pain and all the difficulties that go with it. Within two months of undergoing the six decavitational surgical operations on those involved dental sockets, I was able to return to my podiatry practice and take care of patients once again," confirms Dr. Nordhelm. "Finally, my life has come back to normal. I'm a happy man."

So, what does the American Association of Endodontists (AAE), whose members are the chief implanters of root canals, say about neuralgia-inducing cavitational osteonecrosis lesions? The AAE Research and Scientific Affairs Committee, in an address about NICO-type cavitations, declares: "The practice of recommending the extraction of endodontically treated teeth for the prevention of NICO, or any other disease, is unethical and should be reported immediately to the appropriate State Board of Dentistry."[1]

How Cavitations Look and Why They Occur

Susan Stockton of Winter Haven, Florida, authored and published *Beyond Amalgam: The Hidden Health Hazard Posed by Jawbone Cavitations.*[2] This small, highly informative book is the only text written for the consumer that's currently available on the subject of NICO. Mrs. Stockton's book connects together hidden jawbone pathology with systemic disease.

---

1   American Association of Endodontists, "NICO Lesions," *Communique* (June 1996).

2   Stockton, *Beyond Amalgam*, 56, 57.

As it happens, Mrs. Stockton suffered mightily from cavitation pathology.

In describing the cause of cavitations earlier, I explained that when a root canal is performed or an extraction takes place, incorrect dentistry leaves the periodontal ligament (membrane) intact. Because this ligament attaches the tooth to its jawbone, leaving it in place is a wrong practice. Why? Because a periodontal ligament acts like a kind of hammock in which the tooth sits. Once the tooth is removed, the periodontal ligament no longer serves any purpose and, if left in by the extractionist, will form a barrier to new bone growth. Incomplete healing of the dental socket occurs and the top of this socket tends to seal over with a couple of millimeters of bone. Under the thin bony layer a hole remains. Inside these holes or cavitations, pathological changes take place in the cells and infection develops as a result of restricted blood flow. The site becomes a focal point of ongoing low-grade infection, which definitely perfuses throughout the body. The immune system becomes compromised. This information was provided to me by the excellence of Susan Stockton's literary presentation.[1]

See the address for obtaining the book by Susan Stockton, *Beyond Amalgam,* in appendix B. Also, she is publishing a newsletter for the education of health professionals and the public, especially for dentists and their patients. The Stockton newsletter is called the *Cavitations Plus Quarterly.*

---

1   Ibid., 11, 12.

Fourteen

Fluoridation Brings Hazards
to Human Health

Fluoride, an industrial waste product commonly sold as poison for killing rats and insects, is not good for the human body either. Yet most dentists spouting the American Dental Association's propaganda insist our drinking water must be fluoridated. As this chapter proves, these dentists announcing themselves as proponents of adding fluoride to public water supplies or administering dental fluoride treatments to patients or making fluoride an ingredient of toothpaste are perpetrating evil against all of us, Most especially, they're harming our children.

FDA Warning: Fluoride Toothpaste
Poisons Little Children

The Food and Drug Administration has sent down a ruling. It requires that on all fluoride toothpastes manufactured after April 1997, a printed admonition must appear on the toothpaste package reading:

> "Warning: Keep out of the reach of children under six years of age. If you accidentally swallow more than used for brushing, seek professional assistance or contact a *Poison Control Center* immediately." [emphasis added]

Following that FDA ruling, the manufacturers of fluoride toothpastes either disregarded it altogether, ignored the ruling's voluntary guidelines, or interpreted them overly broadly; consequently, the

FDA has put teeth in its current rules of enforcement. Inasmuch as pharmacies, groceries, convenience stores, health food stores, supermarkets, and other stores have finally sold out old and overstocked inventories of fluoridated toothpastes, now you can read the warning on various, newly distributed toothpaste tubes, boxes, bottles, and cans. For example, Procter and Gamble has included the message inside packages of Crest Multicare, advising customers to stop using the brand if they experience any form of body irritation. The Colgate-Palmolive Corporation prints the FDA warning on its newest toothpaste, Colgate Total. Church and Dwight, the manufacturer of Arm and Hammer toothpaste, provides a new toll-free telephone line for any reports of fluoride poisoning. Unilever PLC, the maker of Mentadent, has put fluoride toxicity information on its web site.

Some toothpaste brands, like Oral B bubble-gum flavor and the Tom's of Maine "Silly Strawberry" formula are so delicious that little children, even as they brush, eat their fluoridated toothpaste like candy. There is danger here, because the kids can die or at the least become very sick from ingesting the fluoride poison. Certainly they may come down with dental fluorosis.

Dental Fluorosis is a condition characterized by mottled tooth enamel, which is opaque and may be stained. Its incidence increases when the level of fluoride in the water supply is above two parts per million. When the drinking water's level of fluoride reaches over eight parts per million, systemic fluorosis may occur, with calcification of ligaments. In general, fluorosis is a bony overgrowth accompanied by neurologic complications and arthritis brought on by long-term fluoride intake, such as occurs in industrial workers.

(Please see the final subsection of this chapter describing the cash payout by Colgate-Palmolive for a legal claim of dental fluorosis occurring in Great Britain.)

If asked, manufacturers do admit that no child could get through a six-ounce tube of fluoridated toothpaste without vomiting. Fluoride causes vomiting because large doses of it, combined with gastric juices, tend to irritate the child's—and even an adult's—stomach and intestines. Of the 4,453 cases of unintended "fluoride exposure" reported to poison-control centers in 1997, 99 percent turned out not to be life-threatening but definitely had the potential to bring on death. In the remaining 1 percent, severe illness, near-death, or actual death did occur.[1]

Harmful Effects Caused by Fluoride Ingestion

In 1974 a three-year-old Brooklyn boy had stannous fluoride gel swabbed over his teeth by a pedodontist (specialist in children's dentistry) as the means of preventing tooth decay. Five hours later this child died from fluoride poisoning because of one fatal mistake. After rinsing his mouth the small boy did not spit out the rinse water but swallowed it instead.[2]

In New York City five years before, another boy, age four, went into violent convulsions and died directly after receiving topical fluoride applications to his teeth. Personnel of the dental clinic claimed this child had sustained a heart attack, even though there was no history of cardiac disease for him or any members of his family. In fact, the ingestion of even small amounts of fluoride is known among cardiologists to be a possible cause of cardiac arrest. It's one of fluoridation's side effects.[3]

On May 23, 1998, in Hooper Bay, Alaska, forty-one-year-old Dominic Smith drank fluoridated well water along with thirty other residents of this Bering Sea coastal village. All of them got sick, but Mr. Smith died. It seems that a broken pump had injected a little more than the usual fluoride quantity into Hooper Bay's water supply. As a result, Dr. Peter Kakamura, director of Alaska's state division of public health, reports: "The man's death occurred by reason of fluoridation." He was poisoned. Dominic Smith's sister almost died, too, and flu-like symptoms struck twenty-nine

---

1   D. Canedy, "Toothpaste a Hazard? Just Ask the F. D. A.," *New York Times*, 24 March 1998, A 18.

2   *New York Times*, 20 January 1979, 16.

3   M. McIvor and others, "Hyperkalemia and Cardiac Arrest from Fluoride Exposure During Hemodialysis," *American Journal of Cardiology* 51 (1983): 901–02.

others who drank from one of the two public wells. Fluoride is routinely added to Alaska's public water supplies, including those in Anchorage and many Eskimo villages, to reduce tooth decay.[1]

From Auckland, New Zealand, nutritionist Toni Jeffreys, Ph.D., asks, "I wonder if the epidemic of osteoporosis and escalating heart disease in women is not due to the current conventional medical advice to take calcium and fluoride tablets? Most of us know that calcium is antagonistic to magnesium, and that it is magnesium that protects our hearts. But also, magnesium is the mineral that provides elasticity in bones. Without magnesium we can build lots of bone but it's a poor grade bone which shatters and fractures at any strain.[2]

"Unfortunately, fluoride is also antagonistic to magnesium and will cancel it out," continues Dr. Jeffreys. "It is therefore quite murderous to give women calcium and fluoride tablets, when we are already overburdened with fluoride in the environment in numerous ways and are deficient in magnesium."[3]

As shown by a scientific study conducted by four prestigious research institutions, Harvard Medical School, Eastman Dental Center, Iowa State University, and Forsyth Research Institute, fluoride has an adverse effect on the brain and central nervous system (CNS). It causes "motor dysfunction, IQ deficits, and/or learning disabilities in humans," say the institutions' cooperating researchers.[4]

At approximately one part per million (1 ppm), fluoride has been added to most public water supplies throughout the United States for over four decades at the urging of dentists. But these four research groups report that the CNS's functional output is vulnerable to fluoride. This scholarly laboratory study indicates that fluoride ingestion's "neurotoxic risks deserve further evaluation."[5]

---

1   "Fluoride Blamed for Death," *Ketchikan, Alaska Daily News*, 1 June 1998.

2   A. Machoy-Mokrzynska, "Fluoride-Magnesium Interactions," *Fluoride* 28 (November 1995): 175.

3   T. Jeffreys, "Fluoride Supplements for Osteoporosis?" *Townsend Letter for Doctors and Patients* 171 (October 1997): 112.

4   P. J. Mullenix, P. K. Denbesten, and A. Schunior, "Neurotoxicity of Sodium Fluoride in Rats," *Neurotoxicology and Teratology* 17 (1995): 169–77.

Taking in fluoride definitely has deleterious consequences for the brain. Pathological conditions of the brain have been studied by Russians, Chinese, the United States Public Health Service (USPHS), and others since 1978. For instance, in their 1978 book *Fluoridation, the Great Dilemma*, three medical authors describe the findings of practicing Soviet physicians. The Russian physicians observed that 79 percent of patients with occupational fluorosis show a series of chalky-white, irregularly distributed patches on the surface of the enamel that become infiltrated by yellow or brown staining or other discolorations on teeth from fluoride ingestion. With these patches, say the Russians, the patients "demonstrate dysfunction of subcortical axial nonspecific structures of the brain."[1]

Moreover, the 1991 review *Fluoride Benefits and Risks*, published by the USPHS, states that there is "relative impermeability of the blood-brain barrier to fluoride." This mineral penetrates the brain's first line of defense against toxins and potentially may be responsible for various brain syndromes such as senile dementia, schizophrenia, and Alzheimer's disease.[2]

Recent studies from China of the relationship between drinking fluoridated water by residents in endemic Chinese dental fluorosis areas and the population's intelligence quotient contain significant references and discussions. They indicate that diminishing IQ for people as a result of residing in dental fluorosis areas has been known since 1989. Chinese studies indicate that the influence of a high fluoride environment on the intelligence of children may occur early in development such as during the stages of embryonic life or infancy when differentiation and growth are more rapid. Ultra-microscopic study of embryonic brain tissue obtained from termination of pregnancy operations in endemic fluorosis regions

---

5   Safe Water Coalition of Washington State, "Fluoride Has Adverse Effect on Central Nervous System," *Townsend Letter for Doctors and Patients* 155 (June 1996): 21.

1   G. L. Walbott, A. W. Burgstahler, and H. L. McKinney, *Fluoridation, the Great Dilemma* (Lawrence, Kan.: Coronado Press, 1978).

2   Department of Health and Human Services, *Fluoride Benefits and Risks*, February 1991.

showed "differentiation of brain nerve cells were poor, and brain development was delayed."[1]

The incidence of thigh bone fractures at the femoral neck in those people sixty-five years of age and older was compared in three communities in the state of Utah. One of the Utah towns had its water artificially fluoridated to one part per million. The other two did not. Measured over a seven-year period, the relative risk of hip fracture for women drinking fluoridated water increased by 1.27, and for men the risk rose to 1.41. As a conclusion to their study, the four medical researchers stated, "We found a significant increase in the risk of hip fracture in both men and women exposed to artificial fluoridation at one ppm, suggesting that low levels of fluoride increase the risk of hip fracture in the elderly.[2]

Commenting on this finding, Seattle, Washington, medical nutritional therapist Alan R. Gaby, M.D., made an observation similar to that of Dr. Toni Jeffreys. Dr. Gaby said: "Hip fracture is the second most common cause of admission to nursing homes, accounting for approximately 60,000 admissions each year. Fluoride apparently causes new bone formation of inferior quality, especially in the femoral head, where there is more cortical bone. Some studies suggest that fluoride is also a carcinogen."[3]

Fluoride as a Carcinogen that Creates Cancer

In 1977 epidemiological studies on fluoridation carried out by Dean Burk, Ph.D., former head of the Cytochemistry Section of the National Cancer Institute, in conjunction with John Yiamouyiannis, Ph.D.,

1   X. S. Li, J. L. Zhi, and R. O. Gao, "Effect of Fluoride Exposure on Intelligence of Children," *Fluoride* 28, no. 4 (1995): 189–92; I. Zhao, G. H. Liang, D. Zhang, and X. Wu, "Effect of High Fluoride Water Supply on Children's Intelligence" (1995).

2   C. Danielson, J. L. Lyon, M. Egger, and G. K. Goodenough, "Hip Fractures and Fluoridation in Utah's Elderly Population," *Journal of the American Medical Association* 258 (1992): 746–48.

3   A. R. Gaby, "Literature Review and Commentary," *Townsend Letter for Doctors and Patients* 113 (December 1992): 1058.

president of the Safe Water Foundation of Delaware, Ohio, were the subject of full-scale U.S. congressional hearings. The Burk/Yiamouyiannis studies showed that fluoridation is linked to about 10,000 cancer deaths annually in this nation. The U.S. Public Health Service, copromoter of fluoridation with the American Dental Association (ADA), opposed the Burk/Yiamouyiannis investigations. The USPHS tried to refute their findings with its own report. But Drs. Yiamouyiannis and Burk evaluated the USPHS findings. Then they explained to the Congress how "conflicting findings of the USPHS are due to the fact that the Service had made mathematical errors by leaving out 80-90 percent of the recorded data. When these errors and omissions are corrected, its method of simultaneously adjusting for age, race, and sex confirm that 10,000 excess cancer deaths per year are linked to water fluoridation in the United States."

To their amazement, officials of the USPHS discovered that their own findings really did coincide with findings from Drs. Burk and Yiamouyiannis. All of the findings from both studies going back a quarter century clearly point to fluoride as a cancer culprit. When added to drinking water fluoride creates a carcinogen. More than this, the following are results released in 1990 by the National Toxicology Program (NTP) under the auspices of the USPHS:[1]

- Precancerous changes occur in human oral squamous cells as a result of elevating the levels of fluoride in drinking water.

- There is an increase in the incidence of tumors and cancers in oral squamous cells as a result of increasing levels of fluoride in the drinking water.

- Osteosarcoma, a rare form of bone cancer, occurs only in animals with fluoride in their drinking water.

- There is an increase in the incidence of thyroid follicular cell tumors as a result of increasing levels of fluoride in the drinking water.

- Hepatocholangiocarcinoma, a rare form of liver cancer, happens in animals with fluoride in their drinking water.

---

1   J. Yiamouyiannis, "Update on Fluoride and Cancer," *Townsend Letter for Doctors and Patients* 89 (December 1990): 864–65.

- The doses of fluoride that are linked to cancer in this NTP study are only one-tenth to one-fiftieth of the amount used to produce cancer by benzene. Thus, fluoride is up to fifty times more carcinogenic than benzene.

- The cancer-causing potential of fluoride is not limited to one type of cancer.

Similar to cancer coverups by cigarette manufacturers in the tobacco industry, Proctor and Gamble, manufacturer of the many Crest fluoridated toothpaste brands, which are endorsed by the American Dental Association, performed carcinogenicity studies with sodium fluoride four years before the above-reported 1990 NTP/USPHS report was released. Dose-dependent increases in cancer were observed in every parameter tested, including squamous cell metaplasias, but the USPHS held back this information and only released it when forced to do so by Dr. John Yiamouyiannis under the Freedom of Information Act.[1]

Added to what's already been said here, the Department of Health and Human Services (HHS) gathered a massive amount of evidence for its own 1991 report, "Review of Fluoride Benefits and Risks." This additional report supports the link between drinking and washing in fluoridated water and the creation of human cancers. Here is what was learned by the HHS:[2]

- Based on rates of 279 cancer cases expected in non-fluoridated areas, 290 people came down with bone and joint cancers when they lived in areas whose water is fluoridated.

- Although 30 to 33 cases were expected, there was an excess of 49 people suffering from Ewing's sarcoma in fluoridated counties.

1   U.S. Public Health Service, "Carcinogenicity Studies with Sodium Fluoride Performed by Proctor and Gamble," *Medical Tribune*, 22 February 1990.

2   Safe Water Coalition of Washington State, Spokane, Washington, "HHS Report on Fluoride," *Townsend Letter for Doctors and Patients* 97/98 (September 1991): 638.

- The observed-to-expected rate of soft tissue cancer for both sexes in Seattle, Washington, increased with the duration of fluoridation of the city's water supply.

- For kidney cancer, the risk ratios for both sexes in Seattle, with its fluoridated drinking water, rose by 10 percent, a trend that the HHS considered statistically significant.

In December 1992 the New Jersey Department of Environmental Protection and Energy and the New Jersey Department of Health released their joint study of November 8, 1992. New Jersey's findings were that bone cancer rates among ten- to nineteen-year-old males living in all New Jersey municipalities having fluoridated drinking water is 6.9 times higher than in other areas of the state. There is no doubt that New Jersey residents drinking from fluoridated public water supplies suffer from a much higher incidence of bone cancer.[1]

Because it continues to fluoridate its public drinking water, New Jersey is a candidate for a class action suit by its residents and by visitors to the state. (See the last subsection of this chapter about legal claims against fluoridation.)

Additional Hazardous Results from Fluoride Ingestion

The poisonous hazards of fluoride ingestion are listed in the United States Pharmacopoeia. They include the less lethal side effects of nausea, vomiting, stomach cramps, tremors, faintness, weakness, unusual psychological excitement, skin rash, sores in the mouth and on the lips, pain and aching of bones, and white, brown, or near-black discolorations of teeth, which I've already identified as dental fluorosis.

Dental or occupational fluorosis is actually a visible sign that

---

1   Safe Water Coalition of Washington State, Spokane, Washington, "Re: Fluoridation," *Townsend Letter for Doctors and Patients* 115/116 (February/March 1993): 206.

fluoride content of the body has caused the enamel-forming cells, the ameloblasts, to produce damaged collagen. Collagen makes up 30 percent of the body's protein. It provides the structural framework for skin, ligaments, tendons, muscles, cartilage, bones, and teeth.

In his well-documented and detailed book, *Fluoride, The Aging Factor,* Dr. John Yiamouyiannis explains that fluoride ingestion causes "increased production of imperfect collagen or collagen-like protein," not just in the teeth but throughout the body. The body's structural components that should not become mineralized, such as ligaments, cartilage, and tendons, turn into hardened tissues. Scleroderma causes not only the skin to harden. The arteries underneath the skin calcify and harden as well.

Fluoride ingestion also affects the structure and strength of bone by causing fused vertebrae, calcified joints, arthritis, and an increase in fractures. It decreases the bone's healing ability. Several studies that evaluate fluoride as a treatment for osteoporosis found that this mineral increases, rather than prevents, skeletal fragility. Only one ppm fluoride in drinking water disrupts collagen metabolism. Yet the U.S. Environmental Protection Agency (USEPA) allows 4 ppm fluoride in our nation's water supply.[1]

Not only does drinking fluoridated water disrupt collagen, it affects other proteins as well, causing widespread dysfunction of enzymes and the immune system, and even chromosomal damage. Fluoride ingestion breaks up existing protein bonds and forms an extremely strong binding to the one particular protein bond H2, disrupting the normal shape and function of other necessary proteins. When the proteins that form enzymes are disrupted in this way, the enzymes themselves become inactivated. Enzymes are the catalysts that cause the biochemical changes in a person's body.

Not only are these enzymatic proteins inactivated, they are rendered unrecognizable to the body's immune system, setting up an autoimmune allergic reaction. Because of this peculiarity,

---

1   J. Yiamouyiannis, *Fluoride: The Aging Factor*, 3d ed. (Delaware, Ohio: Health Action Press, 1993).

fluoride causes a vast variety of ill effects. "The United States National Academy of Sciences (USNAS)[1] and the World Health Organization (WHO),[2] as well as other institutions have published lists of enzymes that are inhibited at fluoride levels of one ppm or less," writes Dr. Yiamouyiannis. Among them, acetylcholinesterase, glutamine synthetase, ATPase, and the DNA Repair Enzyme System are just a few of the known enzymes inhibited by fluoride ingestion at one ppm.

One part per million fluoride in drinking water or other ingested solvents (such as diet cola drinks that contain fluoride) cuts the activity of the DNA repair enzyme by 50 percent, resulting in increased genetic damage. In his 1993 book, Dr. Yiamouyiannis lists nineteen studies since 1973 that show evidence of fluoride-induced genetic damage in mammals, one of which was conducted by Proctor and Gamble (already cited). Scientific studies prove that fluoride levels found in the autopsied brains of persons drinking fluoridated water average 1.5 ppm fluoride; in their autopsied hearts 1.8 ppm was found; and in their thyroid glands there was 4.0 ppm. Fluoride is used, according to the *Merck Index*, to suppress thyroid activity. Clearly, a fluoridated substance taken into the body affects more than teeth.[3]

---

1   "Is Fluoride an 'Essential Element'?" *Fluorides* (Washington, D.C.: National Academy of Sciences, 1971), 66 68, 70 73.

2   World Health Organization, *Fluorides and Human Health* (Geneva, Switzerland: 1970), 183.

3   Yiamouyiannis, *Fluoride: The Aging Factor*, 7.

With All this Danger, Why Are We Fluoridating Ourselves?

Despite so much documentation of fluoride's ill-effects on the body and the outright danger all of us face from its ingestion, we continue to fluoridate ourselves by means of adding it to drinking water, toothpastes, oral rinses, baked goods, prescribed dental treatments, food supplements, soft drinks, beer, wine, fruit juices made from concentrates, and so forth. In one analysis, Coke Classic, bottled in Chicago, is shown to contain 2.56 ppm fluoride. And, as was alluded to, the Chicago-made Diet Coke contains 2.96 ppm. Produce grown with fluorine-containing fertilizers contain from six to twelve times more fluoride than those fruits and vegetables not "fed" with these fertilizers. Not only does fluoride pollute our food and water, but certain manufacturing plants such as aluminum, phosphate, steel, clay, glass, enamel, and many other factory types release high levels of fluoride into the air, soil, rivers, and lakes.[1]

You have every right to ask, why are we continuing to fluoridate ourselves into sickness and death? We do it as a result of media bombardment: emphatic promotions by the United States Public Health Service, propaganda from the American Dental Association, advertising by fluoride toothpaste manufacturers, and other more subtle capitalistic reasons that have nothing to do with dental health. So, allow me to answer your question as to why we are fluoridating ourselves. First, however, you should know the political and capitalistic background of fluoridation that's foisted on our populace in the United States (but not so much in European countries, which mostly know better).

American fluoridation proponents are ever continuing to assert that fluoride is a mineral essential to the body and responsible for preventing tooth decay. But a 1971 review of numerous studies concerning the nutritional value of fluoride, performed by the U.S. National Academy of Sciences, found no evidence to support the claim that fluoride is an essential mineral. Further, both the U.S.

---

1   J. Klotter, "The Fraud of Fluoridation," *Townsend Letter for Doctors and Patients* 145/146 (August/September 1995): 119–120.

Center for Disease Control and Prevention in Atlanta, Georgia, and the British Ministry of Health admit that no laboratory or epidemiological study supports the claim that adding fluoride to the drinking water prevents tooth decay.[1]

Money-Eyed Interests Fluoridate Us

As the aluminum and phosphate fertilizer industries grew in the 1920s and 1930s, manufacturers were faced with ways to get rid of their poisonous by-product, the fluoride waste. They could sell only so much rodenticide and insecticide and desperately needed another means of getting rid of fluoride without incurring public censor. The manufacturers hit on an idea of using it for fluoridating reservoirs, lakes, ponds, rivers, streams, aquifiers and other sources of drinking water. They lobbied the U.S. Public Health Service to introduce this fluoridation measure into the public trough. H. Trendley Dean, M.D., then a bureaucrat with the USPHS, performed surveys of areas in the 1930s that relied for drinking water on fluoride-polluted streams and rivers. In a 1937 report that Dr. Dean published, he found that the higher the content of fluoride in the water, the greater the incidence of mottled teeth (dental fluorosis). He wrote an excellent paper, which clearly made the case against fluoridation.[2]

Then Dr. Gerald J. Cox, an official of the Mellon Institute, pronounced that, while too much fluoride can cause mottling of teeth, low levels of one ppm actually was nutritionally beneficial and prevented tooth decay. Dr. Cox's boss, the Mellon family, owned the Aluminum Company of America (ALCOA), a major fluoride polluter. The Mellons were seeking a way to unload their massive amount of fluoride by-product and maybe even make money from its sale.

---

1   Ibid.

2   H. T. Dean and E. Elvove, "Further Studies on Minimal Threshold of Chronic Endemic Dental Fluosis," *Public Health Reports* 52 (1937): 1249–64.

In 1938, persuaded by a high-paying position provided by the Mellons as the first director of the National Institute of Dental Research, Dr. H. Trendley Dean changed his findings from seven years before. He reversed himself by publishing skewed data to support Dr. Cox's cavity-prevention pronouncement. Then, six years later Oscar Ewing, an ALCOA attorney, was appointed the United States Federal Security Administrator in 1944 and took charge of the USPHS. Mr. Ewing appointed Edward L. Bernays as the "father of public relations" for popularizing ALCOA's water fluoridation campaign. Thus Bernays turned rat poison into "a beneficial provider of gleaming smiles." He did it by getting clinical reports praising the use of fluoride for cavity prevention published in various medical and dental journals.

Mr. Bernays knew that by offering appropriate "under-the-counter" compensation, he could get officials of the American Medical Association, the American Dental association, Proctor and Gamble, independent scientists and laboratories, physicians, dentists, and certain government bureaucrats to proclaim fluoride's safety and advantages for teeth. Mr. Bernays achieved this public relations gambit long before any clinical studies were completed. By accomplishing such positive-sounding publication and declarations, the government officials, physicians, dentists, business executives, scientists, laboratory directors, and others would be too embarrassed and frightened of lawsuits to renege on their well-paid endorsements—regardless of the results of scientific studies.

Those whose scientific research refuted fluoride and showed its toxicity were ignored, labeled crackpots, fired from jobs, denied grants, and stripped of dental and medical licenses. In his very fine book, Dr. Yiamouyiannis contends that the fluoridation campaign still continues under the leadership of New York City psychiatrist, Stephen Barrett, M.D., who is cofounder of the National Council Against Health Fraud (NCAHF).[1] For more information on the NCAHF, see this book's final section of chapter two. To learn how Dr. Barrett and his fellow members of the NCAHF, as advocates of fluoridation, are among the candidates for a class action suit, see the end of this fourteenth chapter.

---

1   Yiamouyiannis, *Fluoride: The Aging Factor*, 99–122.

Does Fluoride Prevent Dental Cavities?

Fluoride, a natural trace mineral in the diet, is found in drinking water naturally in widely varying concentrations from trace amounts to a dozen parts per million. Much like selenium, manganese, and other trace minerals, there is an ideal level of intake. When fluoride's intake is too low, dental caries could possibly occur. Conversely, when intake is too high, dental fluorosis definitely does occur.

Cardiologist/dentologist Thomas Levy, M.D., of Colorado Springs, Colorado, who had worked with Dr. Hal Huggins, tells us about the mottling of teeth by the pathological onset of fluorosis. "Known in the United States since at least 1916, dental fluorosis is sometimes referred to as "Colorado Brown Stain" and "Texas Teeth," as these two states have a high endemic fluoride level in much of their drinking water," states Dr. Levy. "In its advanced stages, affected teeth demonstrate pitting and brittleness. Often chipping, and a yellow, brown, or black appearance [shows up] in different areas [of the teeth]. Earlier stages show a chalky, mottled, inconsistent appearance."[1]

The elegant study in 1937 by Dr. H. Trendley Dean of the USPHS that I described earlier clearly points out that the incidence of dental fluorosis is directly related to fluoride concentration in drinking water, reaching virtually 100 percent when the level exceeds 4.5 ppm. Levels of only 2.2 ppm show a roughly 70 percent incidence of this affliction.[2] Dr. Dean's initial dental fluorosis finding, well after his refutation of it for money, was later supported substantially by another 1984 study published in the *Journal of the American Dental Association*.[3]

Worse, USPHS medical scientists uncovered in 1954 that Bartlett, Texas, with 8 ppm fluoride in its water supply, presented a

---

1   T. Levy, "Fluoridation: Paving the Road to the Final Solution," *Extraordinary Science* (January/February/March 1994), 29–41.

2   Dean and Elvove, "Further Studies."

3   V. A. Segretto and others, "A Current Study of Mottled Enamel in Texas," *Journal of the American Dental Association* 108 (1984): 58–59.

mortality rate among its residents three times greater than that of a neighboring town with a fluoride drinking water level of merely 0.4 ppm.[1] Added to this Bartlett township discovery was another study published in a 1978 issue of the *New England Journal of Medicine* that stated death occurs more frequently among the populace of cities and towns drinking fluoridated water as compared to those folk drinking nonfluoridated water.[2]

Fluoride Weakens Bones and Teeth

Fluoride is not essential for sound teeth and it does not prevent cavities. However, as a result of a 1940s study commissioned by the USPHS that determined one ppm of fluoride in water reduced tooth decay by 60 percent, many countries acted on this erroneous finding. Today, two-thirds of the population of Australia; half the population of the United States, Canada, Ireland and New Zealand; 30 percent of the population of Brazil; and 10 percent of the population of Great Britain, mostly in the west Midlands and northern regions of England, drinks water from municipal supplies that have been artificially fluoridated. Other, more enlightened European nations such as Sweden, Holland, and Germany have reversed their policy and discontinued the practice.[3]

While fluoride ingestion tends to stimulate bone density, the fluoride-stimulated bone is structurally unsound. Restoration of bone mass by use of this mineral not only fails to reduce the risk of fractures in women who suffer with postmenopausal osteoporosis, but it even increases the risk of such fractures.[4] And more disturbing

1   N. Leone and others, "Medical Aspects of Excessive Fluoride in a Water Supply," *Public Health Reports* 69 (1954): 925–36.

2   J. D. Erickson, "Mortality of Selected Cities with Fluoridated and Nonfluoridated Water Supplies," *New England Journal of Medicine* 298 (1978): 1112–16.

3   M. Diesendorf, "Have the Benefits of Water Fluoridation Been Overestimated?" *International Clinical Nutrition Review* 10 (1990): 292–303.

4   R. Lindsay, "Fluoride and Bone-Quantity versus Quality," editorial, *New England Journal of Medicine* 322, no. 12 (1990):845–46.

is accumulating evidence that the fluoridation of public water sup-plies eventually increases the risk of fractures in the community.[1]

Scientific studies are currently reporting higher prevalence of dental fluorosis following the fluoridation of drinking water than had been predicted.[2] Melvyn R. Werbach, M.D., of Tarzana, California, an internationally acclaimed medical journalist, questions the pro-priety of the decision to allow fluoridation to remain for United States drinking water. Dr. Werbach has written, "The fluoride con-troversy is simply another example of the peculiar bias mainstream medicine shows towards apparently powerful new treatments whose dangers are largely unknown, while it continues to show bias against many gentler therapies with safety records far exceeding those of standard treatments."[3]

A University of Arizona study, published in the July 27, 1992 issue of *Chemical and Engineering News* by Cornelius Steelink, Ph.D., professor emeritus in the university's Department of Chemistry, reported that the more fluoride a child drank in its water supply, the more cavities appeared in the child's teeth.[4]

The City of Tucson, Arizona, provided Dr. Steelink with a unique opportunity to test the many fluoridation hypotheses handed out wholesale by proponents of fluoride additives to drinking water. The professor wrote: "Historically, this city has had discrete geographic areas of groundwater with high fluoride contents of 0.8 ppm and areas of low fluoride contents with 0.3 ppm." When Dr. Stelink's evaluation committee plotted the incidence of tooth decay versus fluoride content in a child's neighborhood drinking water, a positive correlation was revealed. As stated above, Professor Steelink's com-mittee reported with this exact summarizing quote: "In other words,

---

1   J. Coquhoun, "Fluoridation: New Evidence of Harm to Young Teeth and Old Bones," *International Clinical Nutrition Review* 12, no. 1 (1992): 1–8.

2   Ibid.

3   M. R. Werbach, "Fluoride," *Townsend Letter for Doctors and Patients* 133/134 (August/September 1994): 853.

4   Safe Water Coalition of Washington State, Spokane, Washington, "The More Fluoride, the More Cavities," *Townsend Letter for Doctors and Patients* 129 (April 1994): 376.

the more fluoride a child drank, the more cavities appeared in the teeth."[1]

David C. Kennedy, D.D.S., of San Diego, California, the author of *How to Save Your Teeth: Toxic-Free Preventive Dentistry,* outright declares that fluorides do not reduce tooth decay.[2]

In a published letter, Dr. Kennedy wrote to the Safe Water Coalition of Washington State: "In Canada, the areas which report the lowest incidence of decay are the unfluoridated areas. Tooth decay is declining worldwide with no statistical difference between fluoridated and unfluoridate areas. Some authors [proponents of fluoridation] attempt to attribute the decline of cavities in unfluoridated areas to a decrease in the consumption of refined sugars. I believe statistics show we are consuming more, not less refined sugar. The latest data from the National Institute of Dental Research (NIDR) found no difference in the incidence of tooth decay in children ages five through seventeen years raised in nonfluoridated, partially fluoridated, and fluoridated communities. NIDR studies show no relationship between fluoridation and tooth decay rates."[3]

Fluoride Reacts with Aluminum to Cause Alzheimer's Disease

Newly declassified documents, obtained under the U.S. Freedom of Information Act, today provide shocking medical facts known but concealed by the U.S. government since the 1940s. During that same period when Dr. H. Trendley Dean changed his laboratory test findings and ALCOA attorney Oscar Ewing won his political appointment, the United States Public Health Service knew that fluoride

---

1   C. Steelink, "Tooth Decay and Fluoride," *Townsend Letter for Doctors and Patients* 135 (October 1994): 1128.

2   D. C. Kennedy, *How to Save Your Teeth: Toxic-Free Preventive Dentistry* (Delaware, Ohio: Health Action Press, August 1993).

3   Safe Water Coalition of Washington State, Spokane, Washington, "Don't Applaud Fluoride Use for Cavities," *Townsend Letter for Doctors and Patients* 82 (May 1990): 286–88.

produces adverse human central nervous system effects. It's true. The USPHS has hidden this horrible information about fluoride as a pollutor and deteriorator of the human brain for over fifty years.

Ellie Rudolph, director of the Pennsylvania chapter of the Health Alliance International, advises that pathological changes in the brain tissue of animals given fluoride and aluminum-fluoride combined are the same changes found in the brains of people dying with Alzheimer's disease and other forms of dementia. Director Rudolph states: "Low levels of fluoride have serious health implications for people and the effect is enhanced in the presence of other neurotoxins like aluminum."[1] (To discuss this hidden aspect of fluoridation pathology, you may contact Ellie Rudolph in person by using communications information furnished in appendix A.)

The peer-reviewed medical journal *Brain Research* reveals that aluminum-induced neural degeneration in rats is greatly increased when the animals are fed low doses of fluoride. The presence of fluoride enhances the bioavailability of aluminum, causing more aluminum to cross the blood-brain barrier and become deposited in the brain. The brain researchers have written: "The aluminum level in the brains of the fluoride-treated group of animals was double that of the controls."[2]

Even worse, the study's authors said, "While the small amount of aluminum fluoride in the drinking water of rats required for neurotoxic effects is surprising, perhaps more significant are the neurotoxic results of sodium fluoride (NaF) at the dose given of 2.1 ppm NaF. This 2.1 parts per million NaF equals 1.0 mg fluoride ion per litre of water *which is the same level found in 1.0 ppm 'optimally' fluoridated drinking water.*"

(Note: The formula for converting NaF to fluoride ion is ppm x 45% so that 2.1 ppm x 45% = .95 ppm [ppm = mgs/litre].)

The present fluoride/aluminum study on the brains of laboratory

---

1   E. Rudolph, "Alzheiner's Disease and Dementia—Important New Study Shows Grave Implications from Interaction of Aluminum and Low Dose Fluoride," *Townsend Letter for Doctors and Patients* 148 (November 1998): 27.

2   J. A. Verner, K. F. Jensen, W. Horvath, and R. L. Isaacson, *Brain Research* 784 (1998).

animals confirms the work of two separate groups of scientists in China, each group publishing their investigations in 1995, which was discussed earlier in this chapter. Both Chinese studies showed that drinking water containing fluoride adversely affects the intelligence quotients (IQs) of children.[1]

Colgate-Palmolive Compensates Brits for Staining Teeth Brown

While selling its fluoridated Colgate toothpaste in the United Kingdom, America's Colgate-Palmolive Corporation paid out the equivalent of US$2,000 to the parents of a ten-year-old British child for fluoride damage to his teeth. It was "good-will" compensation after an independent specialist diagnosed the boy as having developed dental fluorosis from swallowing small amounts of fluoride toothpaste over a period of time. Headlines appeared featuring the November 24, 1996, payout in every major British newspaper, including *The London Times*.

Dental fluorosis, a permanent white and then brown discoloration and mottling of the teeth caused by exposure to fluorides in the drinking water and products such as fluoride toothpaste, is a sign of systemic toxicity. Even though the Colgate case was settled out of court, lawyers said that it set an international precedent, opening the door for future toxic tort litigation related to fluoride-containing products.

Solicitor (attorney) Julian Middleton of the Nottingham, England, law firm Freeth, Cartwright, Hunt and Dickins, said that he represents over two hundred families with children suffering from dental fluorosis. This Colgate payment will help families in their battle for legal aid to file a class action suit. The Nottingham law firm has made several attempts in the past few years to obtain legal aid for the families and have been turned down by the U.K. courts.

---

1   Li, Zhi, and Gao, "Effect of Fluoride Exposure"; Zhao and others, "Effect of High-Fluoride Water Supply."

Unlike the U.S. legal system in which law firms can handle class action suits on a contingency basis, in the U.K. government funding is required for such suits. Also in the United States, only one person is required to file a class action suit on behalf of everyone who has suffered injury from a product or action.

In any country, dental fluorosis is highly litigable for a number of clear-cut legal reasons:

1. Dental fluorosis is the most visible of the adverse effects of fluoride ingestion.

2. Dental fluorosis is the most easily diagnosable.

3. Dental fluorosis occurs from only one cause.

In the United States, an estimated 30 percent of all children in nonfluoridated water areas suffer with some small degree of dental fluorosis from all sources. In contrast, about 62 percent of the children in areas with fluoridated water show obvious signs of dental fluorosis. Therefore, the United Kingdom's attorneys are amazed that numbers of law suits haven't already been filed by American law firms. "Traditionally, in product liability cases, the Americans are ahead of us," said Paul Balen, solicitor for Freeth, Cartwright, Hunt and Dickins, "but for once we appear to be ahead of the Americans."[1]

The key to dental fluorosis litigation involves: failure to adequately warn the public of adverse effects caused from exposure to fluorides. Certainly the ADA and the USPHS have failed miserably in this regard. They declare dental fluorisis as merely a cosmetic effect, but it's not. Such a declaration is illustrative of the big lie—a coverup. Expert witnesses such as toxicologists, physiologists, internists, pediatricians, holistic dentists, anatomists, and other health professionals would prove the lie in such a statement about "cosmetics." Then, malpractice and product liability lawsuits could be leveled at the following groups:

---

1   G. Glasser, "Colgate Pays Out for Fluoride Damaged Teeth," *London Telegraph*, 24 November 1996.

- pediatricians, dentists, and other health professionals who prescribe fluoride supplements,

- fluoride toothpaste manufacturers,

- communities and townships fluoridating drinking water,

- organizations and media outlets such as newspapers endorsing the use of fluoride supplements or water fluoridation,

- manufacturers of fluoridation equipment,

- manufacturers of foods and beverages containing fluorides,

- associations and individuals involved in the promotion of fluorides as a palliative,

- media outlets advertising fluoridated products,

- advertising agencies handling the accounts of fluoridators.

It appears that attorneys have a potential bonanza waiting in the wings, once they pick up on the massive amount of liability that prescribing health professionals, cities, states, and commercial organizations have created for themselves. Such liability is unquestionable because the damage to patients with dental fluorosis is permanent. It's classified into three categories:

1. Mild fluorosis means that there is barely discernable chalky blotching on the teeth.

2. Moderate fluorosis indicates that there is discernable chalky blotching to rust-colored stains on the teeth.

3. Severe fluorosis is shown by brown-stained, pitted, and friable teeth.

Being a permanent condition, there are only costly, temporary remedies to disguise the discolorations. They include dental bleaching, microabrasion, cosmetic bonding, and capping. Most cases of severe dental fluorosis result in loss of teeth or the formation of cavities in fluorosed areas of the teeth. In cases where such teeth have become friable, repairing such cavities is difficult if not impossible.

While some fluoridation litigations have already taken place, as for instance *Feldman v. Lederle Laboratories*, American lawyers have only begun to sue for the enforcement of fluoridation on the public. But now the fluoride proponents and opponents will finally have their day in court. In my opinion, that's a good thing.

Fifteen

Permanent Relief for Periodontal Disease

It has been pretty much confirmed by medical and dental authorities that *advanced periodontitis* was the source of heart disease that killed nationally syndicated TV and newspaper humorist Lewis Grizzard in March 1994. For at least a decade, Grizzard had reigned as a popular celebrity commentator on social, political, and human-interest issues. But difficulties with his teeth and gums became this celebrity's undoing.

Also known as *pyorrhea*, advanced periodontitis is marked by major gum recession, severe bone loss, and loose teeth, all accompanied by tartar with plaque buildup into the gum tissue and on the roots of the teeth. From his early twenties until the day he was struck down, Lewis Grizzard exhibited every one of pyorrhea's signs and symptoms.

Oral surgeon Thomas Boc, D.D.S., of Atlanta, Georgia, says, "Grizzard's heart valve problems stemmed from neglect of his teeth. He wouldn't floss; he wouldn't brush. He was a classic example of somebody whose chronic dental infection led to chronic heart disease, valve failure, and ultimately death."[1]

Grizzard's demise at the premature age of forty-seven was totally unnecessary and quite preventable. Admonitions for tooth cleanliness are offered to the public almost everywhere. They're part of the image-building public relations espoused by the American Dental Association. In fact, "Brush your teeth twice a day and see

---

1   S. Sternberg, "Chronic Tooth Infections Can Kill More Than Smile," *USA Today*, section D, 14 April 1998, D1, 2D.

your dentist twice a year," is the ADA slogan most of us have heard since we were toddlers.

A slight variation on the above dental slogan was recently put out by ADA representative David Mortvedt, D.D.S., when he answered a question from Cindy Ciardello about her three-year-old daughter's teeth. Mrs. Ciardello is a resident of Alpharetta, Georgia, and in the April 16, 1998 issue of *USA Today*, Dr. Mortvedt responded, "Have her brush at least twice a day, and try to get her to floss. Have regular dental checkups for her every six months."[1]

Doesn't Dr. Mortvedt's advice sound familiar? Don't these ADA party-line dentists know anything else? They keep saying the same thing over and over as they've been doing for the past 150 years.

You wouldn't know it from hearing the ADA, but there are numerous techniques for achieving good oral maintenance against gingivitis/periodontitis. However, these useful antipyorrhea techniques certainly are not offered by conventionally practicing dentists. Often, the dental consumer alone makes use of better natural remedies than the conventional allopathic methods blandly mentioned repeatedly by ADA-conforming dentists. In this chapter's next three subsections, I will offer just such useful antipyorrhea techniques that may startle you. Read on.

Medical doctors who ordinarily don't pay much attention to teeth but who do practice using alternative, innovative, or complementary therapies get into the act when it comes to periodontal disease. Holistic physicians, for instance, have some really excellent original methods of periodontal disease prevention and treatment to recommend.

A Holistic Physician Offers Periodontitis Prevention Suggestions

As a means for readers to prevent periodontitis and other gum diseases, from his medical office in Merrillville, Indiana, holistic and

---

1   S. Sternberg, "ADA Members Sink Teeth into Children's Hygiene," *USA Today*, section D, 16 April 1998, D8.

biological physician Arabinda Das, M.D., sent a letter to the editor of the *Townsend Letter for Doctors and Patients*. Dr. Das wrote:

> Mouth, tonsils and gums as the sources of many diseases have been known to physicians for years. Brushing teeth properly with additional simple antiseptic is best for protecting the teeth and gums from diseases.
>
> 1. Brush your teeth about 30 seconds in plain water to remove the food debris.
>
> 2. Brush a second time with hydrogen peroxide and baking soda about 45 seconds to remove the tissue debris and any pus and to make the gum alkaline. This also dissolves the protein debris. Rinse the mouth with plain water.
>
> 3. Buy a scaler from the drugstore. Use the scaler between gum and teeth. If there is discoloration, use slight pressure and apply it between the teeth to remove the debris and hard plaques. You may use a little more pressure to do this like your dental hygienist does. Here you can use dental floss, too, between the teeth.
>
> Chlorox containing sodium hypochlorite is good. Apply it in a dilution of 5.25%. Sodium hypochlorite was used in medicine for several years for its antifungal and antiseptic properties such as in Edinburgh Solution (EUSOL) for wound treatment, including in the intra-abdominal periotoneal cavity.
>
> A. To one ounce of Chlorox add 32 ounces of plain water. Label the bottle "A" for future use.
>
> B. Take one ounce of A solution and add 8 ounces of water. There are many other applications for this solution such as for cleaning plates and utensils. Brush your teeth and gums with this solution for about 45 seconds to kill all organisms. Do this three times a day after eating. Do brush the tongue at the same time.
>
> Results are obtained after one month's time. I have several patients who reported to me that their dentists were happy with their progress. One female patient in her late 60s had three loose teeth. After using this solution, two teeth were not loose after a month. Her holistic dentist examined the fluid between her loose bad teeth microscopically and did not find any bacteria. I have

shown this solution to two dentists who did not have any comment. The best solution for preventing periodontitis is commercially made "Chlorohexiden," but it is not economical and needs a prescription from a medical doctor or dentist. Chlorohexidine also discolors the teeth badly.

Never brush too hard which damages the dental enamel permanently.[1]

Even Long-Dead Edgar Cayce Is More Original than the ADA

Back in the early 1900s, Edgar Cayce, a native of Kentucky with a ninth grade education, accidentally discovered a strange gift. By putting himself in a light hypnotic trance, he could accurately diagnose a wide range of diseases, using precise medical terminology. Following his diagnoses, Mr. Cayce recommended a variety of therapeutic treatments, including a host of specific formulas and products that never failed to bring astounding results. Among his diagnoses and treatments were a few for periodontal disease and gingivitis.

Gingivitis is one of the milder forms of periodontitis. It's a condition in which the gums are red, swollen, and bleeding. Most gingivitis occurs from poor mouth care and from the buildup of bacterial plaque on the teeth. It also may be a sign of another condition, such as diabetes mellitus, leukemia, or vitamin deficiency and is common in pregnancy. Usually painless, gingivitis may come on suddenly or turn serious and be long term as with advanced periodontitis.

Well, in approximately seventy trancelike readings, Edgar Cayce put forth a formula called *Ipsab* as the perfect treatment for gingivitis and periodontal disease. The Ipsab solution contains prickly ash bark, salt, calcium chloride, peppermint, and iodine. Cayce's readings indicated that the cause of periodontal disease

---

1   A. Das, "Hygiene of Gum, Teeth and Mouth," *Townsend Letter for Doctors and Patients* 154 (May 1996): 78–79.

was a particular bacillus, and certain predisposing conditions in the mouth, teeth, and gums, which allowed for attack by the bacillus. According to Cayce, the ingredients in his recommended formula actually destroy this bacillus, which causes gum disease.

And you know what? Ipsab formula works. Modern medical/dental research reveals that its primary active ingredient, prickly ash bark—known to the American Indians as *toothache bark*—does indeed possess antiseptic, disinfectant, and deodorant properties that kill infectious germs.

Santa Barbara, California, dentist Robert Arthur, D.D.S., who uses the Cayce formula, says: "I've seen patients whose gums were so swollen and bleeding that they needed surgery, but Ipsab improved the tonus and health of their gums to the point that they were no longer surgical candidates."

In McLean, Virginia, another holistic-type dentist who wants to remain anonymous out of fear of reprisal by his state's local ADA membership, made Ipsab the subject of a double blind research study. Statistical analysis of the results indicate that 24 percent of the patients using Ipsab showed superior improvement of their gum disease, as contrasted with 5 percent of the patients given conventional treatment using the standard placebo. The McLean dentist is sufficiently impressed with the results that he now recommends the use of Ipsab to all his patients as a prophylactic measure.[1]

Hippie Gum Wash Relieves Sore Gums

Thirty-four-year-old Anthony "Tony" Thomasso, a bricklayer living and working in Rutland, Vermont, was struggling with the decision to undergo periodontal surgery. Out of simple neglect or carelessness with his oral hygiene, Mr. Thomasso had allowed his teeth, gums, and other oral cavity tissues to deteriorate into advanced

---

1   D. S. Taylor, "Research Reveals an Immune System Response to Castor Oil," *Explore More. For the Consumer* 2 (1993): 55–56.

periodontitis. But he wanted no part of the huge expense, the extreme pain, and the long healing time involved with having his teeth, gums, and jawbone scaled or extracted, cut and grafted, and reshaped or splinted by a periodontist.

In *advanced periodontitis*, the gingiva or gum tissue that surrounds the teeth forms a tooth socket with bone and supporting ligaments. Collectively, these three anatomic structures are known as *periodontium*. A variety of problems affecting the periodontium include the discomforts of bleeding, inflammation, swelling, tartar, and mineralized plaque formation, food debris collection, halitosis (bad breath), receding gums, gum pockets, a generalized pyorrhea, bone degeneration, and awful ongoing pain. In fact, so much periodontal pain is present that it can cause emotional anxiety accompanied by depression.[1]

Tony Thomasso's gums were so sensitive that canker sores and other infections became chronic, and that's when he asked members of his family for advice. Even Timothy Thomasso, his twenty-eight-year-old hippie brother, who lives in New York City's Greenwich Village, came up with a suggested solution. It turned out to be an excellent one, for it gave Tony permanent relief for his nearly disabling periodontal problem.

Timmy told his brother about *Hippie Gum Wash*, an herbal elixir that had proved effective for his own pyorrhea. The remedy required diligence on the part of Tony. In my mentioning how it works—much business may be lost to allopathic mainstream periodontists. To apply Hippie Gum Wash, you need to brush and rinse your teeth and gums gently twice a day for three months. Doing so, you must apply two groups of different herbs named in the separate formulations described below.

Once Tony committed himself to the regimen, relief came fast—within the first four weeks. After three months, the periodontal patient returned for another examination by his local periodontist, and that dentist was amazed with the bricklayer's changed oral cavity status. Tony was so improved, in fact, that the periodontist

---

1   F. P. Stay, *The Complete Book of Dental Remedies* (Garden City Park, N.Y.: Avery Publishing Group, 1996), 99–100.

gave him a clean bill of health and announced there was no more need for periodontal surgery. "Come back for a checkup in six months," was the only advice offered.

Yet this ADA-type periodontist never expressed any desire to know what herbs were used in his patient's antipyorrhea remedies. Inasmuch as what you're about to learn is strictly herbal holism (not voodoo), you will possess the two formulations for brushing and rinsing away gum disease. Until he finally reads this chapter, you'll know something that Tony Thomasso's tunnel-visioned allopathic periodontist in Rutland, Vermont, doesn't know.

The following are the double herbal formulations for eliminating the signs and uncomfortable symptoms of periodontal disease:[1]

To make Hippie Gum Wash (which may also be applied as an oral rinse similar to the commercial preparations described later in this chapter), the powdered herbs you should combine and use for required gentle tooth and gum brushing twice daily consist of:

1 part powdered goldenseal root
2 parts powdered myrrh
1 part powdered comfrey root
4 parts powdered baking soda

In a teacup or eggcup, mix these four ingredients together as a small pile of powder, wet your softened toothbrush, dip it in the powder, then brush your teeth and gums for several minutes. Be gentle with the brushing. Do *not* swallow the powder; rather, spit out the residue when finished brushing.

For rinsing all tissues of the oral cavity with Hippie Gum Wash, the liquid herbs you should combine for the rinse twice daily consist of:

5 to 10 drops of tincture of myrrh
5 to 10 drops of tincture of oak bark

Mix the drops together in a shot glass, add a bit of purified water if you have an insufficient amount of liquid, and rinse by swirling the

---

1   D. A. Downs, "Down-Home Remedies: Hippie Gum Wash Relieves Sore Gums," *Country Living's Healthy Living* (1996): 72.

tincture around and about the entire oral cavity (perhaps gargle) but make sure to swirl the mixture well for a couple of minutes.

As a brief explanation of what these herbs accomplish, you'll want to know that the goldenseal herb has antiseptic qualities; myrrh works as an anti-inflammatory to soothe swollen gums; oak bark is an astringent, and comfrey root contains allantoin, a compound that promotes cell growth. Baking soda is a traditional binder for tooth powder and has mildly abrasive qualities. By brushing gently, you are allowing the baking soda to do most of the scrubbing necessary for accomplishing removal of food debris, tartar, and plaque.

I've tried this combination of ingredients and must admit that the rinse of Hippie Gum Wash does taste as if one is chewing on tree bark. It's a similar taste to the wood bark ingredients used for brewing those two effective alternative anticancer remedies, Essiac tea and Pau d' arco tea (also known as lapacho).

Scientists Show Periodontal Disease Is Bad for the Heart

On February 16, 1998, at a meeting of the American Association for the Advancement of Science (AAAS), Mark Herzberg, Ph.D., a researcher at the University of Minnesota, announced that his animal experiments show that some strains of the most common bacteria that coat the teeth can trigger blood clots. Dr. Herzberg said, "Our data suggest that bacteria may cause blood clots that actually obstruct coronary arteries."

Such clots can and do bring on heart attacks by getting stuck within heart arteries already partially clogged by the atherosclerotic plaque substances of cholesterol, collagen, mucopolysaccharides, fibrin, foreign proteins, fat, toxic metals, and calcium. The calcium acts as the glue binding this additional metabolic junk material together.

Other scientists at the same AAAS meeting confirmed that even if the clot-forming dental bacteria are not harmful, the human body's reaction to them could be. People with periodontal disease have a lifelong simmering infection that causes chronic inflammation of the gums. In response, their bodies release a slow but steady stream of potent germ-killing chemicals that are in themselves harmful.[1]

"The ramification of this inflammation can be far-reaching," said bacteriologist Frank Scannapieco, Ph.D., of the State University of New York at Buffalo, who investigates in this area of pathology. The constant low-level infection plays a role in other common conditions, such as hardening of the arteries, valve failure, heart disease, stroke, diabetes, lung diseases, and premature births.

The ADA admits that about three-quarters of all adults over age thirty-five possess some degree of periodontal disease. These people form and retain pockets of infection that contain billions of bacteria. If an individual's oozing mess in the gums was out where it could be observed, it would be a bone-deep sore the size of the palms of both hands. When bacteria build up on the teeth, they form a kind of "crud" also known as *dental plaque,* which is different from the type of plaque inside arteries just described, the *atherosclerotic* plaque.

Dr. Herzberg found that the most common form of microbe in dental plaque is *Streptococcus sanguis,* and 60 percent of all strains of this germ are capable of making the blood clot in a test tube. In experiments the scientist performed on rabbits, one strain of *S. sanguis* created clots that lasted for thirty minutes. Electrocardiograms of these animals showed the clotting was bad enough to slow blood flow in heart arteries and deprive their heart muscles of all the oxygen needed. Large-scale clinical studies on humans suggest that those people with diseased gums and rotting teeth have double the usual risk of dying from heart disease.

Writing in *Let's Live* magazine, University of Minnesota graduate Timothy A. Kersten, D.D.S., says, "The blood that runs through your tooth will run through your toe within one minute. A [dental] infection or abscess and its associated bacteria and toxins are picked up by your bloodstream and carried throughout your body until they are filtered and cleaned out of your cardiovascular system. In the meantime, these circulating toxins from the infected area trigger a

---

1   Associated Press, "Is Flossing Good for Your Heart?" *The Caymanian Compass,* 20 (February 1998): A11.

sensitive, protective mechanism that activates your entire body in the fight against the infection. This is a physical and biochemical interconnection, one that can be observed, detected, and measured."[1]

Armin Grau, M.D., chief of the Neurology Department at the University of Heidelberg, Germany, conducted a study of 166 stroke victims, which was published in the American Heart Association journal *Stroke*. Dr. Grau told his audience, "People who have frequent dental and periodontal infections are more likely than others to suffer a stroke." The reason is that these infections activate blood coagulation, which makes it easier for atherosclerotic plaque to build up inside arteries as the precursor of stroke. Of course, one's appropriate self-defense procedure is to clear up dental infections as quickly as possible.[2]

Holistic Dental Therapies for Periodontal Disease

Typical of the periodontal disease correction programs offered to patients by holistic (biological) dentists, my upstate New York dentist friend reveals the following:

"My periodontal program consists of four to five visits, which include a mechanical removal of plaque, oral hygiene, and nutritional supplementation," he explains. "One cause for periodontal disease to develop is from proliferation of acid-loving bacteria in the mouth, producing inflammation in and about the gingiva. Around this gum tissue bacteria radically increase their population, because they thrive in a mouth that's become excessively acidic. The acidity comes from one's improper eating habits as occurs from giving in to a 'Big Mac Attack.' It also happens from poor food absorption in the gut. An acid mouth, moreover, tends to promote deposits of minerals onto the teeth.

"Since the immune system is weakened during the course of gingivitis or periodontitis, you will need to take nutrients for purposes of supporting immunity. Among these food supplements will be

---

1   T. A. Kersten, "Can Your Teeth Cause an Upset Stomach?" *Let's Live* (July 1990): 69.

2   "Did You Know That . . ." *Bottom Line Personal*, 15 (January 1998): 7.

minerals which aid in rebuilding bone, since loss of supporting bone takes place around the involved teeth," says the New York holistic dentist.

The following description of an attending biocompatible/mercury-free dentist's actions will provide you with an idea of what a program of periodontal or gum disease correction involves in a holistic dental practice.

Visit One: Dedicated to the gathering of periodontal information and for acquiring an education, the patient and biological dentist engage in full disclosure dental discussions together.

A companion to the patient may be present during this gathering of information.

The patient is encouraged to ask questions about his or her underlying pathology and the particular treatment to be administered for its correction.

The attending dentist, when educated in or conditioned to the procedures of holistic (biological) dentistry, collects information from the patient, which usually includes:

- the patient's general health history,

- necessary radiographs (oral X-ray films),

- a full visual and manual periodontal examination,

- a nutritional education for the patient invariably requiring dietary and nutrient recommendations, or the dispensing of specific nutritional supplements (see chapter 16 for Dr. Mike's dental diet and Dr. Mike's Teeth and Gums Support Pack),

- supplementation with nutrients; a dental diet by the patient must begin immediately.

Visit Two: Dedicated to the patient taking instruction from the dentist on the techniques of proper oral hygiene for periodontal disease correction, such teaching usually includes:

- how to use oral cavity irrigators,

- how to effectively remove plaque with a toothbrush and dental floss,

- confirmation and any necessary reinstruction about nutritional supplementation as per the dentist's previous recommendations.

Visit Three: Dedicated to periodontal treatment, there is the commencing of routine or deep cleaning with scaling of teeth and root planing.

Visit Four: Dedicated to the continuation of periodontal treatment, the cleaning, scaling, and planing are brought to a near conclusion.

Visit Five: Dedicated to progress in healing, the dentist checks for any complications. If complications are found, they are corrected. If no complications are found, tooth polishing commences and a recall program for the patient is instituted. If some further treatment becomes necessary, at this time the dentist discusses what therapies are required.

The Holistic Periodontal Cleansing Diet

In addition to Dr. Michael Loquasto's dental diet (created by a chiropractic nutritionist) described in chapter 16, the upstate New York dentist perfected another eating program. It must be followed for one month, after which time you may use it as a guide and add other foods. Thus the diet allows a participating periodontal patient some leeway in following the menu plan. For example, the New York dentist frequently suggests, "If not hungry, skip a meal or two." But this eating program is not a weight loss diet.

As you will discover upon reading the next chapter, the New York dentist's menu plan conforms somewhat with the dental diet put forth by chiropractic nutritionist Michael J. Loquasto, D.C., C.C.N., (Dr. Mike) of Marshalls Creek, Pennsylvania. Dr. Mike recommends strict vegetarianism with no eating of red meat, poultry, dairy, and the limiting of fish to one meal in a week. While Dr. Mike discourages the eating of fruit, because its sugar content stimulates the growth of bacteria in the mouth, the New York dentist allows fruit, especially at breakfast. Both of these diets, recommended by two health professionals who don't know each other, are body detoxifying dining plans. As you eat them, the diets stimulate bowel peristalsis and cleanse the gut of waste products. Large amounts of fiber in these kinds of vegetarian foods provide a dining recipient with good bowel movements.

The New York dentist's Holistic Periodontal Cleansing Diet focuses on two different types of lunches, one on three days of the week and the other on four days during the week. There's a single set form of dinner for all seven days of the week. No suggestion is offered for breakfast except to eat fruit, which contrasts starkly with Dr. Mike's dental diet, described in the next chapter. The sugar in fruit is equivalent to carbohydrates in candy, Dr. Mike believes, and is *verboten*. The holistic dentist isn't persuaded this way.

Dressings for any of the raw salads may be homemade from lemon juice and olive oil or another oil type comprised of omega-3 fatty acids. Moreover, dressings may contain dulce or kelp.

The diet from the holistic New York dentist is an exceedingly healthy, cellular cleansing and gastrointestinal tract detoxifying eating program. It allows the body to become alkaline in a short time and works well against periodontal disease. This diet is found on pages 306 and 307.

As you'll discover when you read chapter 16, although this dietary program may seem restrictive, it's less so than the dental diet advocated by chiropractic nutritionist Dr. Michael J. Loquasto. Dr. Mike eliminates all dairy foods along with all fruit. Yet both diets work to restore dental health, as proven by several hundred patients who praise these two health professionals. They are much loved by their patients. As I mentioned, the two nutritionally oriented health professionals don't know each other at all. They've never even spoken together, and I am the connecting link between them. My feeling of admiration is for them both.

Holistic Periodontal Nutritional Supplementation

The upstate New York dentist begins his patient instructions for the holistic periodontal nutrient supplementation program with homeopathic remedies. They are adjunctive to the larger number of homeopathics discussed at greater length in chapter 17. If you are unfamiliar with the two homeopathic dosage forms, they are explained in chapter 17.

The homeopathic supplements recommended here will help with oral cavity healing during the course of any periodontal treatment. There are four of them, which are:

Arnica 30x	Take two tablets three times a day
Mercurius corrisivus 30x	Take two tablets three times a day
Plantago major 30x	Take two tablets three times a day
Silicea 30x	Take one tablet three times a day

There are standard rules to follow when ingesting homeopathic remedies: do not consume any caffeine such as the drinking of coffee or black tea and don't use mint in any form, not even minted toothpaste. That ruling even includes eating fresh mint from your garden or peppermint, spearmint, and so forth. Furthermore, avoid swallowing raw garlic for two hours after a homeopathic remedy is taken. Any of these particular substances neutralize the homeopathic therapy so that you're just wasting its application.

Particular nutrients taken at certain dosage levels are advantageous in warding off or treating periodontal problems. The following are nutritional supplements often recommended by holistic dentists for helping in the elimination of gum diseases:

Beta carotene complex (precursor for vitamin A):	2500 IU per day
Vitamin B complex:	15 to 25 mg of all twelve B vitamins
Vitamin B1:	50 mg per day
Niacin:	400 mg in divided doses (to avoid flush)
Vitamin B6:	50 mg per day

Vitamin C:	2 to 4 gms per day, taken in four divided doses, but don't take it for twelve hours before a scheduled dental appointment

Decreased levels of vitamin C are associated with periodontal disease. A lack of vitamin C is known to allow greater passage of bacteria into the gums and other tissues surrounding teeth.[1]

Vitamin E:	400 IU per day
Selenium:	200 mcg per day
Multivitamin/mineral:	25 mg per day minimum
Zinc picolinate:	30 mg per day
Magnesium:	600 mg per day
CoEnzyme Q10 :	100 or 200 mg per day

Some significant information about CoEnzyme Q10 is necessary here. It's a nutrient that's often reported as deficient in an amount ranging from 60 to 96 percent in the gingival tissues of people with periodontal disease.[2] When taken as a supplement by patients under periodontal treatment, the degree of their healing speeds up remarkably. In an open clinical study, CoQ10 administration produced "extraordinary" postsurgical healing of up to three times faster than usual in seven patients with advanced periodontitis.[3] The

---

1   T. Wilson and K. Kornman, *Fundamentals of Periodontics* (New York: Quintessence Books, 1996), 250.

2   R. Nakamura and others, "Study of CoQ10-Enzymes in Gingiva from Patients with Periodontal Disease and Evidence for a Deficiency of CoenzymeQ10," *Proceedings of the National Academy of Science* 71 (1974): 1456; I. L. Hansen and others, "Bioenergetics in Clinical Medicine, IX, Gingival and Leukocytic Deficiencies of Coenzyme Q10 in Patients with Periodontal Disease," *Research Communications: Chemistry, Pathology, and Pharmacology* 14 (1976): 729; G. P. Littarru, R. Nakamura, L. Ho, and others, "Deficiency of Coenzyme Q10 in Gingival Tissue from Patients with Periodontal Disease," *Proceeding of the National Academy of Sciences* 68 (1971): 2332; R. Nakamura, G. P. Littarru, K. Folkers, and E. G. Wilkinson, "Deficiency of Coenzyme Q in Gingiva of Patients with Periodontal Disease," *International Journal of Vitamin and Nutritional Research* 43 (1973): 84.

3   E. G. Wilkinson and others, "Bioenergetics in Clinical Medicine, II, Adjunctive

beneficial effect of CoQ10 has been confirmed in dogs, whose experimentally induced periodontal disease was significantly reduced by the nutrient's supplementation.[1]

Oligomeric proanthocyanidins (OPCs)	100 mg per day
Glutathione	150 mg in three divided doses per day
Methionine	600 to 1500 mg in three divided doses per day
Garlic extract	1200 to 2400 mg in two divided doses
Probiotics	1.5 billion organisms of *Lactobacillus acidophilus* and other live cultures friendly to the gut
Flaxseed oil:	up to 2 tablespoons per day
Lecithin:	up to 2 tablespoons per day
Chlorella:	one capsule per day

Cilantro (Chinese parsley) mobilizes mercury and other toxic metals from the gum tissues and pulls it out of the central nervous system, intestines, and liver as well when great quantities are eaten. Mercury from amalgams gets excreted as a waste product in the urine and feces when cilantro is part of one's diet. Common parsley works this way, too, but gastrointestinal upset may occur when massive amounts of the vegetable is eaten for detoxification purposes.[2]

Treatment with Coenzyme Q in Periodontal Therapy," *Research Communications in Chemistry, Pathology, and Pharmacology* 12 (1975): 111.

1   S. Shizukuishi and others, "Therapy by Coenzyme Q10 of Experimental Periodontitis in a Dog-Model Supports Results of Human Periodontitis Therapy," in *Biomedical and Clinical Aspects of Coenzyme Q*, vol. 4, eds. K. Folkers and Y. Yamamura (Amsterdam, Netherlands: Elsevier Science Publications, 1984), 153–62.

2   Y. Omura, "Radiation Injury and Mercury Deposits in Internal Organs,"

Commercial Remedies for Tooth and Gum Diseases

With publication of this book, Swedish experts announce a new gel that painlessly dissolves decayed matter in cavities. In Sweden, this gel, called *Carisolv*, replaces the dental drill in many cases of tooth decay. It dissolves decayed material lying on the cavity surface, while amino acids in the gel form a chemical barrier protecting healthy tissue. The dissolving process takes less than thirty seconds, after which time the dentist scrapes the cavity free of gel. The procedure is then repeated until the gel no longer clouds on contact with the cavity, indicating that all unwanted material has been loosened from the tooth surface. A final cotton swab cleanup prepares the cavity for the application of the mercury-free filling that must follow.

The gel is a remarkable improvement over drilling. As drill usage becomes rarer, "in most cases anesthetics and the pain and discomfort of injections will not be needed," says the manufacturer. Swedish dentists have already applied the gel to over ten thousand patients, and the commercial company has now expanded its domestic use by more than a thousand Swedish dentists.

"Just leave it to the Swedes," writes Schaumburg, Illinois, osteopathic physician Joseph M. Mercola, D.O., in his monthly column for the *Townsend Letter for Doctors and Patients*. "Sweden was one of the first countries to make it a crime to put amalgam ('silver') mercury fillings in anyone's mouth and now they have developed an alternative to the painful dental drill. Most people don't recognize that the high speed drill most dentists use is what is actually responsible for the death of most teeth that eventually require root canals."[1]

All kinds of commercial remedies for tooth and gum disease are coming out of the research facilities of manufacturers to accommodate the demands of dental consumers around the world, especially in the United States and Canada. Long-suffering dental

---

Acupuncture and Electrotherapeutics Research, International Journal 20 (1995): 133–48.

1   J. M. Mercola, "Current Health News You Can Use," *Townsend Letter for Doctors and Patients* 178 (May 1998): 36–39.

patients are becoming aware of dangers from fluoridation, mercury amalgams, periodonture, orthodonture, extractions, cavitations, root canals, and other assaults on their immune systems through the oral cavity.

MistORAL Spray for Gingivitis

Brower Enterprises, Inc. of Canton, South Dakota (see appendix B for the address and telephone numbers), is distributing a new oral spray for overcoming gum disease. The many specific nutrients to prevent and alleviate gingivitis and periodontitis have been placed into one spray-on form for effective application directly to the gums.

Donal Joseph Carter, Ph.D., of Washington, D.C., has formulated a topical mouth spray, MistORAL, which produces significant results for those suffering from periodontal disease. The active ingredients in MistORAL are substantiated in peer-reviewed scientific studies. Its so-called "inactive" ingredients are successfully used by nutritionally oriented dentists to overcome periodontal problems.

Among the MistORAL active ingredients are B complex vitamins such as folic acid to keep the gums healthy and vital; coEnzyme Q10, specific for periodontal wellness discussed earlier; a broad-spectrum antibacterial combination, including green tea extract, to kill the bacteria that are the root cause of gum disease; particular healing agents like aloe vera extract to overcome inflammation; and vitamin K3 to tame excessive bleeding, protect against decay, and facilitate healthy gum metabolism. Ingredients follow:

CoEnzyme Q10	160 mcg/spray
Vitamin K3	16 mcg/spray
Propolis extract	32 mcg/spray
Eucaliptol oil	32 mcg/spray
Menthol	320 mcg/spray
Folic acid	64 mcg/spray
Aloe vera extract	6400 mcg/spray

With each spray, the dosages of seven active ingredients in MistORAL are documented to stop or treat gingivitis/periodontitis, mucous membrane irritation, oral sores, plaque formation, and tooth decay.

Among the oral spray's twenty-one inactive ingredients emulsified into a patented delivery system that guarantees stability and resultant action are the following: purified water, glycerine sorbitan monolaurate, phospholipids, green tea extract, stevia, rebaudiana extract, calcium ascorbate, citrus seed extract, myrrh oil, gotu-kola extract, echinacea extract, calendula extract, chamomile, chapparal extract, lemon grass extract, vitamin E mixed tocopherols, parsley extract, Pau d' arco extract, spearmint oil, peppermint oil, citric acid, goldenseal extract, red thyme oil, tea tree oil, cool cayenne extract, and vitamin B6.

Herbal Mouth and Gum Therapy
from the Natural Dentist

Rinsing twice daily with an oral care mouthwash designed to fight plaque tends to soothe bleeding gums and reduce or prevent swollen gums. As part of a total natural dental care program, it makes sense to choose a mouthwash made from all natural ingredients and not drugs. That way you avoid the harsh chemicals found in mass-produced products. Accordingly, Woodstock Natural Products, Inc. of Englewood Cliffs, New Jersey, makers of *The Natural Dentist Herbal Mouth and Gum Therapy Daily Oral Rinse and Demulcent*, offers the dental consumer herbs for oral care. Highly effective herbal remedies incorporated into the company's rinsing formula are echinacea, goldenseal, and calendula.

Bill Stern, president of Woodstock Natural Products, Inc., advises: "Herbal Mouth and Gum Therapy was formulated to be more than just a breath freshener. In addition to testimonials from dentists and patients, this oral rinse was shown to mitigate periodontal degeneration by fighting plaque and relieving inflamed, edematous, and bleeding gums in a placebo-controlled study of twenty patients with type 1 gingivitis or type 2 periodontitis. Although it contains no alcohol, the product significantly reduces bacterial counts of *Streptococus mutans in vitrol.* Unlike other mouthwashes and rinses, Herbal Mouth and Gum Therapy was developed to be used as a component of a complete oral hygiene program that includes brushing, flossing, and regular visits to the dental office. It can help prevent gingivitis, tooth decay, and minor mouth irritation."

In a report issued by an independent testing laboratory, Mountainview Laboratories of Brainerd, Minnesota, The Natural Dentist Herbal Mouth and Gum Therapy daily oral rinse was found to be 99.9 percent effective in killing the germs that cause gum disease. Also, at the New York University College of Dentistry, three investigating dentists and a supporting scientist proved it is as effective in killing germs that cause gingivitis as the man-made antiseptic, Listerine, which contains alcohol and probably has laboratory-produced substances in it such as preservatives, dyes, or artificial sweeteners.[1]

An additional study by the three dentists and another scientist indicated that Herbal Mouth and Gum Therapy improves oral health in regard to gingivitis and gingival bleeding after three months of use. Its ingredients provide oral health benefits and a natural alternative for those dental consumers who want to avoid chemicals in the mouth.[2]

Finally, still another study from three dentists and another scientist indicated that Herbal Mouth and Gum Therapy produces larger zones of microbial inhibition than Listerine and Scope against three potent bacteria. Tested in this study were *Streptococcus mutans*, *Streptococcus sanguis*, and *Actinomyces viscosus*. The proof was demonstrated when sterile discs treated with mouth rinses were placed on agar plates with controls. Zones of microbial inhibition were measured in millimeters after 48 hours. The natural oral rinse from Woodstock Natural Products, Inc., passed the test and exceeded expectations.[3] (To contact the manufacturer of Herbal Mouth and Gum Therapy, Woodstock Natural Products, Inc., please see appendix B for the company's listing.)

---

1   J. Gulz, J. Kaim, J. Deleo, and W. Scherer, "An *In Vivo* Comparison of the Antimicrobial Activities of Three Mouth Rinses," New York University College of Dentistry, March 1998.

2   J. Gultz, J. Kaim, S. S. Lee, and W. Scherer, "Clinical Efficacy of an Herbal Mouth Rinse," New York University College of Dentistry, March 1998.

3   J. Gultz, L. Do, J. Kaim, and W. Scherer, "The Antimicrobial Activity of an Herbal Mouth Rinse," New York University College of Dentistry, October 1997.

Holistic Periodontal Cleansing Diet

	Breakfast	Lunch	Dinner
Monday	fruit	one or two fresh fruits in season such as berries, kiwi, pineapple, apples, pears, grapes, peaches, and so forth. OR apricots, prunes OR figs, currants (dried fruit may be soaked) AND avocado.	a LARGE *raw* vegetable salad AND a baked potato OR lentils OR peas, AND (if needed out of hunger) one steamed vegetable which may be cabbage, asparagus, broccoli, brussel sprouts, and so forth.
Tuesday	fruit	a small *raw* vegetable salad, which must contain romaine lettuce and sprouts, and two or three other vegetables AND avocado or rice cakes or three ounces of raw nuts such as almonds, filberts, walnuts, or pecans.	a LARGE *raw* vegetable salad AND a baked yam or avocado
Wednesday	fruit	one or two fresh fruits in season such as berries, kiwi, pineapple, apples, pears, grapes, peaches, and so forth. OR apricots, prunes OR figs, currants (dried fruit may be soaked) AND avocado.	a LARGE *raw* vegetable salad AND a baked potato OR corn OR lentils AND (if needed out of hunger) one steamed vegetable.

	Breakfast	Lunch	Dinner
Thursday	fruit	a small *raw* vegetable salad, which must contain romaine lettuce and sprouts, and two or three other vegetables AND avocado or rice cakes or three ounces of raw nuts such as almonds, filberts, walnuts, or pecans.	a LARGE *raw* vegetable salad AND avocado OR beans such as garbanzo, fava, or mung.
Friday	fruit	one or two fresh fruits in season such as berries, kiwi, pineapple, apples, pears, grapes, peaches, and so forth. OR apricots, prunes OR figs, currants (dried fruit may be soaked) AND avocado.	a LARGE *raw* vegetable salad AND a baked potato OR corn OR lentils AND (if needed out of hunger) one steamed vegetable.
Saturday	fruit	a small *raw* vegetable salad, which must contain romaine lettuce and sprouts, and two or three other vegetables AND avocado or rice cakes or three ounces of raw nuts such as almonds, filberts, walnuts, or pecans.	a LARGE *raw* vegetable salad AND brown rice AND beans AND lightly steamed diced vegetables.
Sunday	fruit	a small *raw* vegetable salad, which must contain romaine lettuce and sprouts, and two or three other vegetables AND avocado or rice cakes or three ounces of raw nuts such as almonds, filberts, walnuts, or pecans.	a LARGE *raw* vegetable salad AND six ounces of ricotta cheese OR pot cheese OR cottage cheese AND (if needed out of hunger) one steamed vegetable.

The Toothpaste for Use with Homeopathics

A family owned, publicly listed pharmaceutical company founded in Lyon, France, in 1932, Boiron, offers homeopathic medicines for health care professionals to use in their daily practices. Moreover, consumers have access to these same homeopathics over the counter and without prescription that are sold in health food stores and pharmacies in sixty-one countries. Boiron manufactures more than two thousand five hundred different homeopathic medicines. Among them is Homeodent, an all natural toothpaste, which has been especially designed for people using homeopathic products.

Homeodent's original formula combines fresh plants selected for their soothing and stimulating benefits. They include marigold (*Calendula officianalis*), plantain (*Plantago major*), horse radish (*Cochlearia armoracia*), and witch hazel (*Hamamelis virginiana*). Made in two flavors, delicate anise and lemon, both freshen the teeth and gums without interfering with anyone's homeopathic therapy as do those toothpastes that have some form of mint as part of their ingredients.

Homeodent contains no mint, no saccharin or artificial sweeteners, and no fluoride. (To contact Boiron-Borneman, Inc., the United States distributor of Homeodent, please see the company's listing in appendix B.)

Sixteen

The Dental Diet and Its Supplemental Nutrients

To function at its optimum and hold off or overcome degenerative diseases such as periodontitis, the body requires a ready supply of dietary vitamins, minerals, fatty acids, amino acids, carbohydrates, and other nourishing components like fiber, oxygen, and water. These nutrients are necessary for physiological growth, normal metabolism, and the maintenance of life; they must be supplied by ingestion from the surrounding environment because such items cannot be created within the body. Because what is a suitable diet for one individual or population isn't necessarily healthy eating for another, variations in human biochemistry must be taken into account.

A superior dental diet to achieve optimal health for people living in contemporary society has already been established over eons of evolutionary experience. This chapter offers a general description of the ideal dental diet, all the while bearing in mind that people must adapt aspects of their eating program in accordance with their biochemical individuality.

Based on the research of two nutritional giants I'm about to identify, my recommendation is that Paleolithic nutrition represented by a modified Mediterranean diet should be followed. Despite the difficult-to-resist eating temptations of junk foods, fast foods, sweet foods, meat, and dairy foods, you have the means of staying healthy. Wishing to achieve optimal nutrition will have you sticking to the way populations dined in the primitive past and even today along the Mediterranean coast. This dietary intake of the Paleolithic period involved consuming reduced amounts of saturated fat, fewer milligrams of sodium, moderate quantities of protein, slight increases in cholesterol, more antioxidant vitamins from foods, and elevated milligrams of calcium than what is ordinarily ingested in Western countries today.[1]

One of the two diet and nutrition giants whom I will be quoting in this chapter is certified clinical nutritionist Michael Jude Loquasto, D.C., D.A.B.C.N., C.C.N., clinic director of the Healthplex Medical Center in Marshalls Creek, Pennsylvania. Dr. Loquasto's Healthplex dispenses services relating to dietary counseling, nutritional infusions, sports medicine, clinical testing, and many alternative, innovative, integrative, and complementary medical therapies such as chiropractic, chelation, and nutrition. Another giant in nutritional science to be cited is internist and clinical nutritionist Artemis P. Simopoulos, M.D., president of the Center for Genetics, Nutrition, and Health in Boston, Massachusetts. To offer background for presenting you with new information about the dental diet and its nutritional supplements, I will start off chapter 16 with information furnished by Dr. Artemis Simopoulos.

The Hazardous Trans Fatty Acids

During her May 1996 presentation before the American College for Advancement in Medicine (ACAM) in Orlando, Florida, Dr. Simopoulos discussed the Mediterranean diet as a main reason for the lowered incidence of degenerative diseases among peoples bordering the Mediterranean Sea. She stated, "Dietary changes influence the development of chronic diseases, and diets that are consistent with our evolution, such as the Mediterranean diet, and particularly the Greek diet before 1960, are the most beneficial for

---

1   S. B. Eaton and M. Konner, "Paleolithic Nutrition. A Consideration of Its Nature and Current Implications," *New England Journal of Medicine* 312 (1985): 283–89; A. P.Simopoulos, "Evolutionary Aspects of Diet: Obesity and Reference Standards," in *Obesity: New Directions in Assessment and Management*, eds. T. Van Itallie and A. P. Simopoulos (Philadelphia: Charles Press, 1995).

the prevention of cardiovascular disorders, diabetes, cancer, periodontitis, arthritis, and other degenerative diseases."

As a result of major differences between Paleolithic nutrition and current Western diets in types of fats and oils, it's a fact that ancient peoples actually experienced far less degenerative disease than do those in our modern Western industrialized societies.[1] Fat content was much lower back then; it contained fewer saturated fats and omega-6 fatty acids, but higher amounts of omega-3 fatty acids.[2] While primitive eating might have contained some minimal amounts of trans fatty acids (TFAs) present in nature, in contrast, modern diets eaten by most North Americans and Europeans are loaded with the TFAs of hydrogenated vegetable oils. These TFAs are the hazardous constituents making up, for instance, processed peanut butter and other refined nut butters, margerine, salad dressings, shortenings, and frying oils. The very unhealthy trans fatty acids furnish North Americans, especially, between 5 percent and 15 percent of energy available in the Canadian and United States populations.[3]

Trans fatty acids entered the Western world's food supply shortly after World War I and reached high proportions thereafter. Although margarine is promoted as a healthy substitute for the cholesterol in butter, this promotion is a lie. It's shamefully put forth by the food processors' advertising agencies and has been stupidly advocated by the American Heart Association (AHA). There is nothing healthy about taking margarine into your body. TFAs in margarine and other hydrogenated foods are twice as likely to increase the ratio of total cholesterol to high density lipoprotein (HDL) cholesterol. They do this because TFAs increase low density lipoprotein (LDL) cholesterol while lowering HDL cholesterol. Also TFAs have many other adverse effects, which contribute to gum disease, rotted teeth,

---

1   A. Leaf and P. C. Weber, "Cardiovascular Effects of N-3 Fatty Acids," *New England Journal of Medicine* 318 (1988): 547–49.

2   A. P. Simopoulos, "Omega-3 Fatty Acids in Health and Disease and in Growth and Development," *American Journal of Clinical Nutrition* 54 (1991): 538–68.

3   W. M. N. Ratnayake, R. Hollywood, E. O'Grady, and F. Pelletier, "Fatty Acids in Some Common Food Items in Canada," *Journal of American College of Nutrition* 12 (1993): 651–60.

dental infections, obesity, high blood pressure, diabetes, and worse. To maintain a superior diet, you should avoid consuming any trans fatty acids such as in Jiffy peanut butter, Skippy peanut butter, and Fleishman's margarine.

Inasmuch as there are more than a dozen Mediterranean nations with varied cultures, traditions, and dietary habits, the Mediterranean diet is not a homogeneous nutritional model. But some nutritional properties are common to all or most of the Mediterranean area's eating programs. The results of a European Atomic Energy Community (EURATOM) research study carried out in the 1960s demonstrated that the Mediterranean diet is characterized by being

1. low in saturated fat,

2. high in monounsaturates through the extensive use of olive oil,

3. reduced in animal protein (except fish),

4. rich in complex carbohydrates such as grains,

5. increased in vegetables and leguminous fiber.[1]

The Diet Eaten by Greek People

Two decades after the EURATOM report appeared, another study, published by the Food and Agriculture Organization (FAO) of the United Nations on the dietary intake of fourteen Mediterranean countries, including Portugal, Spain, France, Italy, Yugoslavia, Greece, Malta, Israel, Libya, Algeria, Tunisia, Turkey, Egypt, and Morocco, compared the diets of Mediterranean countries to the diet of the United States for the same period. It showed a startling contrast. People residing in the Mediterranean nations eat in a healthier manner than

---

1   M. Cresta, S. Ledermann, A. Garnier, E. Lombardo, and G. Lacourtly, "Etude des Consommations Alimentaires des Populations de Onze Regions de la Communaute Europeenne en Vue de la Determination des Niveaux de Contamination Radioactive," *Raport etabli au Centre d'Etude Nucleaire de Fotenay-aux-Roses, France:* EURATOM, Commissariat a l'Energie Atomique (CEA), 1969.

do Americans. Of all those people bordering the Mediterranean Sea, the healthiest dietary population is the Greek people.[1]

These Greek people eat more legumes, vegetables, fruits, fish, and cereal grains than do Americans. They drink more wine, eat less meat, or no meat at all, and fewer eggs. As a result of this Grecian way of eating, the Greeks show a life expectancy at age forty-five that is higher than those living in the United States. Dental ill health, coronary heart disease, total cancers, and degenerative diseases in general are less prevalent in Greece.

The Greek diet is considered optimal, although other factors besides diet, genetics, environmental pollutants, and sunlight also differ between Greece and the United States. But diet is the most important factor accounting to a significant extent for the differences in health statistics between the two countries. There's no doubt that Greeks eat proportionately more nutritious food, have fewer diseases, exhibit less incidence of disease, and generally live longer than North Americans and most of the other people bordering the Mediterranean Sea. In fact, despite the emphasis in the United States on sanitation, all people along the Mediterranean coast are healthier than Americans because they eat less commercially prepared and processed foods, almost no fast foods, and near zero amounts of junk foods. They hardly use "convenience" foods at all. Much of the time, the Greek population consumes natural-type edibles.

Fats and Oils Differences between Greece and the U.S.

At an ACAM semiannual meeting, Dr. Simopoulos stated, "A major difference between the diet of the United States and Greece is in the type of fats. Not only is the Greek diet lower in saturated fat, but it is particularly high in monounsaturates, specifically olive oil, whereas the U.S. diet is high in polyunsaturated fatty acids from vegetable oils that are rich in omega-6 fatty acids. Excess amounts

---

1   W. C. Willett, "Diet and Health: What Should We Eat," *Science* 264 (1994): 532–37.

of omega-6 fat is known to lead to tumors in animals and to increased platelet aggregation in humans. Because the U.S. diet is low in omega-3 fatty acids, there is an imbalance between the omega-3 and omega-6 fatty acids, which leads to a proinflammatory and prothrombotic (blood clot) state."

The U.S. food guide pyramid has been criticized for not distinguishing among the various fatty acids, such as trans fatty acids and omega-6 and omega-3 polyunsaturated fatty acids. The United States Department of Agriculture also has failed to emphasize the beneficial effects of olive oil in raising HDL cholesterol and in preventing the oxidation of LDL cholesterol. A low-fat diet has been shown to lead to essential fatty acid deficiency in not less than 5 percent and rising to 25 percent of the Framingham Study population.[1]

Dr. Simopoulos recommends the adoption of "the Greek column" food guide rather than "the U.S. pyramid" food guide, which she describes as symbolically representing "the pharaohs' tomb" or "a Mayan temple."

An excessively high carbohydrate diet leads to people experiencing elevated blood triglycerides (hypertriglyceridemia), especially in middle-aged women and in those men and women who already have elevated blood triglycerides. Any recommendation of two to three servings of meat a day, which has been lobbied for by the U.S. cattle industry, must be considered unhealthy, because red meat has been shown to be associated with cancers of the colon and prostate in epidemiologic studies.[2]

Moreover, later you'll learn something even more surprising from reading about the Mediterranean diet's modifications incorporated

---

1   E. N. Siguel and R. H. Lerman, "Relationship between Fatty Acid Patterns and HDL/Total Cholesterol in Subjects Participating in the Framingham Offspring Heart Study Cycle 4," abstract presented at the 43d annual scientific session of the American College of Cardiology, 14 March 1994, Atlanta.

2   W. C. Willet, M. J. Stampfer, G. A. Colditz, B. A Rosner, and F. E. Spetzer, "Relation of Meat, Fat, and Fiber Intake to the Risk of Colon Cancer in a Prospective Study among Women," *New England Journal of Medicine* 323 (1990): 1664–72; E. J. Giovannucci, E. B. Rimm, G. A. Colditz, and others, "A Prospective Study of Dietary Fat and Risk of Prostate Cancer," *Journal of the National Cancer Institute* 85 (1993): 1571–79.

by Dr. Michael "Dr. Mike" Loquasto. To preserve your teeth, gums, and other aspects of oral health, eating dairy foods is not recommended at all—not ever by Dr. Mike, which will be explained when we arrive at his dietary section in this chapter.

Now, you're going to learn about the Greek column Mediterranean food guide, which is better for your long-term health than the USDA's food pyramid guide. Even before Dr. Simopoulos's research came to fruition, Dr. Mike had set out the foundation for her Greek column food guide.

The Greek Column Mediterranean Food Guide

Dr. Simopoulos is enthusiastic about people returning to their indigenous diets and lifestyles. Indigenous diets of the Mediterranean area differ from the Western diet in types of fats, fiber, antioxidant content, potassium, and protein. Adoption of a Western type of diet and lifestyle has led to increases in heart trouble, stroke, cavitations, dental cavities, rotted teeth, oral infections, periodontal disease, crooked teeth, rheumatism, obesity, diabetes, peripheral vascular diseases, and other American trademarks now appearing in Mediterranean populations. These disorders happen specifically when people have altered the way they've been brought up. In the comparison study mentioned earlier, the original diets of any of the fourteen Mediterranean nations are better than what's eaten in North America. "All these indigenous diets are low in saturated fat; high in essential fatty acids, with plenty of fruits and vegetables; higher in potassium but lower in sodium; and high in antioxidants; with adequate amounts of protein provided by fresh fish, lean meat, eggs, yogurt, and other forms of *fermented* [not regular] milk," says Dr. Simopoulos.

"I have attempted to develop a Mediterranean food guide based on information of Paleolithic nutrition and the dietary habits of the people in the Mediterranean region before 1960, that is, before the onslaught of Western dietary products," she explains. "I have selected a Greek column for the Mediterranean food guide based on genetic variation and nutrition. My guide is consistent with the fact that not everybody is susceptible to chronic diseases to the same extent. And it's predicated on a balanced energy intake and energy expenditure.[1] This is not a low-fat/high-carbohydrate diet, since olive oil is the cooking oil and constitutes a higher source of energy than any other food.

"The concept of the [U.S. Agriculture Department's] 'pyramid' is based on a high-carbohydrate/low-fat diet without any distinction made about the various fatty acids, while promoting grains rather than fruits and vegetables. The Mediterranean food guide excludes vegetable oils and hydrogenated oils and their products. The Greek column is based on foods and not on food groups, and although it excludes certain foods it does not limit the intake of naturally occurring foods nor insist on the inclusion of large numbers of portions," says Dr. Simopoulos. "The first part of the Greek column contains the foods to be added to any meal: olive oil, lemon, vinegar; olives; bread; cheese; yogurt; fruits, fruit juices; nuts, garlic, onions; vegetables, herbs, spices; pasta, rice, potatoes; water and wine. Above that are the basic components of daily meals with emphasis on legumes, fish, and poultry. Meat and eggs, as such, comprise a main meal once a week each." Not much dairy is eaten by the Greeks.

In following the Mediterranean food guide, the foods to be added to any meal are rich in antioxidant vitamins and minerals. They should have a balance of omega-6 and omega-3 fatty acids, with the addition of olive oil and herbs daily and with fish up to three times a week. Margarines rich in trans fatty acids, vegetable oils, and other artificial foods are forbidden altogether. Sweets may not be eaten or may be eaten only rarely just on special occasions. And the same admonition against soft drinks and hard liquor is given. Because olive oil is an absolutely safe oil and definitely nutritious, there is no limit to how much is ingested as long as the consumer's energy intake equals energy expenditure.

The diet described above offers a natural means of preserving the teeth. Dr. Simopoulos' Mediterranean eating program is

---

1   A. P. Simopoulos and B. Childs, eds., "Genetic Variation and Nutrition," *World Review of Nutrition and Diet* 63 (1990): 1–300; A. P. Simopoulos, V. Herbert, and B. Jacobson, "Genetic Nutrition," *Designing A Diet Based on Your Family Medical History* (New York: Macmillan, 1993).

advantageous to adapt for your purposes of dental protection, but olive oil should become an integral part of your food intake.

The Nutritional Desirability of Olive Oil

The backbone of the Mediterranean diet is olive oil, for it provides a larger number of calories than any other single food. Greece, along with Italy, Spain, and Portugal are the major producers of olive oil (see my 1997 Kensington Publishing Corporation paperback book, *Nature's Antibiotic: Olive Leaf Extract*). Greek olive oil is aromatic and high in oleic acid (80 percent) and contains about 11 percent omega-6 fatty acids and 0.8 percent omega-3 fatty acids. Of all other food grade oils, these percentages place olive oil in a unique and superior position when it comes to both taste and health. Here are more olive oil attributes:

- Like all nonanimal fats, olive oil does not contain cholesterol and does reduce LDL oxidation. [1]

- In addition to vitamin E, a known antioxidant, olive oil contains the phenolic antioxidant (with antithrombotic effects *in vitro*), 3,4-dihydroxy-phenyl ethanol. [2]

- Unlike tropical oils, olive oil is very low in saturated fats.

- Olive oil does not raise LDL, but it does elevate HDL, whereas vegetable oils such as corn oil lower both LDL and HDL.

- Making it an integral part of the diet, olive oil replaces omega-6 in phospholipids, cholesterol esters, and triglycerides in the blood serum—a good healthy effect.

1   P. Reaven, S. Parthasarathy, B. J. Grasse, and others, "Effects of Oleate-Enriched and Linoleate-Enriched Diets on the Susceptibility of Low Density Lipoprotein to Oxidative Modification in Hypercholesterolemic Subjects," *Journal of Clinical Investion* 91 (1993): 668–76.

2   A. P. Simopoulos, B. Koletzko, R. B. Anderson, and others, the first congress of the International Society for the Study of Fatty Acids and Lipids (ISSFAL), "Fatty Acids and Lipids from Cell Biology to Human Disease," *Journal of Lipid Research* 35 (1994): 169–73.

- In cultured fibroblasts obtained after an olive oil diet, olive oil (3H) cholesterol efflux was highest in the fraction of HDL.[1]

- Oleic acid found in olive oil increases the incorporation of the omega-3 fatty acids in cell membranes and decreases the oxidation of LDL. Therefore, increasing oleic acid by eating more olive oil tends to reduce the atherogenic (hardening of the arteries) potential of LDL levels.

- Squalene, found in the higher amounts of 136- to 708-mg/100 grams of olive oil, combines easily with oxygen ions, emitting molecular oxygen, especially in tissues short of oxygen, and is very active and effective in the healing of dental trauma, rehabilitation of scars, increasing heart activity, expanding blood vessels, and inhibiting atherosclerosis.

- Olive oil is a truly nutritionally desirable food. There is no scientific reason to restrict its use. In addition to having many health advantages, olive oil is known for its appealing golden emerald color and its aroma and taste.

What Eating Correctly Means

Eating correctly means consuming more natural foods, as much as possible in their raw state. In his book, *Eat Right or Die Young*, osteopathic physician and nutrition educator Cass Igram, D.O., of Des Moines, Iowa, says: "If you follow the standard American diet, your eating habits are creating severe nutritional deficiencies." Dr. Igram advises that eating the American way there's a very good chance you will be deficient in folic acid by 79 percent, niacin by 70 percent, vitamin B6 by 62 percent, thiamine by 70 percent, riboflavin by 40 percent, vitamin B12 by 33 percent, chromium by 100 percent, manganese by 100 percent, calcium by 65 percent, magnesium by 76 percent, selenium by 75 percent, and essential fatty acids by 100 percent.[2]

---

1   Leaf and Weber, "Cardiovascular Effects of N-3 Fatty Acids."

2   C. Igram and J. K. Gray, *Eat Right or Die Young* (Cedar Rapids, Iowa: Literary Visions, Inc., 1989), 10.

In another book, *Native Nutrition: Eating According to Ancestral Wisdom*, naturopathic physician and Jungian psychotherapist Ronald F. Schmid, N.D., of Middleburg, Connecticut, confirms: "The digestive system adapts well to raw foods introduced at a rate appropriate for the individual. . . . While popular wisdom holds that cooking makes foods more digestible, this is true only of grains. The human digestive system is fully capable of digesting a wide variety of foods raw. Many foods may be more easily chewed when cooked, but for the fully functioning human digestive tract, all but the grains are most easily digested raw or lightly cooked."

"Raw food consists mostly of hydrophylic colloids. *Hydrophylic* means water-loving, and a *colloid* is a suspension of solid particles in a gel-like fluid," continues Dr. Schmid. "Eaten uncooked, these colloids absorb large quantities of digestive juices, forming a gelatinous mass that maintains the mucosa of the stomach and digestive tract in a healthy state."[1]

From *Stopping the Clock: Why Many of Us Will Live Past 100—And Enjoy Every Minute*, coauthors Ronald Klatz, D.O., and Robert Goldman, Ph.D., cofounders of the American Academy of Anti-Aging Medicine, tell us what the perfect diet should consist of:

- Raw or lightly cooked whole-grain cereals;

- Raw or lightly steamed vegetables and sprouts;

- Raw fresh fruit, including the skin because of the fiber and pectin it contains;

- Lightly cooked beans, lentils, and peas;

- Raw nuts and seeds (unsalted).[2]

Finally, I direct your attention to intestinal microflora reinforced by the regular ingestion of probiotics as the ultimate preventers of

1   R. F. Schmid, *Native Nutrition: Eating According to Ancestral Wisdom* (Rochester, Vt.: Healing Arts Press, 1994), 41, 42.

2   R. Klatz and R. Goldman, *Stopping the Clock: Why Many of Us Will Live Past 100—And Enjoy Every Minute* (New Canaan, Conn.: Keats Publishing, Inc., 1996), 225.

colon cancer, prostate cancer, breast cancer, and many other degen-erative diseases.

Friendly intestinal microflora when in sufficient quantity—in numbers that are usually supposed to be lodged in the gut—me-tabolize indirect-acting carcinogens and stop them from changing normal body cells into cancer cells. The microflora do this by means of specific microbial enzymes that reduce nitro and azo groups (two cancer-causing agents) or hydrolyze glucuronides (more cancer-causing agents). Five major scientific studies sup-ported by the National Cancer Institute have established that diet can alter the metabolic activity of intestinal flora.[1]

The main focus of these carefully conducted studies has been that bacterial products generated in the large intestine contribute to the induction of colon cancer. Among the fecal bacterial enzymes that stimulate carcinogens ingested from the surrounding environ-ment have been beta-D-glucuronidase, nitroreductase, azoreduc-tase, and steroid 17 alpha-monooxygenase.[2] It was found that Americans eating a mixed "Western" diet had higher levels of fecal bacterial beta-D-glucuronidase than did American vegetarians or the Chinese and Japanese people, both cultures of which also are mostly vegetarians. Shifting the American meat eaters from a high-animal protein Western diet to a vegetarian diet for just four weeks caused them to experience a significant decrease in the enzymatic fecal

---

1   B. S. Reddy, and E. L. Wynder, "Large-Bowel Carcinogenesis: Fecal Constitu-ents of Populations with Diverse Incidence Rates of Colon Cancer," *Journal of National Cancer Institute* 50 (1973): 1437–42; B. S. Reddy, J. H. Weisnurger, and E. L. Wynder, "Fecal Beta-Glucuronidase Control by Diet," *Science* 183 (1974): 416–17; B. R. Goldin and S. L. Gorbach, "The Relationship between Diet and Rat Fecal Bacterial Enzymes Implicated in Colon Cancer," *Journal of the National Cancer Institute* 57 (1976): 371–75; B. R. Goldin and S. L. Gorbach, "Alterations in Fecal Microflora Enzymes Related to Diet, Age, Lactobacillus Supplements, and Dimethylhydrazine," *Cancer* 40 (1977): 2421–26; B. S. Reddy, S. Mangaat, J. H. Weisburger, and E. L. Wynder, "Effect of High-Risk Diet for Colon Carcinogenesis on Intestinal Mucosal And Bacterial Beta-Glucuronidase Activity in F344 Rats," *Cancer Research* 37 (1977): 3533–36.

2   A. Mastromarino, B. S. Reddy, and E. L. Wynder, "Metabolic Epidemiology of Colon Cancer: Enzyme Activity of Fecal Flora," *American Journal of Clinical Nutrition* 29 (1976): 1455–60.

beta-D-glucuronidase levels. Thus they were less predisposed to developing cancer of the colon.

Moreover, it was shown by a team of investigators led by oncologists Barry R. Goldin, M.D., and Sherwood L. Gorbach, M.D., at the Department of Medicine, Infectious Disease Division, New England Medical Center Hospital and Tufts University School of Medicine that lacto-ovo vegetarians had significantly lower activities of the several fecal bacterial enzymes that stimulate the growth of cancer.[1] Most significant was that when probiotic organisms in the amount of 10^{10} administered as *Lactobacillus acidophilus* was added to the subjects' diet each day, there was a marked reduction in fecal enzyme activities. Indeed, the fecal metabolic activity of any omnivores (meat eaters) receiving Lactobacilli resembled that of vegetarians.[2]

Enter Dr. Mike Loquasto, D.C., C.C.N.

Before the Greek column of the Mediterranean diet had been published in a 1994 issue of the *Journal of Lipid Research* and presented to the 1996 Orlando, Florida, ACAM meeting, chiropractic internist and certified clinical nutritionist Michael Jude "Dr. Mike" Loquasto, D.C., C.C.N., had developed his own "dental diet." It is an eating program predicated on similar precepts to those developed by Dr. Simopoulos. Dr. Mike is a diplomat of the American Board of Chiropractic Nutrition, a diplomat of the American Academy of Pain Management, a diplomat and board-certified forensic examiner, a New York State-certified dietitian nutritionist, and, as mentioned, chief of staff of the Healthplex Medical Center in Marshalls Creek, Pennsylvania. (See appendix B for his exact location.)

---

1   B. R. Goldin, L. Swenson, J. Dwyer, M. Sexton, and S. L. Gorbach, "Effect of Diet and *Lactobacillus Acidophilus* Supplements on Human Fecal Bacterial Enzymes," *Journal of the National Cancer Institute* 64 (1980): 255–61.

2   B. R. Goldin and S. L. Gorback, "Alterations of the Intestinal Microflora by Diet, Oral Antibiotics, and *Lactobacillus*: Decreased Production of Free Amines from Aromatic Nitro Compounds, Azo Dyes, and Glucuroides," *Journal of the National Cancer Institute* 73, no. 3 (September 1984): 689–95.

Dr. Mike modified the Dr. Simopoulos concept by focusing his efforts on betterment of the human oral cavity and improvement of permanent dentition. *Dentition* is the development and appearance of a person's teeth, including their arrangement, number, and type as they occur in the mouth. To aid his patients in accomplishing this important aspect of anatomy and physiology, Dr. Mike developed a diet to provide the greatest amount of "living food" and omit the "dead food" of the standard American diet. His dental diet, (which he supplements with Dr. Mike's Teeth and Gum Support Pack) not only promotes excellent oral health, it also detoxifies the body and cleans out accumulated poisons. The Loquasto dental diet helps to restore liver function and normal physiological metabolism.

When following Dr. Mike's Dental Diet you can eat and drink as much as you like, because foods on its menu plan are all quickly and easily digested. As you'll soon learn, this detoxification eating program is very close to the menu plan developed by the ADA-wary upstate New York dentist (discussed in chapter five). The only real difference between them is that the New Yorker permits the consumption of some dairy products and Dr. Michael Loquasto does not. Chapter 5's diet also allows fruit, but Dr. Mike markedly limits its consumption. Both diets are rather strict vegetarian. The idea for both these diets is to aid the body in healing itself.

Included here is the dental diet, an eating program developed by Dr. Mike Loquasto. His patients seldom if ever have dental difficulties. By following the rules for this chiropractic nutritionist's eating plan, here is what they usually take into their mouths:

1. Eat fresh and raw vegetables, especially green salads. Remember to consume only fresh, organic (if possible) vegetables. For your salads, you may splash on apple cider vinegar, olive oil, or natural salad dressing acquired from a health food store.

2. For a beverage, water ("sky juice") is best. You may flavor drinking water with fresh lemon juice, Postum, dandelion coffee or other coffee substitutes such as Roma, Bambue, Pioneer, Piero, Caffix, and so forth, which are very fine. Herb tea is good anytime. Decaffeinated black tea and green tea are allowed, but regular coffee should be avoided under all circumstances.

3. It's OK to eat potatoes, either raw or cooked, but raw potato is a true vegetable and cooked potato furnishes starch. In the cooking, bake or mash them but never eat fried potatoes. Putting a little butter on them is allowed (a rare dairy addition), but a little olive oil is better.

4. Legumes in the form of any or all kinds of beans is fine, and preparation methods may be found in almost any cookbook.

5. For grains, brown or unpolished rice and millet are recommended.

6. As for flour, while corn, rice, or soy flour are fine for this diet, don't eat wheat flour (which rules out many breads).

7. Pasta is standard vegetarian fare, in particular artichoke, spinach, and quinoa pasta. It's best to use these as substitutes for wheat pasta.

8. Eating cold water fish is allowed for one meal per week.

9. Natural sweeteners such as maple syrup or rice syrup are recommended, but aspartame and saccharine must be avoided. They contain factory-made chemicals with the potential for cancer production.

10. You can snack on popcorn and occasionally unsalted potato chips or corn chips, but don't eat pretzels made from white flour wheat.

11. For cooking, use stainless steel, glass, enamel, earthenware, cast iron, or tin utensils. Do not use pressure cookers or aluminum cookware.

On Dr. Mike's dental diet, there are specific guidelines as to what *not* to eat. And this is where Dr. Mike goes into his modification mode as a takeoff from Dr. Simopoulos's Greek column Mediterranean diet. The following listing is what you should *not* eat:

• Avoid dairy products of all types, most especially milk and cheese that come from any animal. Cows' milk is for calves; goats' milk is for kids (not the human kind). Instead, as a substitute for dairy products, you may use soy milk, rice milk, and the cheeses made from these vegetables. (For reasons why everyone should avoid ingesting milk, see below in the section, "The 'Udder' Nonsense of Four Major Milk Myths.")

- Red meat of any kind is forbidden, and that includes fresh-cut or packaged beef, veal, pork, organ meats, tongue, smoked products, tinned products, and so forth. At all costs, avoid eating the meat products of fast food restaurants such as McDonalds, Burger King, Denny's, Wendy's, Roy Rogers, and the many others.

- Don't even think about consuming poultry in any form, and that includes chicken, duck, goose, turkey, pheasant, and the other birds.

- Avoid eggs, even if they're organically raised.

- Discontinue dining on seafood, except for an occasional fish meal, but the fish eaten must have been swimming in cold water and have scales on its body.

- As alluded to in the flour products of the allowable list, white flour products are *not* allowed and that goes for bread, crackers, cookies, pies, doughnuts, spaghetti, macaroni, noodles, pizza, and so forth. Pizza is deceiving with all the toppings applied, but the cheese and wheat crust make it among the worst foods you could eat.

- Never let coffee, black tea, milk cocoa, beer, wine, carbonated beverages, or any and all soft drinks enter your oral cavity. Indeed, the only thing coffee may be useful for is as a rectal enema to help the liver detoxify itself.

- Avoid consuming any kind of frozen food if fresh food is at hand. Make fresh food be your first choice and frozen food a distant second.

- Canned and processed foods are not on Dr. Mike's Dental Diet, and that includes breakfast cereals, packaged mixes, and other such items.

- Stop yourself from eating fruit except for lemon or grapefruit. According to Dr. Mike, any type of fruit contains natural sugar, which feeds the oral bacteria that promote cavities. If you must ingest fruit, limit the amount to perhaps one piece per day of the less sugar-filled type. Better yet, substitute carrots and celery for fruits.

- Don't drink fruit juices. Rather, get your nutrition from live and unprocessed plant products. You'll eat less that way. For example, it takes five apples to make one glass of apple juice. You're not likely to eat five apples at one sitting.

- Additives and preservatives used by food processors are poison for your body and the following are strictly forbidden:

Benzoate of Soda	Polysorbate 60
BHA	Polysorbate 80
BHT	Sodium nitrate
Carageenan	Sodium nitrite
Dipotassium phosphate	Sodium silica aluminate
Monosoidum glutamate	Sorbitol monostearate
Oxygen interceptor	U.S. certified food color
Disodium dehydrogen phosphatase	

The "Udder" Nonsense of Four Major Milk Myths

Dr. Michael Loquasto is dead set against anyone considering dairy products as viable food. Dairy just doesn't fit into Dr. Mike's Dental Diet, and the editor of that broadly distributed monthly newsletter, *Health & Healing,* is fully in accord. Julian Whitaker, M.D., in his October 1998 newsletter issue headlines milk as "'Udder' Nonsense," and cites four major myths attached to milk by the commercial interests of the dairy industry.[1]

The first milk myth is that drinking it helps build strong bones and teeth. In reality, Dr. Whitaker says, milk and other dairy products weaken the bones to accelerate osteoporosis. And it probably causes the teeth to loosen, develop caries, and rot.

---

1   J. Whitaker, "Food Safety: Milk Is 'Udder' Nonsense," *Dr. Julian Whitaker's Health & Healing* 8 (October 1998): 1–4.

"That's right," Dr. Whitaker states, "consumption of milk causes the very condition it's advertised to prevent . . . osteoporosis results from calcium loss, not insufficient calcium intake. And dairy products, because of their high protein content, promote calcium loss. Studies examining the incidence of osteoporosis have found that a high consumption of dairy products is associated with high rates of osteoporosis. If you want strong bones [and teeth], don't drink milk."

The second milk myth is that drinking milk is a healthy thing to do. Not only are dairy products clearly linked to osteoporosis causation, they also produce heart disease, promote obesity, cause cancer, excite allergies, and stimulate diabetes. "Dairy products are anything but 'health' foods," affirms Dr. Whitaker. "Their association with heart disease is particularly strong. . . . Nonfat milk is a major player in heart disease. It's very low in B vitamins. The metabolism of [milk] protein in the absence of B vitamins contributes to the buildup of homocysteine, a marker for heart disease."

The third milk myth is that growing children need it. Not true. "Milk is the leading cause of iron-deficiency anemia in infants," says Dr. Whitaker. "The American Academy of Pediatrics now discourages giving children milk before their first birthday. . . . Milk consumption in childhood contributes to the development of type I diabetes. Certain proteins in milk resemble molecules on the beta cells of the pancreas that secrete insulin. . . . The immune system makes antibodies to the milk protein that mistakenly attack and destroy the beta cells.

"Milk allergies are very common in children and cause sinus problems, diarrhea, constipation, and fatigue. They [milk allergies] are a leading cause of the chronic ear infections that plague up to 40 percent of all children under the age of six," Dr. Whitaker assures us. "Milk allergies are also linked to behavior problems in children and to the disturbing rise in childhood asthma." Even the late Dr. Benjamin Spock changed his recommendation in his later years and discouraged parents from giving milk to their children.

The fourth milk myth is that it's pure and wholesome. Perhaps at some time in the past it might have been but now milk is neither pure or wholesome at all. Recombinant Bovine SomaToropin (rBST), a genetically engineered hormone manufactured and sold to farmers by the chemical giant, Monsanto Company, has elevated growth hormone factors in milk. Drinking this genetically altered stuff coming from cows treated with rBST offers people massive amounts of Insulin-like Growth Factor-1 (IGF-1). What's the result? There is a 700 percent increase of breast cancer in women with elevated IGF-1 levels and a 400 percent increase in prostate cancer in men with high IGF-1 levels. You're ingesting a hormone-laden beverage when drinking milk that's rBST-produced, and hormonal cancers are possibly being stimulated in your body.

Besides all this, the udders of rBST-treated cows come down with infections so that they must be treated with antibiotics in massive dosages. Higher traces of these drugs are in their milk, accompanied by pus and bacteria. Dr. Whitaker tells us this, and he backs up Dr. Mike's admonition to never consume dairy products. Certainly, if you follow Dr. Mike's Dental Diet, you won't be doing so. (To subscribe to Dr. Julian Whitaker's *Health & Healing* newsletter, see the subscription information in appendix A.)

Dr. Mike's Teeth and Gum Support Pack

Nutritional supplementation works effectively to prevent or correct a variety of oral illnesses and traumas. The list of discomforts or even life-threatening problems involved with the mouth is lengthy, but nearly all of them respond positively to adjunctive nutrition using food supplements. The following alphabetically listed mouth problems are just some of the oral pathologies that may be lessened or eliminated by taking nutritional supplementation:

AIDS-related dental problems	endodonture problems
anesthesia-related troubles	facial pain
antibiotic-related disorders	facial paralysis
anxiety and dental fear associations	fractured tooth
bad breath	gingivitis
braces-related problems	glossitis
bridge-related difficulties	gum disease
broken, cracked, or chipped teeth	gums receding

cancer in the mouth	headaches related to teeth
candidiasis (thrush)	herpes infections
cavitations from pulled teeth	herpetic stomatitus
cavities	impacted teeth
cracked lips	infection
cracked tooth	jaw fracture
crowns	knocked-out tooth
cysts and tumors	lip- and cheek-biting
dental caries	periodontitus
dentures	pyorrhea
dry socket	receding gums
	stomatitis in general

Stomatitis is inflammation of lips, palate, insides of the cheeks, gums, the tongue, and other tissues surrounding the teeth.

By eating a varied diet of leafy salad greens and other fresh vegetables and whole grains, especially brown rice, you'll be following closer to Dr. Mike's Dental Diet recommendations, but there is something even more therapeutic you can do for oral health. Dr. Mike's Teeth and Gum Support Pack is vital for nutritional supplementation to insure oral health. That's because the nutrients in such a pack focus specifically on the tissues so listed: the teeth and gums. Every pack contains seven groups of nutrients. Each group is described below.

CoEnzyme Q10 with Vitamin C. Inasmuch as in at least four clinical and laboratory studies report CoQ10 deficiency being present in the gingival tissue of patients with periodontal disease, this specific nutrient is exceedingly important for overcoming periodontitis.[1] A total of 25 mg of CoQ10 is incorporated

---

1   R. Nakamura and others, "Study of CoQ10-Enzymes in Gingiva from Patients with Periodontal Disease and Evidence for a Deficiency of CoenzymeQ10," *Proceedings of the National Academy of Sciences* 71 (1974): 1456; I. L. Hansen and others, "Bioenergetics in Clinical Medicine, IX, Gingival and Leukocytic Deficiencies of Coenzyme Q10 in Patients with Periodontal Disease," *Research Communications: Chemistry, Pathology, and Pharmacology* 14 (1976): 729; G.

into Dr. Mike's Teeth and Gum Support Pack to increase blood flow to all of the dental tissues and to improve immune system defenses for the destruction of pathological bacteria. Additionally, vitamin C (ascorbic acid) has been added to provide for a reduction of tissue inflammation and to strengthen those tissues surrounding the teeth.

Super C 1000. Among all nutrients having significant benefit for the body, vitamin C at an elevated Percentage (%) of Daily Value (%DV) served up in quantity is vital for maintaining homeostasis. And the 1000 mg (1667 %DV) of vitamin C present in Dr. Mike's Teeth and Gum Support Pack works synergistically with its accompanying components: 90 mg (9 %DV) of calcium, 125 mg (9 %DV) of magnesium, 60 mg (2 %DV) of potassium, 100 mg of pectin, and 100 mg of bioflavonoids.

Vitamin C. In combination with other nutrients, vitamin C forms complexes that have proven to be effective against any sort of infection, particularly in elderly patients. For example, a double-blind study of fifty-seven older individuals admitted to St. Luke's Hospital in Huddersfield, England, for dental infections complicated with bronchitis and pneumonia demonstrated the value of this recommendation. The patients received 200 mg of vitamin C a day or a placebo, were assessed by clinical and laboratory methods, and were evaluated. Those patients receiving the modest dosage of vitamin C demonstrated significantly faster healing. This study shows that even a fractional dosage of vitamin C has value in healing dental and respiratory infections.[1]

P. Littarru, R. Nakamura, L. Ho, and others, "Deficiency of Coenzyme Q10 in Gingival Tissue from Patients with Periodontal Disease," *Proceedings of the National Academy of Sciences* 68 (1971): 2332; R. Nakamura, G. P. Littarru, K. Folkers, and G. Wilkinson, "Deficiency of Coenzyme Q in Gingiva of Patients with Periodontal Disease," *International Journal of Vitamin and Nutritional Research* 43 (1973): 83.

1   C. Hunt and others, "The Clinical Effects of Vitamin C Supplementation in Elderly Hospitalized Patients with Acute Respiratory Infections," *International Journal of Vitamin and Nutritional Research* 64 (1994): 212–19.

In the present instance vitamin C has been combined with calcium ascorbate complex, potassium chloride, pectin, bioflavonoids, cellulose, alfalfa, magnesium, magnesium stearate from a vegetable source, and silica. Altogether they form complexes which synergize each other for a more effective healing result.

Calcium 6 + Magnesium. Having a further quantity of vitamin C as ascorbic acid in the amount of 50 mg (83 %DV), this Cal 6 + Mg is combined with 400 IU (100 %DV) of vitamin D, 750 mg (75 %DV) of calcium from many calcium sources, including citrate, gluconate, carbonate, lactate, scorbate, and the rarer microcrystallin hydroxyapatite. Added to these are 375 mg (94 %DV) of magnesium from magnesium chelate, 3 mg (3 %DV) of Boron from Boron aspartate citrate, 60 mg (94 %DV) of glutamic acid from 75 mg of glutamic acid hydrochloride (HCl), 29 mg (94 %DV) of L-lysine from 36 mg of L-lysine HCl, and cellulose, vegetable stearate, and silica.

As it happens, Cal 6 + Mg is an exclusive six-source calcium chelate complex of calcium citrate, calcium gluconate, calcium ascorbate, calcium carbonate, calcium lactate, calcium microcrystalline hydroxyapatite, and the amino acids Lysine hydrochloride and glutamic acid to supply a readily available amount of calcium for the body's requirements. Cal 6 + Mg strengthens teeth and ligaments to tighten loose teeth.

Nutri A 25. Consisting of the nutrients, vitamin A 25,000 IU (500 %DV), vitamin C 60 mg (100 %DV), vitamin E 30 IU (100 %DV), zinc 20 mg (133 %DV) derived from the ingredients cellulose, gelatin, calcium ascorbate, vitamin E, vitamin A, zinc chelate, and magnesium stearate, Nutri A 25 increases the human immune system's ability to kill bad bacteria that cause gingivitis.

Tri B 100. Comprised entirely of those healing vitamins coming from the B complex, Tri B 100 consists of thiamin (vitamin B1) 100 mg (6.667 %DV), riboflavin (vitamin B2) 100 mg (5.882 %DV), niacinamide (vitamin B3) 100 mg (500 %DV), pyridoxine (vitamin B6) 100 mg (5 %DV), folate (folic acid) 400 mcg (100 %DV), cobalamin (vitamin B12) 100 mcg (1.667

%DV), biotin 100 mcg (33 %DV), pantothenic acid (vitamin B5) 100 mg (1 %DV), and numbers of other ingredients.

The additional nutrients in Tri B 100 are choline 100 mg, inositol 100 mg, and para amino benzoic acid (PABA) 100 mg in a base designed to provide prolonged (sustained or timed) release over a six to eight hour period, thiamin, riboflavin, pyridoxine HCl, niacinamide, calcium, pantothenate, choline bitartrate, inositol, PABA, cellulose, biotin, cobalamin, magnesium stearate, silica, and folic acid.

This Tri B 100 combination of nutrients improves nerve function to reduce nerve pain and to so strengthen the nerves that it prevents them from dying even when injured.

Proteozyme. With the ability to reduce inflammation and actually strengthen ligaments for the tightening of loose teeth, proteozyme consists of vitamin A 1000 IU (20 %DV), vitamin C 500 mg (833 %DV), thiamine 10 mg (667 %DV), riboflavin 10 mg (588 %DV), niacin 10 mg (50 %DV), vitamin B6 50 mg (2500 %DV), folate 200 mcg (50 %DV), vitamin B12 50 mcg (833 %DV), pantothenic acid 50 mg (500 %DV), calcium 150 mg (15 %DV), magnesium 75 mg (19 %DV), zinc 75 mg (500 % DV), manganese 150 mg (7500 %DV), and potassium 75 mg (2 %DV).

Proteozyme's active ingredients are combined with a huge number of other ingredients for massive nutritional benefit. These additional components consist of bioflavonoids 250 mg, bromelain (enteric coated) 200 mg, trypsin (enteric coated) 100 mg, chymotrypsin (enteric coated) 200 mcg, glucosamine sulfate 125 mg, papain (enteric coated) 100 mg, bovine cartilage 100 mg, pepsin (1:3000) 60 mg, raw veal bone 50 mg, aspartic acid 50 mg, hesperidin complex 50 mg, rutin 50 mg in a base of shave grass, valerian root, passiflora, and dried pineapple juice, calcium (freeze-dried veal bone), manganese sulfate, vitamin C, glucosamine sulfate, bromelain, cellulose, bioflavonoids, potassium, magnesium, zinc, trypsin, bovine cartilage, rutin, veal bone powder, hesperidin, aspartic acid, calcium pantothenate, pyridoxine HCl, magnesium stearate (vegetable source), pepsin, papain, niacinamide, riboflavin, thiamine, silica, vitamin B12, vitamin A, and folic acid.

STD Chamomile Extract. In a strength of 400 mg, this ancient herb, STD Chamomile Extract, reduces gum inflammation by its natural, built-in anti-inflammatory action and calming effect.

Dr. Mike's Teeth and Gum Support Pack is taken in a dose or serving of one packet a day for oral maintenance and disease prevention. For disorders of a severe or advanced nature such as those listed at the beginning of this section, take three packs a day. To acquire Dr. Mike's Teeth and Gum Support Packs, contact Dr. Michael J. Loquasto at his Healthplex Medical Center as in appendix B.

More of Dr. Mike's Suggestions for Healthy Gums and Teeth

- Brush with tea tree oil tooth paste produced by Dessert Essence. (See appendix B under "Periodontal Remedy Suppliers.")

- Use Sulcabrush with replaceable tips to clean between the teeth. Sulcabrush has proven to be more effective than dental floss for the removal of plaque and reduction of gingivitis.

- Use the Oral B electric tooth brush.

- Use the water pic with the following active ingredients:
  2 ounces of George's Aloe Vera liquid;
  2 ounces of hydrogen peroxide;
  2 drops of Dessert Essence tea tree oil;
  2 heaping tablespoonsful of baking soda;
- Fill the balance of the water pic reservoir with purified water.

- Avoid the use of chlorinated or fluorinated water.

Seventeen

Homeopathic Medical Remedies for Dental Discomforts

Remember, it is the patient who has to cure himself; the drug cannot cure him; the drug is only the stimulus which starts the vital [healing] reaction.

The above statement made by Sir John Weir, HOM, dean of all practicing British homeopathic physicians, the personal doctor-healer to the present queen of England and her entire royal family, best sums up the full essence of homeopathy, including its many drug, herbal, energetic, and nutrient therapies.

Homeopathic treatment is dedicated to reestablishing an ailing, afflicted, or otherwise impaired patient's physiological equilibrium. To bring about this restoration of body balance (known as *homeostasis*), an energy medicine, a toximolecular drug, a healing herb, or some orthomolecular nutrient is carefully chosen by the homeopath for application to the patient. The therapeutic agent, whether a nutrient or another substance, is selected because it is known to have an effect on the biochemistry and cells of the sick person's dysfunctional body system. Such a specially selected medicinal substance, in the tiniest dosage, invariably has an effect that is similar to the known disease-provoking agent that caused the patient's distress. Given in sufficiently small doses, the chosen homeopathic formula will likely stimulate a strong reaction from the defense mechanisms of the ill person. The body's reaction will then automatically bring about healing and restore a patient's physiological balance.

This sort of body response, as described, may seem strange to someone who is oriented only to modern allopathy (orthodox medicine the way it's conventionally practiced in most Western industrialized nations). As is obvious, homeopathy works in direct contrast to modern allopathy.

There are, in fact, two main schools of therapeutics being practiced in the West: allopathy, which applies medical opposites, and homeopathy, which employs medical similars. Both work. But allopathy's remedies fall into the *toximolecular* class because of their frequent unwanted adverse side effects. And homeopathy's remedies may be considered *orthomolecular* because of their highly diluted concentration, which provides desirable therapeutic effects. (Please return to chapter 1 for clear definitions of the two types of remedies, orthomolecular and toximolecular.)

Homeopathy therefore provokes a patient's immune response that's counterbalancing the illness by the doctor's administration or the patient's usage of some orthomolecular drug, herb, enzyme, nutrient, or energy. In contrast, allopathy resorts to drugs, surgery, radiation, chemotherapy, or immunotherapy rather exclusively (almost never herbs, energy therapy, or nutrients) to produce physiological responses that directly oppose or mask disease symptoms.[1]

The administering practitioner of homeopathic medicine may be a doctor of homeopathic naturopathy (HND), a wholistic-type homeopathic medical doctor (HMD), a doctor of homeopathic osteopathy (HDO), or another form of certified homeopathic professional (HOM). Nurse practitioners, chiropractors, podiatrists, acupuncturists, and even dentists may practice homeopathy.

Narrow-minded American allopaths often condemn homeopaths as "quacks" without considering that allopathy is only one type of medical patient care among dozens practiced around the world. When an allopath arrogantly condemns homeopathy or any other practice as quackery, most of the time this medical conventionalist is actually ignorant of the science being condemned. As Garry F. Gordon, M.D.,

---

1   M. Walker, "Consumer Education Series: Homeopathy," *Health Food Business* (October 1989): 62, 63.

of Payson, Arizona, president of the International College of Advanced Longevity Medicine, points out, "Invariably, the condemning allopath will be down on what he is not up on."

The Law of Similars

Homeopathy is exceedingly popular in Europe as the preferred means of bringing about the healing of illness and restoration of health. There, homeopathic therapies are readily available to consumers, not only in pharmacies and health food stores but even in supermarkets. Most Europeans have a full understanding of the way homeopathy helps to overcome disease.

Professsor Spiro Diamantidis, M.D., M.A., general director of the Medical Institute for Homeopathic Research and Application in Athens, Greece, states that the basic law of homeopathy is the Law of Similars or *Similia Similibus Curantur* ("like cures like"). Dr. Diamantidis writes: "When a specific form of medicine is given to the patient, it is as if we are administering an entity which, by being similar to that of the illness, repels and expels it from the organism."[1]

The homeopathic rule or formula expressing the *Law of Similars* declares: "any drug which is capable of producing morbid symptoms in the healthy will remove similar symptoms occurring as an expression of disease." Another version of the law of similars formula, a defining rule employed, in 1796, by the founding father of homeopathy, Samuel Christian Friedrich Hahnemann, M.D., states: "Let likes be cured by likes."

Thus, *homeopathy* is a holistic therapeutic medical science based on the teachings of Dr. Samuel Hahnemann. His *homeopathic law of similars* requires that minute doses of potentized substances prepared from plant, animal, or mineral kingdoms be employed to treat illnesses and inherent constitutional problems. While written down only about two centuries ago, homeopathic principles are among the most ancient on earth. In time long past, Moses was a

---

1   S. Diamantidis, *Homeopathic Philosophy and Hippocratic Medicine* (Athens, Greece: Medical Institute for Homeopathic Research and Application, 1989).

healer who used homeopathic principles, and the Bible does describe his application of homeopathy.

The Bible states: "The Hebrew came to Mara, where the water was bitter. Some complained: 'What shall we drink?' Moses prayed and after the prayer he threw a bitter branch into the bitter water; and the water turned sweet. For God is not like the humans, who can soothe the bitter only with sweet: with the bitter He makes the bitter sweet."[1]

Incidentally, for biblical quotations or detailed definitions relating to anything in homeopathy, the finest book of interpretations available for substantiation is *Yasgur's Homeopathic Dictionary and Holistic Health Reference* by licensed pharmacist Jay Yasgur, R.Ph., M.Sc. of Greenville, Pennsylvania. (See appendix B for the book's acquisition address.)

Rules by Which Homeopaths Practice

A health professional employing homeotherapeutics follows a series of rules or principles consisting of the following:[2]

1. Disease is manifested by symptoms.

2. Knowledge of the biological response to drugs, herbs, energy, enzyme, or nutrients must be obtained by experimentation on the normal human body.

3. The application of principle B (above) depends on introduction of a similar, but controlled, iatrogenic illness by administration of some drug, herb, energy, enzyme, or nutrient.

4. For the swiftest and longest lasting healing, the selected drug, herb, energy, enzyme, or nutrient should be administered alone and uncombined; this single remedy rule is the one followed in

---

1   J. Yasgur, *Yasgur's Homeopathic Dictionary and Holistic Health Reference*,4th ed. (Greenville, Pa.: Van Hoy Publishers, 1998), 105, 112, 113.

2   Walker, "Homeopathy."

the administration of *classical homeopathy* which does not countenance combining remedies.

5. In the practice of modern *antihomotoxicology*, based on the two hundred-year-old classical homeopathic practice of Dr. Samuel Hahnemann, German physician, Hans-Heinrich Reckeweg, M.D., *does* combine numerous single-constituent homeopathic drugs and combination preparations for the treatment of different diseases. (See the various types of homeopathic dental remedies described in two following sections.)[1]

The three essentials of homeotherapeutics require that homeopaths be self-regulated by some additional principles, which state:

1. Prescribe according to the law of similars,

2. Administer the smallest remedial dose that will actuate homeostasis for the patient,

3. Avoid repeating the efficacious drug, herb, energy, enzyme, or nutrient as long as improvement continues.

Finally, certain requirements for homeopathic medical practice prevail for the prescribing health professional. These requirements are:

1. Restore health in a prompt, mild, and permanent manner.

2. At all costs, avoid homeopathic-caused (iatrogenic) side effects.

3. Recognize health and disease states.

4. Determine whether the patient's disease state is reversible.

5. From practical healing experience or by homeopathic medical repertory study, know the appropriate homeopathic remedies for most of the conditions affecting patients.

---

1   C. F. Claussen, *Homotoxicology* (Baden-Baden, Germany: Aurelia-Verlag GmbH, 1988), 69; H. H. Reckeweg, *Homotoxicology: Illness and Healing through Anti-homotoxic Therapy*, 2d ed. (Albuquerque, N.Mex.: Menaco Publishing Co., Inc., 1984), 39.

6. Be aware of the body's probable reaction to the homeopathic medicine to be employed.

7. Identify idiosyncracy or iatrogenic symptoms as they appear from use of the selected homeopathic remedy or remedies.

8. Realize that intensification of symptoms with the onset of iatrogenic illness or increased severity of the disease often is a favorable drug, herbal, energy, enzyme, or nutrient reaction manifested by the patient who is healing.

9. Know the precise indication for the drug, herb, energy, enzyme, or nutrient and its optimal dose, effective duration of effect, when to repeat it, when to stop it, and when to change to another remedy.

The State of Homeostasis

Homeostasis is the homeopath's goal, which often gets achieved by use of homeopathic therapeutics. Homeostasis is a property of humans and other living organisms that operates to maintain functional health. It consists of physiological equilibrium produced by a balance of functions and of chemical composition within an individual. When sickness does occur, homeostasis balancing makes the major contribution toward a person's recovery. All organic systems automatically adjust to disturbances resulting from changes in their surroundings.

Essential to maintenance of health and recovery from illness is this state of homeostasis, which may be acquired by application of classical homeopathy or homeopathic antihomotoxicology. Dr. Hans-Heinrich Reckeweg has told us that inhibition of homotoxicologic agents is vital, for the living organism must protect itself against toxic substances called *homotoxins*. They include poisons of many types, chemotherapeutics (drugs), and multiple ecological toxins.[1]

Adaptation of ecology depends on the ability of the regulating

---

1   Recheweg, *Homotoxicology*, 9.

mechanism to maintain its homeostatic ability. And *ecology* is the study of the environmental relations of organisms. If the internal ecology has gone awry, as may occur when conventionally practicing dentists make oral adjustments, patients are likely to suffer from pathological processes not only in their mouths but throughout their bodies as well.

Then, classical homeopathy or homeopathic antihomotoxicology can come to the rescue and bring about healing of the oral cavity and the body of which it is a part.

Successful Treatment of Dental Problems Using Homeopathy

Classical homeopathy specifies *single* medicines and homeopathic. *Antihomotoxicology* offers *combination* medicines. Each discipline is invaluable in reducing dental discomforts and alleviating dental disease. But only a rare few dentists have invested time, effort and brain power in acquiring the healing skills exhibited by both types of homeopathy. These would be mercury-free, biocompatible, biological, or holistic dentists who use homeopathy for the successful treatment of dental problems.

Without attempting to be facetious, Bill Wolfe, D.D.S., HND, of Albuquerque, New Mexico says: "More dentists are recognizing that attached to the teeth is a human being, and that in treating a localized manifestation of disease in the mouth, it is imperative that due consideration be given to the general physical state of the patient. Only when the dentist understands the relationship that oral disease has to the physical and mental reactions of the patient can that health professional offer a fully therapeutic service."

In rendering what has been designated as "constitutional homeopathy," a dentist engaged in homeopathic dental practice, analyzes a patient's body type, temperament, disposition, and behavioral tendencies. He or she then prescribes one remedy or a combination of them to suit the general temperament or psychological state of the patient and another type for the particular problem the patient is experiencing. The remedies selected with their specific indications, contraindications, potencies, and dosages may be found in modern reference books such as the *Homeopathic Medical Repertory* by naturopathic physician Robin Murphy, N.D., of Pagosa Springs, Colorado. Using his twenty-five years of homeopathic research and practice, Dr. Murphy designed his book in an alphabetical format to be a modern, practical, and easy to use reference guide to the homeopathic materia medica. (See appendix B for the book's acquisition address.)[1]

Using the *Homeopathic Medical Repertory*, it is possible for any dentist investing a little time and study to carry out usual constitutional homeopathic prescribing as part of his biological dental practice. With such prescribing, patient success in the elimination of systemic symptoms arising from oral pathology is sure to follow. Necessary to remember, however, is that the potency of a homeopathic remedy is expressed in either the decimal, or X system, or in the centissimal, or C system. The X system is more commonly used in the United States. In this decimal system, the number preceding the X is equal to the number of zeros in the dilution. Hence, a potency of 3X is a dilution of 1:1,000. The number before the C is equal to half the number of zeros in the dilution. A strength of 3C means a dilution of 1:1,000,000.[2]

Effects of Single-Constituent Homeopathic Remedies

As mentioned earlier, since the time of Hippocrates, two schools of therapeutics have existed, one using opposites (allopathic medicine) and the other using similars (homeopathic medicine).[3] This second therapeutic practice had been neglected for centuries until Dr. Samuel

---

1   R. Murphy, *Homeopathic Medical Repertory* (Pagosa Springs, Colo.: Hahnemann Academy of North America, 1993).

2   K. Siegel-Maier, "Research Shows Americans 'Like' Homeopathy," *Better Nutrition* (October 1998): 12.

3   Ibid.; J. Tyler, *Kent's Repertory of the Homeopathic Materia Medica* (New Delhi, India: B. Jain Publishers, 1987); W. Boericke, *The Materia Medica with Repertory* (New Delhi, India: B. Jain Publishers, 1990).

Hahnemann rediscovered it, subjected it to experimentation, and codified it as the healing science of homeopathy.[1]

For the treatment of approximately one dozen dental problems, some thirty different homeopathic remedies have shown themselves efficacious. Listed below is a curtailed description of those homeopathics and what they can accomplish in the oral cavity. However, the listing is far from complete, so that the following is a partial list of homeopathic dental remedies for use individually in the classical homeopathic manner; and, included are the various separate pathological dental conditions for which these remedies are recommended. My acknowledgement goes to Dr. Bill Wolfe who educated me about the remedies for treating dental problems.

To Relieve Dental Abscess:

- *Belladonna* for infection accompanied by redness and throbbing;

- *Bryonia* for acute inflammation or if pricking pain is relieved by firm pressure;

- *Hepar sulphuris* for abscess accompanied by pus formation;

- *Myristica* for swelling accompanied by numbness;

- *Pulsatilla* for pain accentuated by heat and relieved by cold;

- *Pyrogenuium* for pus present without drainage;

- *Silicea* for hastening the discharge when pus is draining.

To Relieve Apprehension:

- *Aconite* for panic, fright, and general mental and physical restlessness, or sudden violent panic attacks;

---

1   de Prevost, *A Homeopathic Approach to Dentistry and Oral Biology* (Newtown Square, Pa.: Boiron S. A., 1992), 9.

- *Calcarea carbonica* for fear, weariness, hopelessness, and for the person who worries toward evening;

- *Coffea cruda* for tranquilizing;
- *Chamomilla* for tranquilizing, to promote restful sleep, and to raise the pain threshold;

- *Nux vomica* for high strung, nervous, and irritable people with stomach problems;

- *Pulsatilla* for states of anxiety.

To Relieve Bruxism

(gnashing, grinding, or clenching of teeth that is usually performed during sleep, perhaps while dreaming):

- *Belladonna* for tooth grinding with pain;

- *Podophyllum* for night grinding with burning tongue sensation;

- *Tuberculinum* for childhood grinding.

To Relieve Gingivitis, Periodontitis, and Alveolitis:

- *Arsenicum album* for unhealthy bleeding gums;

- *China* for gum bleeding;

- *Hypericum* for tender gum tissue;

- *Kali chloricum* for acute ulcerative tissue;

- *Naturium muriaticum* for tissue integrity;

- *Hepar sulphuris* for suppuration and chronic abcesses;

- *Silicea* for periodontal abscess with swollen glands;

- *Staphysagria* for loose teeth and pressure pain;

- *Symphytum* for periosteum injury and to stimulate epithelium growth on ulcerated surfaces;

- *Mercurius solubilis* for acute ulcerative tissue with coated tongue and metallic taste;

- *Nux vomica* for swollen painful gums with whitish tongue coating and for excess stimulant use (for example, coffee or black tea drinking);

- *Phosphorous* for swollen gums that bleed easily and for over-production of saliva;

- *Ruta graveoalens* for dry socket and injured bone and alveolitis.

To Relieve Hemorrhage:

- *Arnica* for bleeding accompanied by bruised soreness;

- *Ferrum phosphoricum* for bright red bleeding;

- *Phosphorus* for persistent bleeding.

To Relieve Neuralgia:

- *Aconite* for trigeminal neuralgia;

- *Aranea diadema* for radiating pain on the right side of the face aggravated by cold—also for sudden tooth pain at night after retiring;

- *Cuprum metallicum* for cramping of muscles;

- *Gelsemium sempervirens* for headache and upper back pain extending over the neck and head—also for dizziness and numbness;

- *Ignacia* for headache as if a nail were being driven through the head;

- *Lachesis* for left-sided oral complaints;

- *Lycopodium* for right-sided oral complaints;

- *Magnesia phosphorous* for spasmodic pains made worse by cold and made better by heat with rubbing;

- *Sanguinaria* for right-sided oral neuralgia and facial migraine;

- *Spigelia* for pain in the eye, cheek, and left temple areas;

- *Sincum phosphoricum* for right-sided sharp head pain;

- *Zincum valerian* for left-sided sharp head pain.

To Relieve Postoperative Discomfort:

- *Apis mellifica* for postinjection soreness after dental work;

Elements of Danger

- *Chamomilia* for a predental appointment to elevate the patient's pain threshold;

- *Hypericum* for an injured nerve;

- *Ledum* for puncture wounds and soreness after dental injection;

- *Magnesia phosphorica* for stiff and sore jaws after prolonged dental care;

- *Staphysagria* for incision-type wounds after soft tissue surgery;

- *Symphytum* for trauma to bone and periosteum.

To Relieve Excessive Salivation:

- *Baryta carbonica* for excessive saliva during sleep;

- *Bryonia alba* for dry mouth and dry mucous membranes with great thirst;

- *Phosphorous* for hypersalivation and for swollen and bleeding gums;

- *Pulsatilla* for diminished saliva with no thirst.

To Relieve Temporomandibular Joint (TMJ):

- *Arum triphyllum* for joint pain upon swallowing;

- *Calcarea flourica* for hypermobile joints;

- *Calcarea phosphorica* for a mouth locked shut;

- *Carbo vegetabilis* for vertigo with nausea and tinnitus;

- *Chamomilla* for low pain threshold and spasms of pain radiating to the ear;

- *Cuprum metallicum* for trismus of muscles;

- *Granatum* for painful cracking of joints;

- *Magnesium phosphorica* for muscle spasms;

- *Phyltolacca decanda* for earaches with pain in the teeth, jaw, and throat;

- *Rhus toxicodendron* for joint stiffness improving with movement and for "popping" of the TMJ.

To Relieve Toothache:

- *Antimonium crudum* for toothache worsening at night and aggravated by heat;

- *Aranea diadema* for sudden severe tooth pain after lying down;

- *Belladonna* for throbbing tooth worsened by pressure;

- *Calcarea carbonica* for toothache worsened by hot or cold air;

- *Chamomilla* for intolerable tooth pain worsened by warmth and not improved by cold;

- *Coffea cruda* for toothache worsened by heat but relieved by ice;

- *Ferrum metallicum* for toothache relieved by ice water;

- *Magnesia carbonica* for toothache worse at night that's relieved by walking about;

- *Magnesia phosphorica* for toothache worsened by cold and improved by warmth;

- *Plantago major* for toothache improved by pressure and worsened without cold air;

- *Pulsatilla* for toothache relieved by cold water in the mouth;

- *Staphysagria* for pain from major decay of teeth.

To Relieve Tooth Eruption:

- *Calcarea carbonica* for delayed eruption;

- *Chamomilla* for difficult teething;

- *Zincum metallicum* for gritting teeth during difficult dentition with loose teeth and bleeding gums.

To Relieve Ulcerations:

- *Natrum muriaticum* for cold sores and fever blisters and cracked lips;

- *Nitricum acidum* for ulcers with irregular edges and raw appearance.

Any of the individual healing remedies mentioned above may be purchased from the homeopathic product suppliers listed alphabetically in appendix B.

Homeopathic Antihomotoxic Dental Remedies

Selecting from the prior remedies list, certain homeopathics may be combined to create dental homeopathic antihomotoxicologic drops or tablets or spantules (tiny balls of remedy) for holding and absorbing into the oral mucous membranes under the tongue (sublingual). The following discomforting conditions respond positively to the ingredient combinations put together by certain homeopathic remedy manufacturers in a single liquid, tablet, or spantule. Not all the manufacturers of homeopathics have acquaintanceship with dental problems, and they may consider themselves unqualified for producing the combinations of homeopathic antihomotoxic dental remedies.

1. Toothache: To relieve minor toothache and discomfort arising from trapped food between the teeth, a cavity, a gum infection, a crack in the tooth, pressure from orthodontic treatment, or the reaction to a recent dental adjustment, particular groups of homeopathics work synergistically when put together. Toothache may radiate from one specific tooth or be more generalized, affecting a wider area of the mouth. Homeopathic antihomotoxicologic drops, tablets, or spantules should be held under the tongue for absorption over approximately a four-minute period.

Instruction: take the combination remedy for toothache three or four times daily. As required for relief, the homeopathics may be taken as often as every five to fifteen minutes. Children ages two to six usually receive just one half the adult dosage recommended by the manufacturer on the product label.

The constitutional homeopathic remedies joined together against toothache include *Arnica montana* for the relief of neuralgia and the healing of wounds; *Asafoetida* for inflammation of the jawbone (osteitis); *Belladonna* to relieve an excess of blood in the tooth pulp, which produces a throbbing that feels worse with pressure; *Coffea cruda* for comforting pain seemingly relieved only by the application of cold; *Hekla lava* to reduce facial neuralgia from decayed teeth or that comes on after surgery; *Hypericum perforatum* for the relief of nerve pain; *Magnesia phosphorica* to comfort pain seemingly relieved only by the application of heat; *Staphysagria* for overcoming the pain of a penetrating wound.

2. Dental infection: To relieve minor jaw infections and discomfort arising from gum involvement, tooth abscess, or a localized collection of pus anywhere in the mouth, some biological dentists suggest that the patient hold sublingually homeopathic antihomotoxicologic drops, tablets, or spantules. For common symptoms, take a few drops, a few spantules or one tablet of the combination remedy three or four times daily. As required for relief, remedy may be held for four minutes under the tongue as often as every fifteen minutes. Children ages two to six receive only one-half the adult dosage.

The constitutional homeopathic remedies against infection include *Arnica montana* to comfort neuralgia and heal wounds; *Belladonna* to relieve an excess of blood in the tooth pulp that produces a throbbing that's worse with pressure; *Carduus marianus* for stimulation of the liver and its portal circulation as an enhancement of detoxification; *Echinacea purpurea* to reduce inflammation and septic processes; *Hepar sulphuris calcareum* to drain any abscess accompanied by pus; *Mercurius solubilis* to diminish the inflammation of tissues and sinuses; *Ruta graveolens* to comfort injuries to the bone and to cause blood flow in a circumstance of venous stasis; *Silicea* for strengthening the weakness of connective tissue and to stop acute and chronic suppuration; *Sulphur* to reduce irritating and weeping skin eruptions.

3. TMJ syndrome: While the following combination of homeopathic remedies doesn't correct the misalignment arising from derangement between the upper and lower jaw, to relieve minor headaches and jaw pain connected with TMJ (Temporomandibular Joint) syndrome, a victim will find certain homeopathic antihomotoxicologic remedies useful for counteracting pain and discomfort in the head, ears, eyes, and sinuses. The available homeopathic antihomotoxicologic drops, spantules or

tablets composing this remedy are held under the tongue. For common symptoms, take the combination remedy three or four times daily. As required for relief, the homeopathic remedy may be self-administered sublingually as often as every fifteen minutes. Children ages two to six receive only one half the adult dosage.

The constitutional homeopathic remedies for TMJ discomfort include *Aranea diadema* to dispel neuralgia of the upper jaw; *Bryonia* for reducing inflammation of the membranes; *Causticum* to stop grinding (crepitation) of the joints; *Coffea cruda* for comforting pain seemingly relieved only by the application of cold; *Condurango* for diminishing tissue growths and inflammation; *Gelsemium sempervirens* to overcome vertigo and headache coming from pain in the occiput; *Humulus lupulus* that stops a dull, heavy headache accompanied by dizziness; *Lachesis mutus* that acts as a remedy for afflictions on the left side of the head and body; *Lycopodium clavatum* that acts as a remedy for affliction on the right side of the head and body; *Magnesia phosphorica* to comfort pain seemingly relieved only by the application of heat; *Mecurius praecipitatus ruber* to end fistulae of the bone and bone inflammation; *Nux vomica* to assist in balancing the stomach meridian which courses alongside of the TMJ; *Petroleum* to ease a joint that's easily dislocated; *Rhus toxicodendron* for stopping joint stiffness and subluxation that produces a popping of the TMJ; *Symphytum officinale* for neuralgia of the TMJ, especially after trauma has occurred.

4. Dentist-created trauma: For relief of discomfort after dental treatment (iatrogenic injury) in a traumatized oral area, the homeopathic antihomotoxicologic combination remedy of either drops, spantules, or tablets are taken under the tongue. For common symptoms, take one homeopathic three or four times daily. As required for relief, the product may be held sublingually as often as every fifteen minutes. Children ages two to six receive just one half the adult dosage.

The constitutional homeopathic remedies for oral trauma include *Aconitum napellus* for the reduction of fear and anxiety; *Arnica montana radix* for the relief of neuralgia and the healing of wounds; *Calendula officianalis* to treat contusions and lacerated wounds; *Carbo vegetabilis* for an emergency to neutralize severe toxic states;

Chamomilla for its tranquilizing action; *Echinacea purpurea* as a lymphatic drainage stimulant; *Hekla lava* to reduce facial neuralgia after extractions; *Hypericum perforatum* for the relief of nerve pain; *Ledum palustre* for puncture wounds created with a sharp instrument; *Magnesia phosphorica* to comfort pain seemingly relieved only by the application of heat; *Mercurius solubilis* for the reduction of suppuration accompanying the inflammation of tissues and sinuses; *Phosphorous* for stopping hemorrhage; *Rhus toxicodendron* to overcome neuralgia; *Ruta graveolens* as an offset to injuries to bone and stagnant blood flow in the veins; *Staphysagrie* as a healer for penetrating wounds; *Symphytum offcianale* to heal fractures of all kinds.

5. Oral cavity pollution: The internal cleansing homeopathic antihomotoxicologic combination remedy is taken under the tongue to detoxify dental and environmental pollutants and the poisonous properties of chemical substances used in dental manipulation and for other toxic agents created by the immune system as a defense mechanism. For common symptoms, take the homeopathic remedy three or four times daily. As required for relief, drops, spantules or tablets may be taken sublingually as often as every fifteen minutes. Children ages two to six receive one half the adult dosage.

The constitutional homeopathic remedies include *Alumina* for the treatment of weakness, exhaustion and irritability; *Apis mellifica* to bring about drainage and lymphatic stimulation; *Aranea diadema* to stop neuralgia of the jaw; *Argentum metallicum* is homeopathic silver, which produces an antimicrobial effect; *Cantharis* acts as a kidney stimulant; *Curum metallicum* is the homeopathic version of copper for joints; *Galium aparine* works to offset various poisons; the quadruple poisonous mercurial compounds consisting of *Mercurius auratus*, *Mercurius corrosivus*, *Mercurius solubilis*, and *Mercurius vivus* act to heal you against the mercury amalgam poisons placed by dentists; *Niccolum metallicum* acts to neutralize nickel poisoning from "stainless steel" mouth appliances, *Plumbum metallicum* acts to neutralize poisoning from lead; *Stannum metallicum* acts to neutralize poisoning from tin (in amalgams); *Sulphur* is used for general detoxification; *Thymus serpyllum* is a stimulator of the human thymus gland; *Thyroidinum* is a stimulator of the human thyroid gland;

Uranium nitricum works to quench the free radicals related to radiation; *Vaccinum myrtillus* is the neutralizer of vaccination poisons; *Zincum metallicum* is homeopathic zinc for the normalization of the prostate and other organs.

Dental Consumer Organizations and Information Sources

For Education about Mercury Toxicity and Detoxification

DAMS, Inc. (Dental Amalgam Mercury Survivors)

Terresa Kaiser, executive director, telephone (757) 721-2039
Bernice Rudelice, president, telephone (704) 541-6037
P.O. Box 64397, Virginia Beach, Virginia 23467-4397
telephone answering device (800) 311-6265
The DAMS newsletter editor in Madison, Alabama, is
Murlene Brake, telephone (205) 830-0662;
teleFAX (205) 830-6847

Foundation for Toxic-Free Dentistry (FTFD)

Nonprofit and totally staffed by volunteers, FTFD was formed to research and disseminate information on biocompatible dental materials and the adverse effects of mercury amalgam fillings on general health. (See the recommended reading list on mercury amalgams in appendix B for *The Bio-Probe Newsletter*.)

P.O. Box 608010, Orlando, Florida 32860-8010;
telephone (407) 298-2450

Toxic Element Research Foundation (TERF)

Lodged in the Huggins Diagnostic Center
5080 List Drive, Colorado Springs, Colorado 80919
telephone (800) 331-2303 or (719) 548-1600;
teleFAX (719) 522-0563

American Academy of Environmental Medicine (AAEM)

P.O. Box CN 1001-8001, New Hope, Pennsylvania 18938
telephone (215) 862-4544; teleFAX (215) 862-4583

American College for Advancement in Medicine (ACAM)

Edward A. Shaw, Ph.D., executive director
23121 Verdugo Drive, Suite 204, Laguna Hills, California 92653
telephone (800) 532-3688 or (949) 583-7666;
teleFAX (949) 955-9679

For Education about Fluoridation

Health Alliance International, Pennsylvania Chapter

Ellie Rudolph, director of the Pennsylvania chapter
telephone/teleFAX (412) 828-5096 or on the Internet, see the
"Report of the Expert Panel for Water Fluoridation Review"
at http://www.cadvision.com/fluoride/report.htm

Safe Water Coalition of Washington State

Betty Fowler, spokesperson
West 5615 Lyons Court, Spokane, Washington 99208
telephone (509) 328-6704

For a Subscription to Dr. Julian Whitaker's Newsletter
Phillips Publishing, Inc.

Dr. Julian Whitaker's monthly *Health & Healing*
(ISSN 1057-9273)
7811 Montrose Road, Potomac, Maryland 20854-3394
telephone (800) 539-8219.

Homeopathic/Isopathic or Pleomorphic/Enderlein

Medical-Dental Seminars
for Health Professionals

Enderlein Enterprises, Inc.

Chrystyne Jackson, president
International seminars are conducted twice annually, generally in January and June; Darkfield Microscopy seminars are held separately; also seminars are conducted regionally (inquire by telephone or teleFAX for times and locations). For Pleomorphic/Enderlein information or technical support, contact:
(headquarters) P.O. Box 11510, Prescott, Arizona 86304-1510
telephone (520) 541-1920; cell phone (520) 713-0814;
teleFAX (520) 541-1906
or
(warehouse) P.O. Box 82430, Phoenix, Arizona 85071-2430
telephone (602) 439-7977; teleFAX (602) 439-7996
for either address, E-mail: sanumlit@aol.com
Website: http://www.euderlein.com
E-mail: Euderlein@aol.com
Website: http://www.pleomorp.com
E-mail: pleomorp@aol.com

Suppliers of Body Detoxification Agents, Oral Remedies, and Nutrition Products

Where to Acquire DMPS (Dimaval)

(R,S)-2,3-Dimercaptopropane-1-sulfonic acid, sodium salt (DMPS), a chelating agent from vicinal dithiols, with a high affinity for heavy metals, forming stable complexes with them, may be acquired by health professionals from the

Heyltex Corporation

Robert Z. Martin, vice president of operations
10655 Richmond Avenue, Suite 170, Houston, Texas 77042
telephone (800)237-6793 or (713) 784-6258;
teleFAX (713) 781-0960

Where to Acquire DMSA

2.3-Dimercaptosuccinic Acid (DMSA), a chelating agent, binds mercury in a provocative oral dose, which burden is determined by analyzing a six-hour collection of the patient's urine. Acquire DMSA by prescription from

Hopewell Pharmacy and Compounding Center

James Palmieri, R.P., and Gene Ragazzo, R.P.,
compounding pharmacists
1 West Broad Street, Hopewell, New Jersey 08525
telephone (800) 792-6670 or (609) 466-1960;
teleFAX (609) 466-6222

Lakeside Pharmacy

4632 Highway 58, Chattanooga, Tennessee 37416
telephone (800) 523-1486 or (423) 894-3222;
teleFAX (423) 499-8435

Hazle Drugs Apothecary Compounding Pharmacy

20 North Laurel Street, Hazleton, Pennsylvania 18201
telephone (800) 439-2026 or (717) 454-2670;
teleFAX (800) 400-8764

College Pharmacy

833 North Tejon Street, Colorado Springs, Colorado 80903
telephone (800) 888-9358 or (719) 634-4861;
teleFAX (800) 556-5893 or (719) 634-4513

Wellness Health and Pharmacy, Inc.

2800 South 18th Street, Birmingham, Alabama 35209
telephone (800) 227-2627 or (205) 879-6551;
teleFAX (800) 369-0302 or (205) 871-2568

Central Florida Pharmacies

1724 South Orange Avenue, Orlando, Florida 32806
telephone (407) 422-4495; teleFAX (407) 236-9900

Women's International Pharmacy

5708 Monona Drive, Madison, Wisconsin 53716-3152
telephone (800) 279-5708; teleFAX (800) 279-8011

Medquest Pharmacy

6955 Union Park Center, Suite 360, Salt Lake City, Utah 84047
telephone (888) 222-2956 or (801) 566-5350;
teleFAX (801) 569-4632

Medical Center Compounding Pharmacy

3675 South Rainbow Boulevard, #103, Las Vegas, Nevada 89103
telephone (800) 723-7455 or (702) 873-8455;
teleFAX (800) 238-8239

Apothecare

604 Grove Road, Greenville, South Carolina 29605
telephone (888) 276-2483 or (864) 241-0477;
teleFAX (864) 241-0479

Where to Acquire Dr. Mike's Teeth and Gum Support Pack

Accompanying Dr. Mike's Dental Diet is his Teeth and Gum Support Pack to provide the finest in nutritional supplementation for oral health. To acquire a full month's supply (30 packs) of Dr. Mike's Teeth and Gum Support Pack at a cost of US$39.95 and US$4.55 for shipping & handling = US$44.50, send your check or money order or offer your credit card by phone or FAX (sorry no CODs) to

Healthplex Medical Center

Michael J. Loquasto, D.C., D.A.B.C.N., C.C.N., clinic director
P.O. Box 1380, Marshalls Creek, Pennsylvania 18335
telephone (570) 223-0140; teleFAX (570) 223-7355
Websites: http://www.healthplexmedicalctr.com or
http://www.naturallyrite.com

Where to Acquire MistORAL Spray for Mouth, Gum, and Tooth Restoration

Brower Enterprises, Inc.

P.O. Box 277, 102 South Main Street, Canton, South Dakota 57013
telephone (800) 373-6076 or (605) 987-2405;
teleFAX (605) 987-2613
E-mail: brower.ent@dtg.net.com

Where to Acquire the Natural Dentist Herbal Mouth and Gum Therapy

Woodstock Natural Products, Inc.

William M. Stern, president
140 Sylvan Avenue, Englewood Cliffs, New Jersey 07632
telephone (800) 615-6895 or (201) 944-0123;
teleFAX (201) 944-1717
E-mail: natdent@worldnet.att.net

Periodontal Remedy Suppliers Listed Alphabetically

- Albrite, Inc., P.O. Box 1095, Crystal Beach, Florida 34681; telephone (800) 533-1821 (Dental self-care programs).

- Auromere Ayurvedic Imports, 2621 West Highway 12, Lodi, California 95242; telephone (800) 735-4691 (Ayurvedic dental care).

- Dental Herb Company, P.O. Box 687, Northampton, Massachusetts 10611; telephone (800) 747-HERB [747-4372] (All-Natural mouthwash and toothpaste).

- Desert Essence, 101 Corporate Drive, Hauppauge, New York 11788; telephone (800) 645-5768 (Toothpastes, dental floss, dental pics, breath freshener, and mouthwash).

- Dr. Tungs, 3593A Alain Drive, Honolulu, Hawaii 96822; telephone (808) 988-3161 (Tongue scraper and ayurvedic tooth powder).

- Eco-Dent International, Inc., 3130 Spring Street, Redwood City, California 94063; telephone (888) ECO-DENT [326-3368], (Toothpowders, mouthwashes, dental floss, and tooth whitener).

- Nathan Export, P.O. Box 7138, McLean, Virginia 22106, no phone listing; (Herbal breath freshener).

- Perfect Breath, 4701 Marion, Suite 303, Denver, Colorado 80216; telephone (303) 293-0290 (Breath freshener and toothbrush).

- Tea Tree Therapy, 230 South Olive Street, Ventura, California 93001; telephone (800) 990-4221; (Toothpaste, whitener, and mouthwash).

- Woodstock Natural Products, 2337 Lemoine Avenue, Fort Lee, New Jersey 07024; telephone (800) 615-6895 (Mouthwashes and toothpastes).

Where to Acquire Boiron Homeodent Toothpaste

Boiron USA Corporate Headquarters

Fabienne Pugnetti-Boiron,
pharmacist and public relations manager
6 Campus Boulevard, Building A,
Newtown Square, Pennsylvania 19073
telephone (800) 258-8823 or (610) 325-8326;
teleFAX (610) 325-7480
E-mail: boiron@worldnet.att.net

Where to Acquire Homeopathic/Isopathic Plemomorphic/Enderlein Therapies (by Sanum)

Pleomorphic Product Sales, Inc.

Chrystyne Jackson, president
Colonel Felix J. Muller (Ret.), vice president and general manager
P.O. Box 11510 (executive offices),
Prescott, Arizona 86304-1510
telephone (520) 541-1920; teleFAX (520) 541-1906;
E-mail: sanumlit@aol.com

For a detailed information packet on *Pleomorphism* and its highly effective counteracting Enderlein Therapies, teleFAX your request to (520) 541-1906 or

P.O. Box 82430 (warehouse mail drop),
Phoenix, Arizona 85071-2430
telephone (602) 439-7977
teleFAX (602) 439-7996, or Toll free (888) 439-7980
No telephone orders please; ask for order form and
send by teleFAX instead or
5160 West Phelps Road, Suite B (warehouse),
Glendale, Arizona 85306

Homeopathic Remedy Suppliers Listed Alphabetically

- Apex Energetics, 700 North Central Avenue, #420, Glendale, California 91203; telephone (800)736-4381 or (818) 243-5336.
- Arnica, Inc. (Staufen-Pharma Homeopathics), 144 East Garry Ave. Santa Ana, California 92707; telephone (714) 545-8203.
- Biological Homeopathic Industries (BHI), 11600 Cochiti Southeast, Albuquerque, New Mexico 87123; telephone (800) 621-7644.
- Boericke and Tafel, 2381 Circadian Way, Santa Rosa, California 95407; telephone (800) 876-9505.
- Boiron-USA, 6 Campus Blvd., Bldg. A., Newtown Square, Pennsylvania 19073; telephone (800) 258-8823.
- D. L. Thompson Homeopathic Supplies, 844 Yonge Street, Toronto, 5, Ontario Canada M4W 2H1; telephone (416) 922-2300.
- Dolisos-USA Homeopathics, 3014 Rigel Avenue, Las Vegas, Nevada 89102; telephone (800) 824-8455.
- Hahnemann Homeopathic Pharmacy, 828 San Pablo Avenue, Albany, California 94706; telephone (888) 427-6422.
- Homeopathic Educational Services, 2124 Kittredge Street, Berkeley, California 94704.
- Humphrey's Pharmacal Co., 63 Meadows Road, Rutherford, New Jersey 07070; telephone (201) 933-7744.
- Longevity Pure Medicines, 9595 Wilshire Boulevard, #706, Beverly Hills, California 90212.
- Luyties Pharmacal, 4200 Laclede Ave., St. Louis, Missouri 63108; telephone (800) 325-8080.
- National Center of Homeopathy, 1500 Massachusetts Ave., Northwest, Washington, D.C. 20005; telephone (202) 223-6182.
- Standard Homeopathic, 210 West 131 Street, P O Box 61067, Los Angeles, California 90061; telephone (800) 624-9659.
- Washington Homeopathic Products, 4914 Delray Avenue, Bethesda, Maryland 20814; no phone listed.
- Weleda, Inc., Route N-9W, Congers, New York 10920; telephone (914) 268-8572.

Recommended Reading on Root Canals and Cavitations

Root Canal Cover-Up (ISBN 0-945196-19-9, US$19.95 and US$3.05 postage and handling) by George E. Meinig, D.D.S., F.A.C.D., Bion Publishing, 323 East Matilija Street, #110-151, Ojai, California 93023.

Beyond Amalgam: The Hidden Health Hazard Posed by Jawbone Cavitations (ISBN 0-9640539-7-7, US$11.95 and US$3.05 postage and handling) by Susan Stockton, M.A., Nature's Publishing, 88 Ridge Avenue, Winter Haven, Florida 33880; telephone/teleFAX (941) 295-9076; E-mail: Npath1@aol.com

Cavitations and Quarterly newsletter (US$26 per annual subscription), Editor/Publisher Susan Stockton, M.A., 88 Ridge Avenue, Winter Haven, Florida 33880; telephone/teleFAX (941) 295-9076.

Recommended Reading on Oral Cavity Pain Relief

Instant Pain Relief: A Proven Method of Immediate Resolution of Pain and Dysfunction (ISBN 0-1-879361-00-0, US$12.95 and US$3.05 postage and handling) by William J. Faber, D.O., and Morton Walker, D.P.M., published by Biological Publications and distributed by Freelance Communications, 484 High Ridge Road, Stamford, Connecticut 06905-3020; telephone (203) 322-1551; teleFAX (203) 322-4656; E-mail: mortwalk@compuserve.com

Recommended Reading on Mercury Amalgam Fillings

The Holistic Dental Digest PLUS bimonthly newsletter (US$13.25 per annual subscription), edited by Jerry Mittelman, D.D.S., F.P.P.M., and Beverly Mittelman, B.S., C.N.C., published by The Once Daily, Inc., 263 West End Avenue, #2A, New York, New York 10023; telephone/tele-FAX (212) 874-4212.

The Bio-Probe Newsletter (US$65 per year subscription rate), published bimonthly by Bio-Probe, Inc., the Ziff family company, P.O. Box 608010 or 5508 Edgewater Drive, Orlando, Florida 32810-8017 (see this appendix for the same address as the Foundation for Toxic-Free dentistry); telephone (407) 290-9670.

It's All in Your Head (ISBN 0-89529-550-4, 1993, US$10.95 and US$3.05 postage and handling) by Hal A. Huggins, D.D.S., Avery Publishing Group, Inc., 120 Old Broadway, Garden City Park, New York 11040; (800) 548-5757 or (516) 741-2155 ; teleFAX (516) 742-1892.

Beating Alzheimer's: A Step Towards Unlocking the Mysteries of Brain Diseases (ISBN 0-89529-488-5, 1991, US$12.95 and US$3.05 postage and handling) by Tom Warren, Avery Publishing Group, Inc., 120 Old Broadway, Garden City Park, New York 11040; (800) 548-5757 or (516) 741-2155; teleFAX (516) 742-1892.

Chronic Mercury Toxicity: New Hope against an Endemic Disease (ISBN 0-9620479-1-0, 1988, US$67.50 and US$12.00 postage and handling) by H.L. Queen, M.A., Queen and Company Health Communications, Inc., P.O. Box 49308, Colorado Springs, Colorado 80919-9938; telephone (800) 243-2782.

The Mercury in Your Mouth: The Truth about "Silver" Dental Fillings (ISBN 0-9643870-0-X, 1994, US$14.95 and US$3.05 postage and handling) by Lydia Bronte, Ph.D., Quicksilver Press, 10 East 87th Street, New York, New York 10128; telephone (212) 289-1365; teleFAX (212) 289-3046.

Mercury-Free: The Wisdom behind the Global Consumer Movement to Ban "Silver" Dental Fillings (ISBN 0-9649801-0-2, 1996, US$16.95 and US$3.95 postage and handling) by James E. Hardy, D.M.D., published by Gabriel Rose Press, distributed by STCS Distributors, P.O. Box 246, Dept. BK, Glassboro, New Jersey 08028-0246; telephone (800) 266-5564; teleFAX (609) 881-8042.

How to Save Your Teeth (ISBN 0-913571-04-0, 1993, US$10.00 and US$3.05 postage and handling) by David Kennedy, D.D.S., published by Health Action Press, 6439 Taggart Road, Delaware, Ohio 43015.

The Key to Ultimate Health (no ISBN advertised, 1998, US$19.95 and US$4.00 postage and handling) by Richard T. Hansen, D.M.D., and Ellen Brown, J.D., published by Advanced Health Research Press, 1943 Sunnycrest Drive, Suite 183, Fullerton, California 92835; telephone (888) 792-1102 or (714) 870-0310; teleFAX (714) 870-0153; E-mail: drhansen@advancedental.com

Thriving in a Toxic World: Tools for Flourishing in the 21st Century (ISBN 0-9636491-1-6, 1996, US$29.95 and US$5.05 postage and handling) by William Randall Kellas, Ph.D., and Andrea Sharon Dworkin, N.D., published by Professional Preference Publishing, 27701 Murrieta Road, Suite 30, Sun City, California 92586-2348; telephone (888) 244-4420.

Surviving the Toxic Crisis: Understanding, Preventing and Treating the Root Causes of Chronic Illness (ISBN 0-9636491-2-4, 1996, US$29.95 and US$5.05 postage and handling) by William Randall Kellas, Ph.D., and Andrea Sharon Dworkin, N.D., published by Professional Preference Publishing, 27701 Murrieta Road, Suite 30, Sun City, California 92586-2348; telephone (888) 244-4420.

Recommended Reading on Chelation Therapy

The Chelation Way: The Complete Book of Chelation Therapy (ISBN 0-89529-415-X, 1990, US$12.95 and US$3.05 postage and handling) by Morton Walker, D.P.M., published by Avery Publishing Group, Inc., 120 Old Broadway, Garden City Park, New York 11040; telephone (800) 548-5757 or (516) 741-2155; teleFAX 742-1892.

The Healing Powers of Chelation Therapy: Unclog Your Arteries, An Alternative to Bypass Surgery (ISBN 094 5498-01-2, 1998, US$3.95 and US$3.05 postage and handling) by John Parks Trowbridge, M.D., and Morton Walker, D.P.M., published by New Way of Life, Inc., 484 High Ridge Road, Stamford, Connecticut 06905-3020; telephone (203) 322-1551 or (203) 329-3394; teleFAX (203) 322-4656; E-mail: 102760.2071@compuserve.com or mortwalk@compuserve.com

The Chelation Answer: How to Prevent Hardening of the Arteries and Rejuvenate Your Cardiovascular System (ISBN 0-9626646-7-7, 1994, US$16.95 and US$3.05 postage and handling) by Morton Walker, D.P.M., in consultation with Garry Gordon, M.D., published by Second Opinion Publishing, Inc. and distributed by New Way of Life, Inc., 484 High Ridge Road, Stamford, Connecticut 06905-3020; telephone (203) 322-1551 or (203) 329-3394; teleFAX (203) 322-4656; E-mail: mortwalk@compuserve.com or 102760.2071@compuserve.com

Toxic Metal Syndrome: How Metal Poisonings Can Affect Your Brain (ISBN 0-89529-649-7, 1995, US$14.95 and US$3.05 postage and handling) by H. Richard Casdorph, M.D., Ph.D., and Morton Walker, D.P.M., published by Avery Publishing Group, Inc., 120 Old Broadway, Garden City Park, New York 11040; telephone (800) 548-5757 or (516) 741-2155; teleFAX 742-1892.

Everything You Should Know About Chelation Therapy: Unclog your Arteries and Rejuvenate Your Cardiovascular System without Surgery and Other Invasive Procedures (ISBN 0-87983-730-6, 1997, US$14.95 and US$3.05 postage and handling) by Morton Walker, D.P.M., and Hitendra Shah, M.D., published by Keats Publishing, Inc., a division of NTC Contemporary Publishing, Inc., 4255 Touhy Ave., Lincolnwood, Illinois 60646; telephone orders (800) 323-4900, Ext. 2

Recommended Reading on Flouridation

Fluoride: The Aging Factor (ISBN 0-913571-00-8, 1983, US$11.95 and US$3.05 postage and handling) by John Yiamouyiannis, Ph.D., Health Action Press, 6439 Taggart Road, Delaware, Ohio 43015; no telephone available.

Recommended Reading on Homeopathy

Yasgur's Homeopathic Dictionary and Holistic Health Reference, 4th ed. (ISBN 1-886149-04-6, 1998, US$19.95 and US$3.05 postage and handling) by Jay Yasgur, R.Ph., M.Sc., Van Hoy Publishers, P.O. Box 636, Greenville, Pennsylvania 16125; no telephone available.

Homeopathic Medical Repertory, 1st ed. (ISBN 0-9635764-0-2, 1993, US$80.00 and US$5.00 postage and handling) by Robin Murphy, N.D., published by the Hahnemann Academy of North America, 60 Talisman Dr., Suite 4028, Pagosa Springs, Colorado 81157; telephone (303) 264-2460.

Four Dental Professional Organizations
Offering the Names, Addresses, and Telephone Numbers of Mercury-Free, Biocompatible, Holistic, or Biological Dentists

For Referrals to Dentists in Your Area Who Are Mercury-Free/Biocompatible/Holistic/Biological

American Academy of Biological Dentistry

Edward Arana, D.D.S., president and executive director
107 Quiensabe, Carmel Valley, California 93924
telephone (813) 659-5385

Holistic Dental Association (HDA)

Richard Shepard, executive director;
Robert B. Stephan, D.D.S., president
Offers a biological dentist list for US $2.50 and
stamped SA envelope for 2 ounces
P.O. Box 5007, Durango, Colorado 81301
telephone/teleFAX (970) 259-1091; E-mail: hdd@frontier.net

Members of the HDA who have given their permission to have their names and addresses provided to prospective patients are listed on the Internet. They can be identified by downloading them from the HDA home page at http://www.holisticdental.org

International Academy of Oral Medicine and Toxicology (IAOMT)

Michael F. Ziff, D.D.S., executive director; Walter Jess Clifford, president; P.O. Box 60851, Orlando, Florida 32860-8531
telephone (407) 298-2450; teleFAX (407) 298-3075

Environmental Dental Association (EDA)

Joyal W. Taylor, D.D.S., president
Offers a biological dentist list for US$3.00 and stamped SA envelope for 2 ounces, P. O. Box 2184, Rancho Santa Fe, California 92067
telephone answering device (800) 388-8124; to order books (619) 586-7626

Professional Dental Testing Laboratories

Oral and Systemic Pathology Laboratory Testing

Head and Neck Diagnostics of America

A Division of The Maxillofacial Center for Diagnostics and Research
Jerry E. Bouquot, D.D.S., M.S.D., laboratory director
165 Scott Avenue, Suite 101, Morgantown, West Virgina 26505
telephone (304) 292-4429; teleFAX (304) 291-5649

Huggins Diagnostic Center

Hal A. Huggins, D.D.S., M.S., laboratory director
P.O. Box 2589, Colorado Springs, Colorado 80901
telephone (303) 473-4703; or outside Colorado,
telephone (800) 331-2303

Biocompatible Dental Materials Testing

Clifford Consulting and Research

Walter Jess Clifford, M.S., R.M. (AAM),
president and laboratory director
P.O. Box 17597, Colorado Springs, Colorado 80935
telephone (719) 550-0008; teleFAX (719) 550-0009

Body Tissue/Fluids Testing and Hair Mineral Analysis

Doctor's Data, Inc.

James T. Hicks, M.D., Ph.D., F.C.A.P., medical director
P.O. Box 111, 170 West Roosevelt Road
West Chicago, Illinois 60186-0111
telephone (800) 323-2784 or (630) 231-3649;
teleFAX (630) 231-9190
E-mail: inquiries @ doctorsdata.com
Web site: www.doctorsdata.com

Toxicity Testing of Avital Teeth, Cavitational Materials and Microbial Proteins

Affinity Labeling Technologies, Inc.

Boyd Haley, Ph.D., laboratory director and professor
University of Kentucky
A-215 ASTeCC Building, Lexington, Kentucky 40506-0286
telephone (606) 257-2300, ext. 291;
teleFAX (606) 252-9029

Index

B

C

D

T

About the Author

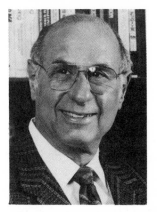

Morton Walker, D.P.M., who discontinued more than sixteen years of practice as a doctor of podiatric medicine in 1969, has since written full time as a professional freelance medical journalist. Dr. Walker is the author of seventy-three published books, including fourteen worldwide best-sellers, each distributed with more than a hundred and fifty thousand copies. His titles are marketed in thirty-two countries and have been translated into twelve languages.

Each month Dr. Walker writes columns for American holistic medical journals and consumer health magazines. In all, he has had more than twenty-two hundred magazine, newspaper, and clinical journal articles published.

Dr. Walker has presented his magazine article and book concepts during no less than two thousand media events, including national, international (by satellite), and local radio and TV talk shows, press interviews, lectures, videofilms, audiotapes, and news conferences. He specializes in researching and writing in those health care sciences referred to as orthomolecular (proper or correct element) nutrition, holistic health, biological medicine, and alternative methods of healing.

The winner of twenty-three medical journalism awards and medals, Dr. Walker was recognized with the 1992 Humanitarian Award from the Cancer Control Society, which named him "the world's leading medical journalist specializing in holistic medicine." He received the 1981 Orthomolecular Award from the American

Institute of Preventive Medicine, which states: "For outstanding achievement in orthomolecular education." He was presented with the 1979 Humanitarian Award from the 1,250 physician members of the American College for Advancement in Medicine: "For informing the American public on alternative methods of healing."

This author-lecturer received two prestigious Jesse H. Neal Editorial Achievement Awards from the American Business Press, Inc., for creating the best series of magazine articles published in any audited United States magazine in both the years 1975 and 1976.

From his home in Stamford, Connecticut, U.S.A., for three decades, this health reporter has combined medical knowledge and writing ability in his second highly successful career as a professional medical journalist and author. The Avery Publishing Group, Inc., of Garden City Park, New York, U.S.A., has produced twelve of his titles and provides him with his own imprint. Newly published titles coming from his word processor and contracted by Avery are marketed with the designation, "A Dr. Morton Walker Health Book." He is ever expanding his publishing horizons.

Hampton Roads Publishing Company

. . . for the evolving human spirit

Hampton Roads Publishing Company
publishes books on a variety of subject including
metaphysics, health, complementary medicine,
visionary fiction, and other related topics.

For acopy of our latest catalog,
call toll-free, 800-766-8009,
or send your name and address to

Hampton Roads Publishing Company
134 Burgess Lane
Charlottesville, VA 22902
email: hrpc@hrpub.com
www.hrpub.com